A PRACTICAL MANUAL OF
Diabetic Retinopathy Management

A PRACTICAL MANUAL OF
Diabetic Retinopathy Management

SECOND EDITION

Edited by

Peter H. Scanlon MD FRCP FRCOphth
Consultant Ophthalmologist, Gloucestershire and Oxford Eye Units
Senior Research Fellow, Harris Manchester College, University of Oxford
Visiting Professor of Medical Ophthalmology, University of Gloucestershire, UK

Ahmed Sallam MD PhD FRCOphth
Staff Surgeon, Jones Eye Institute
Assistant Professor of Ophthalmology
University of Arkansas for Medical Sciences, USA

Peter van Wijngaarden MBBS PhD FRANZCO
Consultant Ophthalmologist, Centre for Eye Research Australia,
Royal Victorian Eye and Ear Hospital, Australia; Ophthalmology,
Department of Surgery, University of Melbourne, Australia

WILEY Blackwell

This edition first published 2017 © 2009, 2017 by John Wiley & Sons Ltd

Registered office: John Wiley & Sons Ltd, The Atrium, Southern Gate, Chichester, West Sussex, PO19 8SQ, UK

Editorial offices: 9600 Garsington Road, Oxford, OX4 2DQ, UK
The Atrium, Southern Gate, Chichester, West Sussex, PO19 8SQ, UK
111 River Street, Hoboken, NJ 07030-5774, USA

For details of our global editorial offices, for customer services and for information about how to apply for permission to reuse the copyright material in this book please see our website at www.wiley.com/wiley-blackwell

The right of Peter H. Scanlon, Ahmed Sallam and Peter van Wijngaarden to be identified as the author of this work has been asserted in accordance with the UK Copyright, Designs and Patents Act 1988.

All rights reserved. No part of this publication may be reproduced, stored in a retrieval system, or transmitted, in any form or by any means, electronic, mechanical, photocopying, recording or otherwise, except as permitted by the UK Copyright, Designs and Patents Act 1988, without the prior permission of the publisher.

Designations used by companies to distinguish their products are often claimed as trademarks. All brand names and product names used in this book are trade names, service marks, trademarks or registered trademarks of their respective owners. The publisher is not associated with any product or vendor mentioned in this book. It is sold on the understanding that the publisher is not engaged in rendering professional services. If professional advice or other expert assistance is required, the services of a competent professional should be sought.

The contents of this work are intended to further general scientific research, understanding, and discussion only and are not intended and should not be relied upon as recommending or promoting a specific method, diagnosis, or treatment by health science practitioners for any particular patient. The publisher and the author make no representations or warranties with respect to the accuracy or completeness of the contents of this work and specifically disclaim all warranties, including without limitation any implied warranties of fitness for a particular purpose. In view of ongoing research, equipment modifications, changes in governmental regulations, and the constant flow of information relating to the use of medicines, equipment, and devices, the reader is urged to review and evaluate the information provided in the package insert or instructions for each medicine, equipment, or device for, among other things, any changes in the instructions or indication of usage and for added warnings and precautions. Readers should consult with a specialist where appropriate. The fact that an organization or Website is referred to in this work as a citation and/or a potential source of further information does not mean that the author or the publisher endorses the information the organization or Website may provide or recommendations it may make. Further, readers should be aware that Internet Websites listed in this work may have changed or disappeared between when this work was written and when it is read. No warranty may be created or extended by any promotional statements for this work. Neither the publisher nor the author shall be liable for any damages arising herefrom.

Library of Congress Cataloging-in-Publication Data

Names: Scanlon, Peter H., editor. | Sallam, Ahmed, editor. | Wijngaarden, Peter van, editor.
Title: A Practical manual of diabetic retinopathy management / edited by Peter H. Scanlon, Ahmed Sallam, Peter van Wijngaarden.
Description: 2nd edition. | Chichester, West Sussex ; Hoboken, NJ : John Wiley & Sons, Ltd, 2017. | Includes bibliographical references and index.
Identifiers: LCCN 2016055390 (print) | LCCN 2016056036 (ebook) | ISBN 9781119058953 (cloth) | ISBN 9781119058960 (pdf) | ISBN 9781119058977 (epub)
Subjects: | MESH: Diabetic Retinopathy–therapy | Diabetic Retinopathy–diagnosis
Classification: LCC RE661.D5 (print) | LCC RE661.D5 (ebook) | NLM WK 835 | DDC 617.7/35–dc23
LC record available at https://lccn.loc.gov/2016055390

A catalogue record for this book is available from the British Library.

Wiley also publishes its books in a variety of electronic formats. Some content that appears in print may not be available in electronic books.

Cover design: Wiley

Typeset in 9.25/11.5pt MinionPro by SPi Global, Chennai, India
Printed and bound in Singapore by Markono Print Media Pte Ltd

1   2017

Contents

List of contributors, vii

Prologue, ix

Acknowledgements, xv

About the companion website, xvii

1 Introduction, 1
Peter H. Scanlon

2 Diabetes, 15
Jonathan Shaw & Peter H. Scanlon

3 Lesions and classifications of diabetic retinopathy, 26
Peter H. Scanlon

4 Screening for diabetic retinopathy, 40
Peter H. Scanlon

5 Imaging techniques in diabetic retinopathy, 54
Peter van Wijngaarden & Peter H. Scanlon

6 The normal eye, 86
Stephen J. Aldington

7 Diabetic macular oedema, 93
Ahmed Sallam & Abdallah A. Ellabban

8 Mild non-proliferative diabetic retinopathy, 116
Peter H. Scanlon

9 Moderate and severe non-proliferative diabetic retinopathy, 120
Peter H. Scanlon

10 Proliferative and advanced diabetic retinopathy, 128
Ahmed Sallam & Peter H. Scanlon

11 Proliferative diabetic retinopathy with maculopathy, 150
Ahmed Sallam & Peter H. Scanlon

12 The stable treated eye, 160
    Peter H. Scanlon

13 Vitrectomy surgery in diabetic retinopathy, 171
    Charles P. Wilkinson

14 Cataract surgery in the diabetic eye: Pre-, intra- and postoperative considerations, 183
    Abdallah A. Ellabban & Ahmed Sallam

15 Pregnancy and the diabetic eye, 197
    Peter H. Scanlon

16 Low vision and blindness from diabetic retinopathy, 207
    Peter H. Scanlon

17 Future advances in the management of diabetic retinopathy, 219
    Peter van Wijngaarden

18 Other retinal conditions in diabetes, 228
    Stephen J. Aldington & Peter H. Scanlon

19 Conditions with appearances similar to diabetic retinopathy, 247
    Stephen J. Aldington & Peter H. Scanlon

Glossary, 255

Index, 259

List of contributors

Stephen J. Aldington
Retinopathy Research and Professional Development Manager, Gloucestershire Hospitals NHS Foundation Trust, UK
Honorary Associate Professor, University of Warwick Medical School, UK

Abdallah A. Ellabban
Lecturer, Department of Ophthalmology, Suez Canal University, Egypt

Ahmed Sallam
Staff Surgeon, Jones Eye Institute
Assistant Professor of Ophthalmology
University of Arkansas for Medical Sciences, USA

Peter H. Scanlon
Consultant Ophthalmologist, Gloucestershire and Oxford Eye Units
Senior Research Fellow, Harris Manchester College
University of Oxford
Visiting Professor of Medical Ophthalmology
University of Gloucestershire, UK

Jonathan Shaw
Associate Professor, Baker IDI Heart and Diabetes Institute, Melbourne, Australia

Peter van Wijngaarden
Consultant Ophthalmologist, Centre for Eye Research Australia, Royal Victorian Eye and Ear Hospital
Australia Ophthalmology, Department of Surgery
University of Melbourne, Australia

Charles P. Wilkinson
Professor of Ophthalmology, Johns Hopkins University
Emeritus Chairman, Department of Ophthalmology
Greater Baltimore Medical Center, USA

Prologue

Peter H. Scanlon

THE SCOPE OF THE PROBLEM OF THE EPIDEMIC OF DIABETES

There is currently an epidemic of diabetes in the world, principally type 2 diabetes, that is linked to changing lifestyle, obesity and increasing age of the population. The International Diabetes Federation (IDF) publishes the Diabetes Atlas[1] and has forecast a rise from the current level of 387 million people worldwide in 2014 to 592 million by 2035. The current level in 2014 is equivalent to 1 in 12 people in the world having diabetes, and 48.3% of these people are believed to be undiagnosed.

In 2000, Karvonen et al.[2] reported a global variation in the incidence in different populations; the overall age-adjusted incidence of type 1 diabetes varied from 0.1/100,000 per year in China and Venezuela to 36.8/100,000 per year in Sardinia and 36.5/100,000 per year in Finland. The 2014 estimates[1] for the prevalence of type 1 diabetes are 500,000 children aged under 15 years with type 1 diabetes worldwide, the largest numbers[3] being in Europe (129,000) and North America (108,700), with the numbers have increased in most of the IDF regions.

The International Diabetes Federation has estimated[1] the prevalence of diabetes in 2014 in 20–79 age groups and projected this to an estimate in 2035 (Fig. 1).

Individual publications[4–10] from each region have described how these figures were arrived at. The report from the Western Pacific region was noteworthy because this region is home to one-quarter of the world's population, and includes China with the largest number of people with diabetes (98.41 million) as well as the Pacific Islands countries with the highest prevalence rates (Tokelau 37.49%, Federated States of Micronesia 35.03%, Marshall Islands 34.89%).

THE PREVALENCE OF SIGHT-THREATENING DIABETIC RETINOPATHY WORLDWIDE

It is difficult to compare the many studies that have recorded the incidence and prevalence of diabetic retinopathy (DR) or sight-threatening or vision-threatening diabetic retinopathy (STDR or VTDR) because of the difference in examination techniques and the different definitions, particularly of STDR and VTDR (see Fig. 2).

The map in Figure 2 uses data from the following studies.

1. In 2012, Yau et al.[11] reviewed a total of 35 studies (1980–2008) which provided data from 22,896 individuals with diabetes, and found that the overall prevalence was 34.6% (95% CI 34.5–34.8) for any DR, 6.96% (6.87–7.04) for proliferative DR, 6.81% (6.74–6.89) for diabetic macular oedema and 10.2% (10.1–10.3) for VTDR.
2. In the USA, Zhang et al.[12] reported that the estimated prevalence of diabetic retinopathy and vision-threatening diabetic retinopathy was 28.5% (95% CI, 24.9–32.5%) and 4.4% (95% CI, 3.5–5.7%) among US adults with diabetes, respectively.
3. In Saudi Arabia, Ghamdi et al.[13] reported that the prevalence of any DR was 34.6% but what was noticeable was the high level of STDR of 17.5%, which was mostly due to high levels of referable maculopathy (15.9%) and may be related to the high number with poor glycaemic control.
4. Burgess et al.[14] reported a systematic literature review of studies of diabetic retinopathy and maculopathy in Africa. A total of 62 studies from 21 countries were included. In population-based studies, the

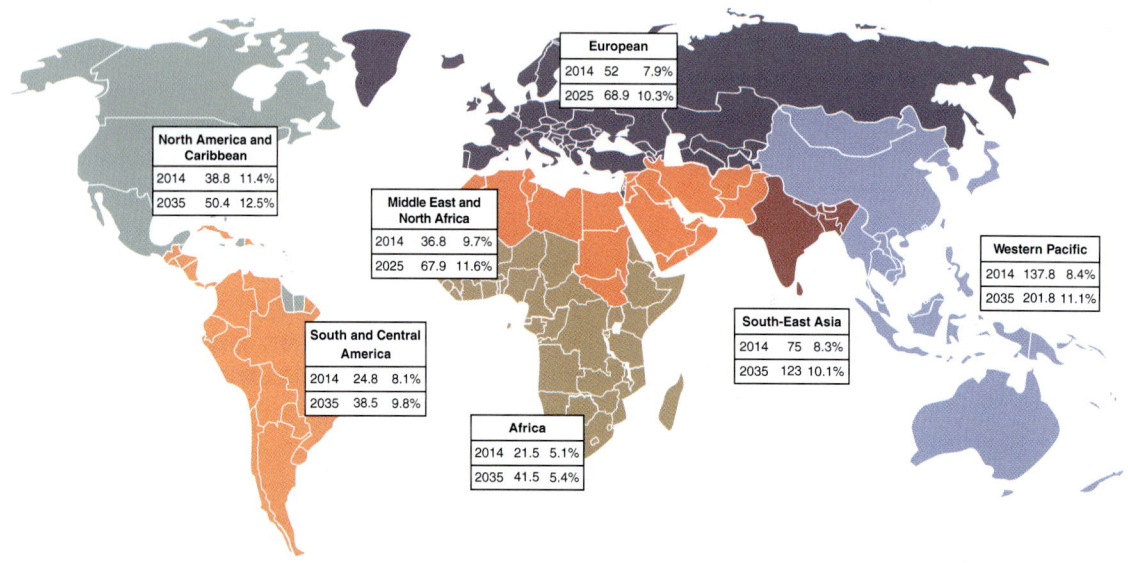

Fig. 1 World map showing rising incidence and prevalence of diabetes.

Table 1

International Diabetes Federation Prevalence estimates of Diabetes in 2014 and 2035 in 20-79 age group

		Number with diabetes in millions	% of adult population with diabetes
Africa	2014	21.5	5.1%
	2035	41.5	5.4%
Middle East and North Africa	2014	36.8	9.7%
	2025	67.9	11.6%
European	2014	52	7.9%
	2025	68.9	10.3%
North America and Caribbean	2014	38.8	11.4%
	2035	50.4	12.5%
South and Central American Region	2014	24.8	8.1%
	2035	38.5	9.8%
South-East Asian Region	2014	75	8.3%
	2035	123	10.1%
Western Pacific Region	2014	137.8	8.4%
	2035	201.8	11.1%

reported prevalence range in patients with diabetes was 30–31.6% for any DR, 0.9–1.3% for PDR and 1.2–4.5% for any maculopathy.

5. Thomas et al.[15] reported results from the Welsh Screening Programme in the UK. The prevalence of any DR and sight-threatening DR in those with type 1 diabetes was 56.0% and 11.2%, respectively, and in type 2 diabetes was 30.3% and 2.9%, respectively.

6. Wu et al.[16] reported on the prevalence of diabetic retinopathy in mainland China. The prevalence of

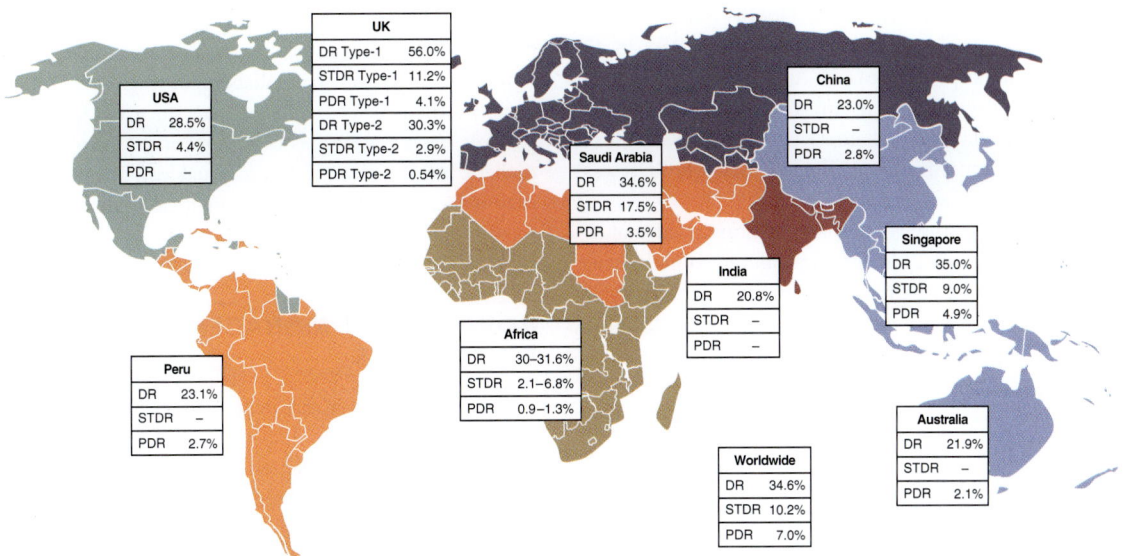

Fig. 2 World map showing high prevalence of diabetic retinopathy (DR) and proliferative DR.

Table 2

	Any DR	Sight threatening or Vision Threatening (STDR or VTDR)	Proliferative DR (PDR)
Worldwide	34.6%	10.2%	7%
USA	28.5%	4.4%	–
Saudi Arabia	34.6%	17.5%	3.5%
Africa	30–31.6%	2.1–6.8%	0.9–1.3%
UK Type 1	56.0%	11.2%	4.1%
UK Type 2	30.3%	2.9%	0.54%
China	23%	–	2.8%
Singapore	35.0%	9.0%	4.9%
India	20.8%	–	–
Peru	23.1%	–	2.7%
Australia	21.9%	–	2.1%

DR, non-proliferative diabetic retinopathy (NPDR) and proliferative diabetic retinopathy (PDR) was 23% (95% CI: 17.8–29.2%), 19.1% (95% CI: 13.6–26.3%), and 2.8% (95% CI: 1.9–4.2%) in people with diabetes.

7. Wong et al.[17] reported from the Singapore Malay Eye Study that the overall prevalence of any retinopathy was 35.0% (95% CI, 28.2–43.4%), the overall prevalence of macular oedema was 5.7% (95% CI, 3.2–9.9%), PDR 4.9% (95% CI, 2.7–8.8%) and the overall prevalence of vision-threatening retinopathy was 9.0% (95% CI, 5.8–13.8%).

8. Rema et al.[18] reported that the overall prevalence of DR in the population of known diabetic subjects in Chennai, India was 20.8% (95% CI: 18.7–23.1%) and 5.1% (95% CI: 3.1–8.0%) in subjects with newly detected diabetes.

9. Villena et al.[19] reported from a hospital-based photographic screening programme in Peru that DR was detected in 282 patients (23.1%) (95% CI: 20.71–25.44%); 249 patients (20.4%) (95% CI: 18.1–22.6%) had non-proliferative DR and 33 (2.7%) (95% CI: 1.8–3.6%) had proliferative DR.

10. In the Australian Diabetes, Obesity and Lifestyle study (AusDiab) of 11,247 adults > 25 years in 42 randomly selected areas of Australia, Tapp et al.[20] showed a prevalence of any DR of 21.9% in those with known type 2 diabetes (KDM) and 6.2% in those newly diagnosed (NDM). The prevalence of PDR was 2.1% in those with known DM.

Of note, three studies[21-23] have demonstrated that, if one screens for type 2 diabetes in different populations, the prevalence of diabetic retinopathy in screen-positive patients (7.6%, 6.8% and 9%) is much lower than the prevalence in the known population of people with diabetes.

In 1997, Kernell et al.[24] reported the youngest child in the literature (11.8 years) at that time with pre-proliferative DR from Sweden.

In 1999, Donaghue et al.[25] described the youngest child reported in the literature to have background diabetic retinopathy at that time (1999): 7.9 years (duration 5.6 years, HbA1c 8.9%) from Australia.

INCIDENCE OF DR

In 2008 and 2009, Klein et al.[26,27] reported on the 25-year cumulative progression and regression of diabetic retinopathy and cumulative incidence of macular oedema (MO) and clinically significant macular oedema (CSMO) in type 1 patients in the Wisconsin Epidemiologic Study of Diabetic Retinopathy. The 25-year cumulative rate of progression of DR was 83%, progression to proliferative DR was 42%, and improvement of DR was 18%; the 25-year cumulative incidence was 29% for ME and 17% for CSME.

In 2009, Wong et al.[28] conducted a systematic review of rates of progression of diabetic retinopathy in people with both type 1 and type 2 diabetes during different time periods. The article concluded that, since 1985, diabetic patients have lower rates of progression to proliferative diabetic retinopathy and severe visual loss. These findings may reflect an improvement in medical management of the diabetes and associated risk factors.

ADVANCES IN MANAGEMENT OF DIABETES

Advances in the management of diabetes have had a substantial impact on diabetic retinopathy. These are discussed in detail in Chapter 2 on diabetes.

The demonstration by the Diabetes Control and Complications Trial[14] that retinopathy in type 1 diabetes could be reduced by intensive treatment of blood glucose has led to much better control and retinopathy progression has been reduced. Studies[29,30] in the early 1990s showed the link between hypertension in type 1 diabetes and a higher occurrence of retinopathy and of progression of pre-existing retinopathy.

A similar demonstration in the United Kingdom Prospective Diabetes Study[31] (UKPDS) that in type 2 diabetes the development of retinopathy (incidence) was strongly associated with baseline glycaemia and glycaemic exposure, and progression was associated with hyperglycaemia (as evidenced by a higher HbA1c), has led to better control in type 2 diabetes and in a reduction in retinopathy progression. The UKPDS[32] also demonstrated that high BP is detrimental to each aspect of

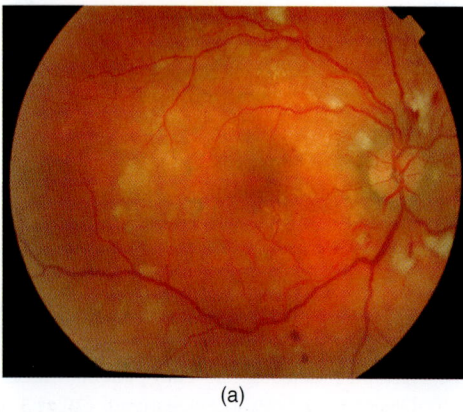
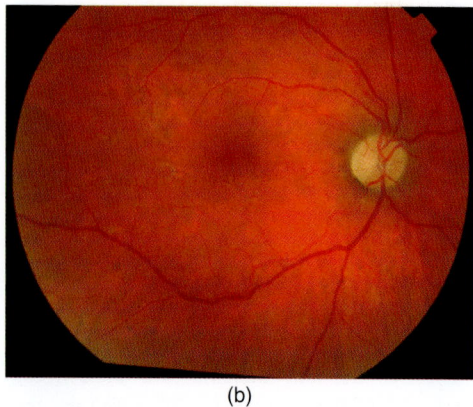

(a) (b)

Fig. 3 (a) Uncontrolled hypertension in a person with diabetes: right macula colour photo showing flame haemorrhages and cotton wool spots. (b) The result of treating the hypertension in this person.

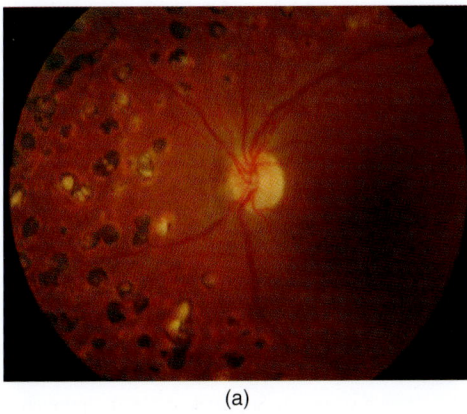
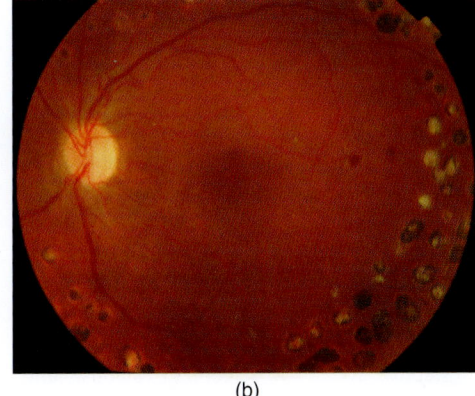

(a)   (b)

Fig. 4 Stable treated eye after panretinal photocoagulation for NVD.

diabetic retinopathy in type 2 diabetes and that a tight BP control policy reduces the risk of clinical complications from diabetic eye disease (Fig. 3).

ADVANCES IN MANAGEMENT OF DIABETIC RETINOPATHY

Since Spalter[33] described the photocoagulation of circinate maculopathy in diabetic retinopathy, clear evidence for the efficacy of laser treatment for diabetic eye disease has been shown from the Diabetic Retinopathy Study[34-38] and the Early Treatment Diabetic Retinopathy Study[39-47]. In 1981 they reported[36] that photocoagulation, as used in the study, reduced the two-year risk of severe visual loss by 50% or more (Fig. 4).

In 1985, a report[39] from the Early Treatment Diabetic Retinopathy Study showed that focal photocoagulation of 'clinically significant' diabetic macular oedema (CSMO) substantially reduced the risk of visual loss. Smiddy and Flynn[48] wrote an excellent review in 1999 when they noted that, according to the Early Treatment Diabetic Retinopathy Study, at least 5% of eyes receiving optimal medical treatment will still have progressive retinopathy that requires laser treatment and pars plana vitrectomy. They also noted that, although vitrectomy improves the prognosis for a favourable visual outcome, preventive measures such as improved control of glucose levels and timely application of panretinal photocoagulation are equally important in the management. Vitrectomy clearly does have a place in the management of diabetic eye disease. Evidence of improving visual results during the last 20 years following vitrectomy have been shown in studies reported by Blankenship and Machemer[49], Thompson et al.[50-53], Sigurdsson et al.[54], Flynn et al.[55], Nakazawa et al.[56], Karel and Kalvodova[57], Harbour et al.[58], Pendergast et al.[59], La Heij et al.[60], Yamamoto et al.[61], Amino and Tanihara[62], Lewis[63], Lahey et al.[64], Treumer et al.[65], Schrey et al.[66], Diolaiuti et al.[67], Haller et al.[68], Tao et al.[69], Gupta et al.[70] and Ostri et al.[71]. However, a restriction in driving field has been reported in over two-thirds of patients in a small series of patients by Barsam and Laidlaw[72].

Improved postoperative outcomes have recently been reported[73-75] using VEGF inhibitors preoperatively.

Developments in techniques of laser treatment are discussed Chapter 10 and treatments for DME (e.g. corticosteroids and anti-vascular endothelial growth factor drugs) are described in Chapter 7. Laser photocoagulation remains the standard of care for proliferative diabetic retinopathy, but the anti-vascular endothelial growth factor drugs are now used as a first line of treatment in many centres for centre-involving diabetic macular oedema.

Despite the available treatments, many patients present late in the course of the disease when treatment is more difficult. There have been considerable advances in early detection in the last 10 years with the advent of systematic screening programmes for diabetic retinopathy.

The St Vincent Declaration, a joint initiative on diabetes care and research of the World Health Organisation (Europe) and the International Diabetes Federation (Europe), included 5 year targets for improvement in diabetes outcomes. One of these targets was to reduce diabetes-related blindness by one-third or more over the next 5 years.

In Liverpool, UK on 17–18 November 2005 a conference took place to review progress in the prevention

of visual impairment due to diabetic retinopathy in Europe. The conference recommended the following steps in the development of systematic screening programmes for sight-threatening DR.
- Step 1: Access to effective treatment: minimum number of lasers per 100,000 population; equal access for all patient groups; and maximum time to treatment from diagnosis 3 months.
- Step 2: Establish opportunistic screening: dilated fundoscopy at time of attendance for routine care; annual review; and national guidelines on referral to an ophthalmologist.
- Step 3: Establish systematic screening: establish and maintain disease registers; sytematic call and recall for all people with diabetes; annual screening; test used has sensitivity of ≥80% and specificity of ≥90%; and coverage ≥80%.
- Step 4: Establish systematic screening with full quality assurance and full coverage: digital photographic screening; all personnel involved in screening will be certified as competent; 100% coverage; quality assurance at all stages; and central/regional data collection for monitoring and measurement of effectiveness.

The establishment of systematic screening in the UK, combined with better management of diabetes and its associated risk factors, has resulted in a report[76] demonstrating that diabetic retinopathy is no longer the leading cause of blindness in England and Wales.

PRACTICE POINTS

There is an epidemic of diabetes worldwide. The prevalence of diabetic retinopathy is rising as a consequence of the epidemic of diabetes. Effective treatments are available, but are dependent on the stage of diagnosis. Systematic screening programmes can be set up to detect diabetic retinopathy at an appropriate stage to reduce the incidence and prevalence of blindness.

REFERENCE

Please visit www.wiley.com/go/scanlon/diabetic_retinopathy

Acknowledgements

I am grateful to my colleagues in Gloucestershire and Oxford who have assisted in identifying and imaging patients that have provided very useful examples of conditions that have enhanced the quality of this book. In particular, thanks are due to: Lisa Collins (Senior Optometrist), Quresh Mohammed, Emily Fletcher, Rob Johnston, Victor Chong and Samia Fatum (Ophthalmologists), Mike Taylor, Emily Arthur, Seren Stacey-Jones (Medical Photographers), Gwen George, Scott Vallance, Jenny Mason, Tracey Scott, Lewis Smith (Ophthalmic Photographers) and Steve Chave (Informatics Lead).

I am grateful to Professor David Matthews who wrote the draft of the diabetes chapter for the first edition that has subsequently been edited, and to Dr Bahram Jafar-Mohammadi from the Oxford Centre for Diabetes and Endocrine Medicine for providing a case history of a patient with HNF-1α MODY.

I am also grateful to Professor Ogura from Nagoya, Japan and Associate Professor Fred Chen from Perth, Australia for providing images on OCT angiography and swept-source OCT.

We thank the editors for their support.

We are very grateful to all the patients who have allowed photographs of their eyes and some case histories to be included in this book.

Finally, we are grateful to our long-suffering wives and partners for their patience and understanding, and I am particularly grateful to my wife Sally for her support.

Peter H. Scanlon

About the companion website

This book is accompanied by a companion website:

www.wiley.com/go/scanlon/diabetic_retinopathy

The website includes:
- References cited in the chapters
- Figures used in the book.

1 Introduction

Peter H. Scanlon

Harris Manchester College, University of Oxford; Medical Ophthalmology, University of Gloucestershire, UK

In this book the fundamental approach is to describe the classification of diabetes, risk factors for diabetic retinopathy and lesions of diabetic retinopathy, and explain the significance of these lesions in terms of progression of the disease, recommended treatment and consequences to vision. Methods of screening for diabetic retinopathy and other retinal conditions that are more frequent in diabetes, or have similar appearances to diabetic retinopathy, are also discussed.

The four main themes in this introductory chapter are: (1) practical assessment consisting of history and examination; (2) multidisciplinary management; (3) investigative techniques to assess diabetic retinopathy; and (4) the use of lasers in diabetic retinopathy.

PRACTICAL ASSESSMENT

History

The history of the patient can be divided into the following sections: presenting complaint; past ocular history; diabetic history; past medical history; family history; drug history; and psychosocial history.

Presenting complaint

Many patients with diabetic retinopathy are asymptomatic until the more advanced stages of the disease. When symptoms do occur they are usually a gradual blurring of vision in diabetic maculopathy and a sudden onset of visual symptoms with a vitreous haemorrhage. Patients notice a streak or a sudden onset of floaters in one eye, which increases with progressive visual loss over the next hour as the vitreous haemorrhage progresses. The amount of visual loss depends on the amount or position of the vitreous haemorrhage. If the vitreous or preretinal haemorrhage is in the visual axis of the eye, then visual loss is usually quite marked.

Past ocular history

The past ocular history of patients covers: (1) visual symptoms; (2) cataract or strabismus surgery; (3) laser treatment; and (4) vitrectomy.

Diabetic history

The diabetic history of a patient includes: (1) type of diabetes; (2) duration of diabetes; and (3) treatment of diabetes (e.g. diet, oral hypoglycaemics, insulin or a combination).

Complications of diabetes

The complications of diabetes can fall within three categories: (1) nephropathy (renal impairment, peritoneal dialysis, haemodialysis); (2) cardiovascular (angina, myocardial infarction, coronary artery bypass); and (3) cerebrovascular (transient ischaemic attack, stroke).

Past medical history

Past medical history can include serious illnesses and operations.

Drug history

Patients should disclose drug history such as present medication and any allergies.

Family history

Any history of diabetes or other illnesses in the family should be discussed.

Psychosocial

The patient's physosocial factors, such as occupation, number of cigarettes smoked per day, units of alcohol consumed per day, history of psychiatric illness and home circumstances (e.g. type of accommodation, whether lives alone, etc.), must be considered.

A Practical Manual of Diabetic Retinopathy Management, Second Edition.
Edited by Peter Scanlon, Ahmed Sallam, and Peter van Wijngaarden.
© 2017 John Wiley & Sons Ltd. Published 2017 by John Wiley & Sons Ltd.
Companion Website: www.wiley.com/go/scanlon/diabetic_retinopathy

Eye examination

Assessment of visual acuity

The first part of the eye examination is an assessment of visual acuity (VA). A Snellen or LogMar chart is used and should be back surface illuminated in order to provide accurate measurements (see Figs 1.1 and 1.2).

The unaided VA is recorded first. The VA with current distance spectacle correction is then recorded. Finally, the VA with current distance spectacle correction and a pinhole is recorded. The best of these three measurements is recorded as the best corrected visual acuity. A refraction may be performed if required.

Assessment of colour vision

People with diabetes can develop an acquired colour vision defect (typically a blue loss initially) prior to showing any significant features of diabetic retinopathy. I have seen one patient who appeared to have mild non-proliferative diabetic retinopathy who had developed pronounced loss of colour vision; this meant that he was unable to continue in his current employment as a train driver.

The most appropriate test for identifying and quantifying acquired colour vision loss is the Farnsworth-Munsell 100 hue discrimination test (see Fig. 1.3). In clinical practice, however, this test is often not available and the Ishihara test, which is designed for detecting congenital (red/green) colour vision defects, is applied. If the Ishihara test is used for the assessment of acquired colour vision defects, clinicians need to be cautious when interpreting test results since it produces a high false-negative rate; passing the test is not necessarily consistent with normal colour vision.

Inspection of external structures

An inspection of external structures includes comparing one eye with the other to detect unilateral abnormalities and to determine whether the opening between the lids is symmetrical. The margins of the eyelids are inspected for ingrowing eye lashes, inversion or eversion, mucus, discharge, scales or lumps. The conjunctival lining is inspected in each eye and the area over the lacrimal sac at the medial corner of the lower lids and nose on each side.

Visual fields to confrontation

The patient must cover one eye and stare at the examiner's eye. The examiner's finger/hand or an object such as a hat pin with a white or coloured head will then be moved out of the patient's visual field and be brought back in, and the patient asked to indicate when the finger/hand

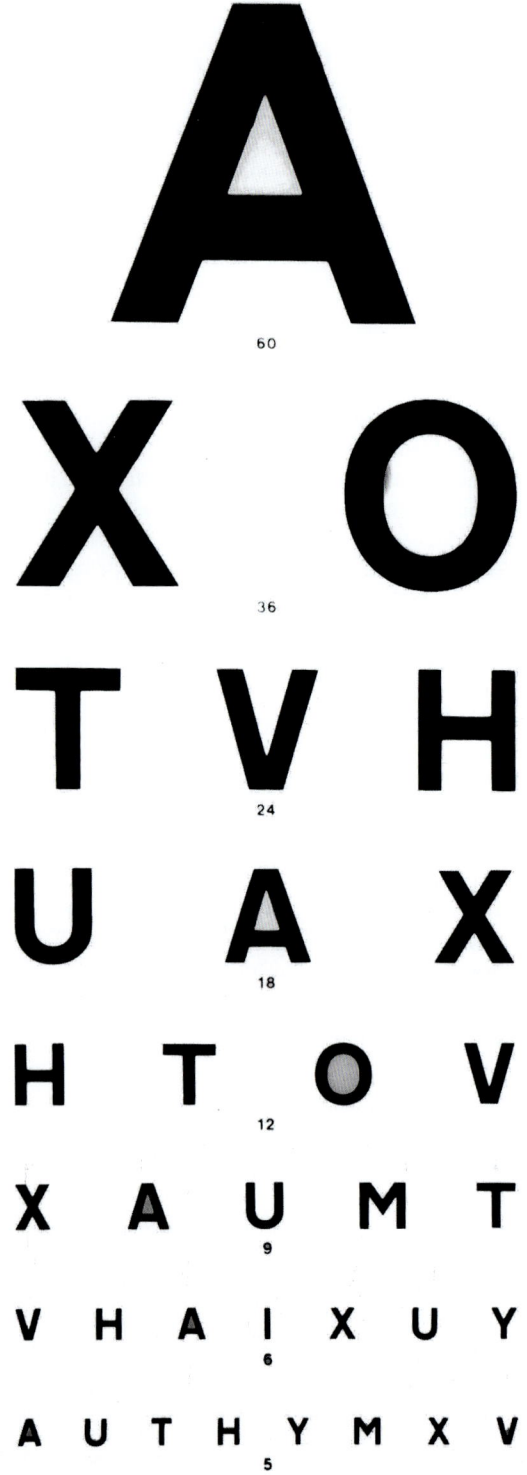

Fig. 1.1 Snellen visual acuity chart.

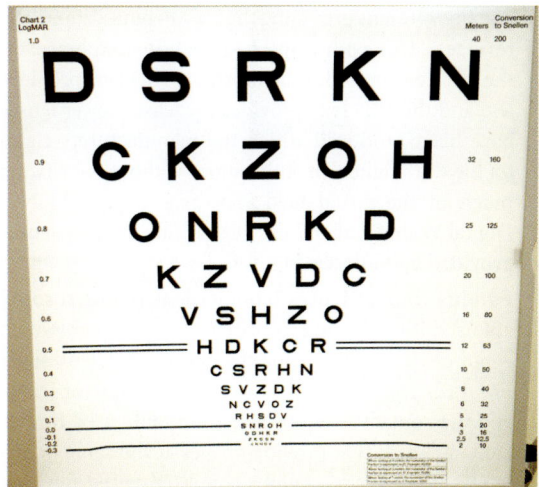

Fig. 1.2 LogMar visual acuity chart.

or object comes back into view. This can be used as a simple preliminary test and can be useful particularly if a hemianopia is suspected. More minor degrees of field loss usually require formal testing using automated perimetry or a tangent screen examination.

Ocular movement
Patients with diabetes do develop nerve palsies that affect ocular movement, but this is usually apparent from the history of sudden onset of diplopia.

Pupillary reactions to light and accommodation
The pupils should be inspected to check that they are equal in size and shape and that they react equally to light and accommodation.

Red reflex with an ophthalmoscope
This helps to determine if a media opacity is present, for example, a cataract or vitreous haemorrhage.

Slit-lamp biomicroscopy of the eye
1. **Check that a clear binocular image of the slit beam can be obtained.** First check that clear monocular images can be obtained from each eyepiece. A frequent cause of blurred vision is that the previous operator may have left these eyepieces at an unusual focus. The eyepiece construction allows for the distance between both eyepieces to be modified to reflect the interpupillary distance of the user. A sharply defined single image of the slit should be seen.
2. **Patient instructions and positioning.** Clear instructions need to be given to the patient and the patient needs to be comfortable. This may require: adjusting the patient height; adjusting the height of the chin rest so that the outer canthus of the patient's eye is aligned with the marker; ensure that the patient's head is central; and a fixation target may be used for the eye not being examined.
3. **Illumination.** Controlling the light levels falling on the eye is also an important part of any slit-lamp routine. This can be achieved by altering the power, adding a filter or altering the slit width and height.
4. **Magnification level.** The magnification can be adjusted depending on the type of slit lamp used.

Routinely undertaken examinations
Examination of the following structures is routinely undertaken: (1) lids and lashes; (2) conjunctiva, cornea and sclera; (3) tear film assessment; (4) anterior chamber; (5) iris (it is important in diabetic retinopathy to check the iris for rubeosis); and (6) lens (a cataract is more common in people with diabetes).

Intraocular pressure
Measurement of intraocular pressure is often undertaken using the Goldmann tonometer.

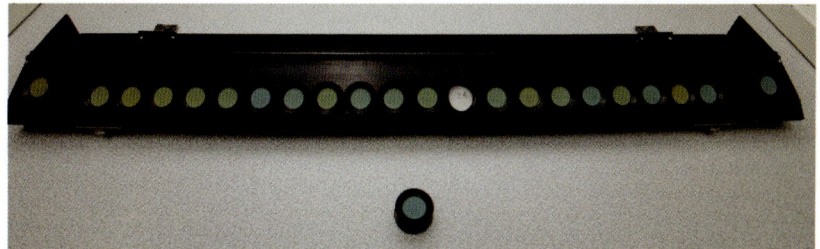

Fig. 1.3 Farnsworth-Munsell 100 hue discrimination test.

Pupil dilation

Both pupils are dilated with G Tropicamide 1% and, in most patients, also G Phenylephrine 2.5%.

Direct ophthalmoscopy

Direct ophthalmoscopy is an examination method which is commonly used by physicians and general practitioners. It provides magnified views of retinal details such as the optic disc, individual retinal vessels and the fovea. It is fast and easy to perform and images appear upright and in normal orientation. It has a limited two-dimensional (2D) field of view and has been shown to have a limited sensitivity and specificity for the detection of sight-threatening diabetic retinopathy. It is, however, useful for ad hoc detection of diabetic retinopathy (see Fig. 1.4).

Slit-lamp biomicroscopy of the retina

Slit-lamp biomicroscopy is the most common method employed by ophthalmologists to diagnose and monitor retinal disease. A well-dilated pupil is very important for obtaining an adequate view of the posterior segment with the slit-lamp biomicroscope. Several condensing lenses enable the desired magnification to be achieved. These lenses fall into two categories.

1. **Non-contact lenses**, such as the 60D, 78D and 90D, provide a magnified stereoscopic view and an inverted, reversed image of the retina. The 60D lens provides the most magnification, with the 78D lens providing less and the 90D lens providing the least magnification. The reverse is true with respect to field of view, however; the 90D lens provides the most, the 78D lens provides less and the 60D lens provides the least. Newer lenses have been produced which the manufacturers claim to have a higher magnification without sacrificing much of the visual field view (e.g. Superfield NC, Digital Wide Field and the Digital 1.0x imaging lenses provided by Volk; see Fig. 1.5).

2. **Fundus contact lenses (contact lens biomicrosopy)** are used if thickening or oedema is suspected (which is not obvious when using the non-contact lenses; see Fig. 1.6). The Goldmann three- or four-mirror lenses and the contact ruby lens are commonly used fundus contact lenses that provide images at the same orientation as the retina. Lenses commonly used for laser such as the Volk Area Centralis and the Ocular Mainster (Standard) focal/grid lens provide an inverted image.

For scanning the retina, moderate illumination and a wider slit-lamp beam are used. For evaluating retinal thickness in the macular area and elsewhere, a thin, elongated slit-lamp beam with bright illumination is used. Patients who are sensitive to light can be examined using a red-free filter. When a red-free filter is used, choroidal naevi are more difficult to visualise but haemorrhages, intraretinal microvascular abnormality (IRMA) and neovascularisation are usually easily visible.

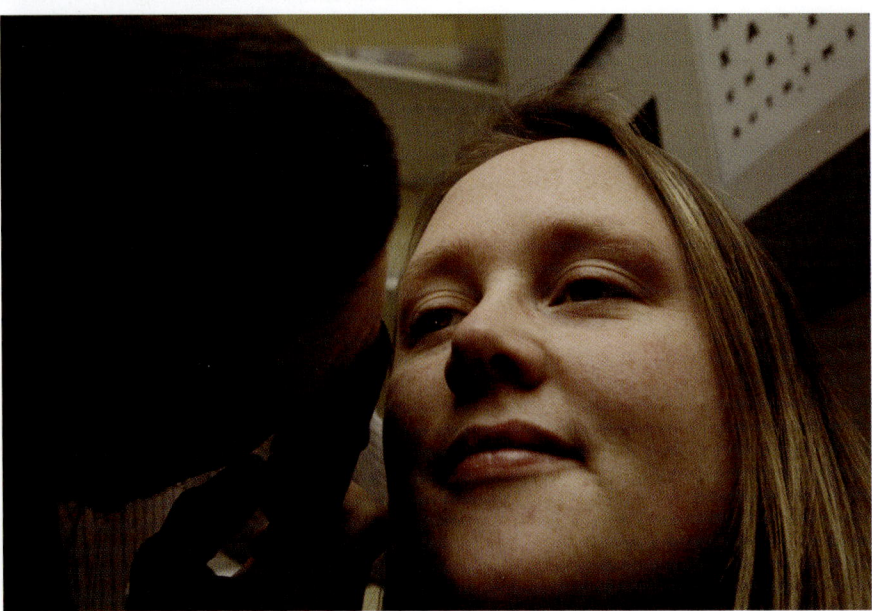

Fig. 1.4 Direct ophthalmoscopy.

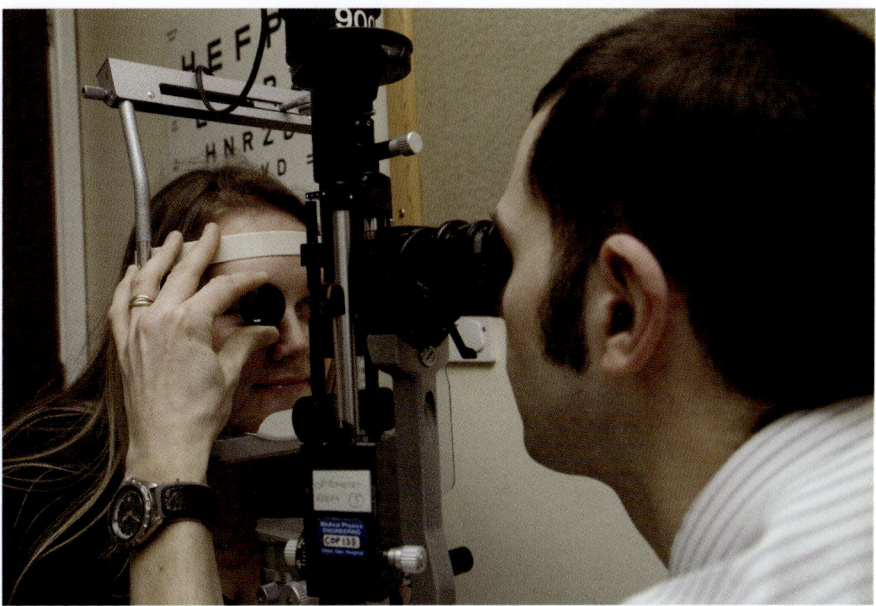

Fig. 1.5 Slit-lamp biomicroscopy with 78D lens.

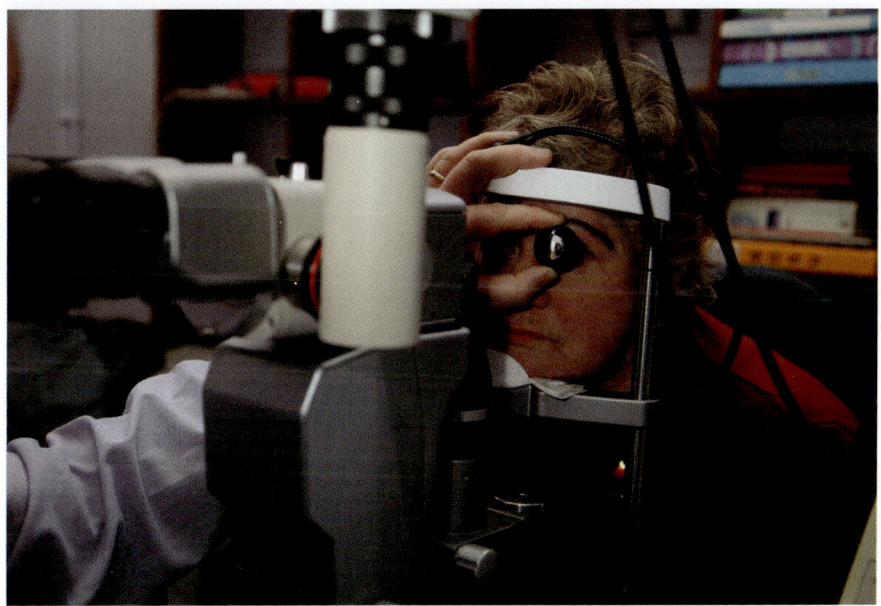

Fig. 1.6 Contact lens biomicroscopy.

Binocular indirect ophthalmoscopy

Binocular indirect ophthalmoscopy (BIO) is useful for evaluating the posterior segment and retinal periphery (see Figs 1.7 and 1.8). A larger area can be viewed than with slit-lamp biomicroscopy, but this view is less magnified.

The BIO is adjusted for the operator's interpupillary distance; the illumination system is usually placed in the upper one-third of the field for the superior retina examination and lower one-third for the inferior retina. Lens powers used for binocular indirect ophthalmoscopy vary from +14D to +40D lenses. The 20D lens is often

6 A practical manual of diabetic retinopathy management

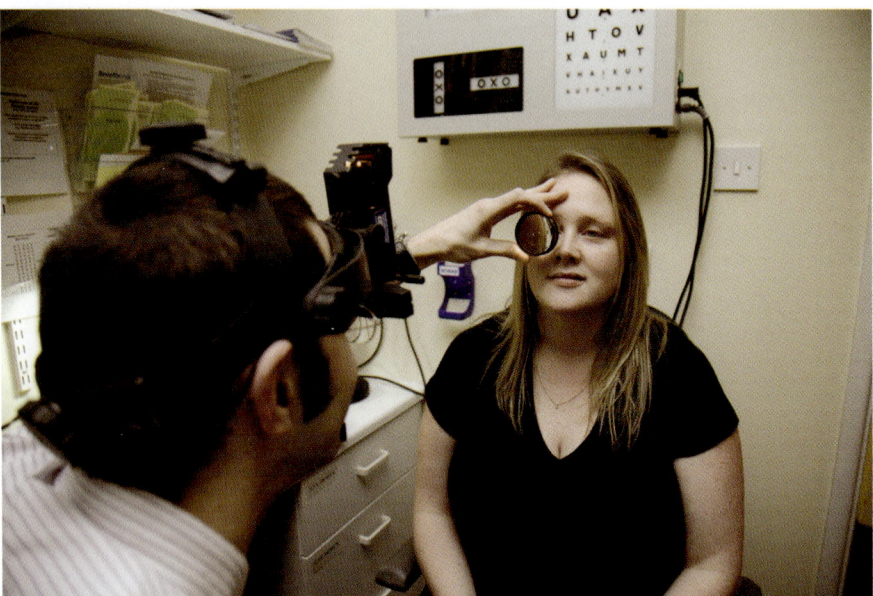

Fig. 1.7 Binocular indirect ophthalmoscopy.

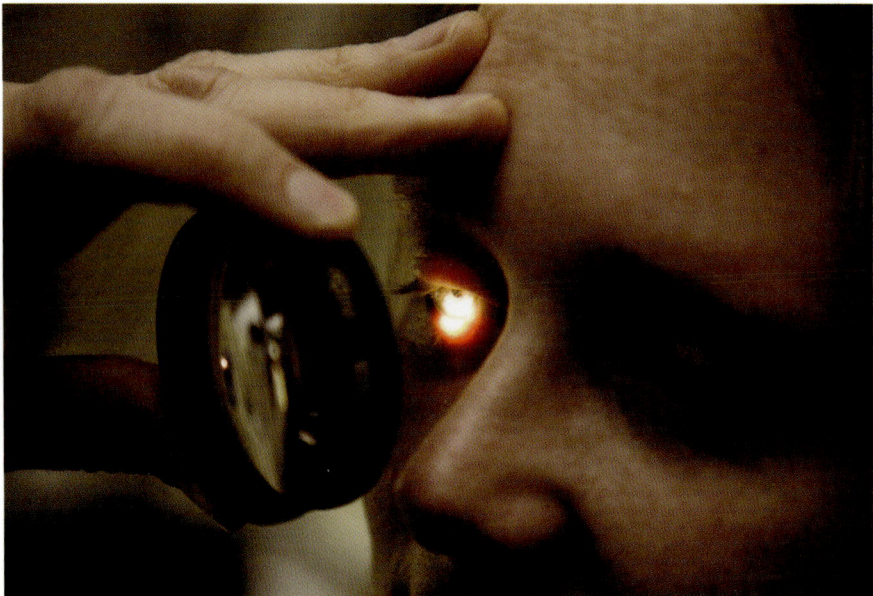

Fig. 1.8 Binocular indirect ophthalmoscopy.

used as it provides adequate magnification and field of view in most situations. As the lens dioptre increases, the width of the field of view increases. The lower the power of the condensing lens, the further from the eye it must be held. The stronger the power of the condensing lens, the closer it must be held towards the eye. To achieve high magnification with any lens, the lens is kept stationary and the operator should move closer to it.

When performing binocular indirect ophthalmoscopy, the best position for the patient is reclined. The addition of scleral depression enables one to further evaluate the retinal periphery when required.

MULTIDISCIPLINARY MANAGEMENT

There are a number of risk factors for progression of diabetic retinopathy that do not usually come within the remit of the ophthalmologist's management of the patient, such as control of blood glucose, blood pressure (BP) and lipids. It is very important for the ophthalmologist to be aware of the control of these risk factors in the individual patient and to have good communication with the diabetic physician or general practitioner who is looking after this aspect of the patient's management.

A rapid improvement in diabetic retinopathy can sometimes be seen when a previously uncontrolled hypertensive receives adequate treatment for their BP. Similarly, a patient who has had poor renal function who commences renal dialysis nay show an improvement in their diabetic retinopathy independent of their BP control.

It is important for the ophthalmologist to be involved when a patient who has had poor glucose control and high HbA1c values for a number of years suddenly decides to dramatically improve their control with the assistance of their diabetic physician. Monitoring for a deterioration of their diabetic retinopathy in the first 6–12 months following the rapid improvement of diabetic control caused by the 'early worsening phenomenon' (described in Chapter 7) is required, particularly if any diabetic retinopathy is present at baseline.

INVESTIGATIVE TECHNIQUES TO ASSESS DIABETIC RETINOPATHY

Retinal photography, fundus fluorescein angiography, ocular coherence tomography and ultrasound B-scan examination are described in Chapter 5.

Perimetry

Perimetry is the systematic measurement of differential light sensitivity in the visual field by the detection of the presence of test targets on a defined background in order to map and quantify the visual field. There are two main methods for undertaking perimetry: (1) kinetic stimulus presentation; and (2) static stimulus presentation.

Goldmann kinetic perimetry

The most common visual field equipment used for kinetic assessment is the Goldman perimeter. It is a large hemispherical bowl of radius 30 cm with a standardized white interior brightness onto which stimuli of various sizes and brightness are projected. Patients are required to maintain fixation on a central target while a stimulus of specified size (from 1 mm to 5 mm diameter) and brightness is moved slowly from the patient's peripheral area of 'non-seeing' into the area of 'seeing'. When the patient first detects the light stimulus, they respond by pressing a buzzer to alert the operator (Fig. 1.9a and b).

The stimulus is moved systematically by the perimetrist to examine areas of the visual field. Points of equal retinal sensitivity are mapped onto a chart, which when joined together produce a contour line called an 'isopter'. Any contraction of the visual field, area of reduced sensitivity or blind spot becomes evident as they are mapped out (Fig. 1.10).

Goldmann perimetry is particularly helpful in the detection and diagnosis of neurological visual field defects, for example quadrantinopia and hemianopia. Due to the subjectivity and versatility of the examination procedure, the assessment requires an experienced and skilled perimetrist.

Automated static perimetry

Automated perimeters use static light stimuli, of various intensities at fixed locations within a hemispherical bowl, to provide an accurate measurement of retinal sensitivity. Automated perimeters are particularly effective in identifying and quantifying defects within the central visual field and are used routinely for screening for abnormality and for quantifying progression of defects. The equipment employs various testing strategies which are selected by the clinician based on the underlying pathology, suspected pathology and the level of detail required (screening or detailed quantification of defects).

The testing procedure involves presenting single- or multiple-patterned, static light stimuli in a pre-selected, random order to minimize patient prediction. Once the stimulus is observed, the patient responds either verbally or via means of a buzzer. The pattern of stimuli presented and the time taken to complete the test is dependent on the strategy selected. Visual field examination can be time-consuming for the patient who may be required to concentrate for long periods of time. Optimizing the length of testing time to reduce patient fatigue and to maximize performance is an important factor in test selection and in obtaining reliable results.

The Humphrey visual field analyser is generally considered to be the most common visual field equipment in use in UK ophthalmology departments (see Fig. 1.11). Normal visual field examination requires each eye to be tested

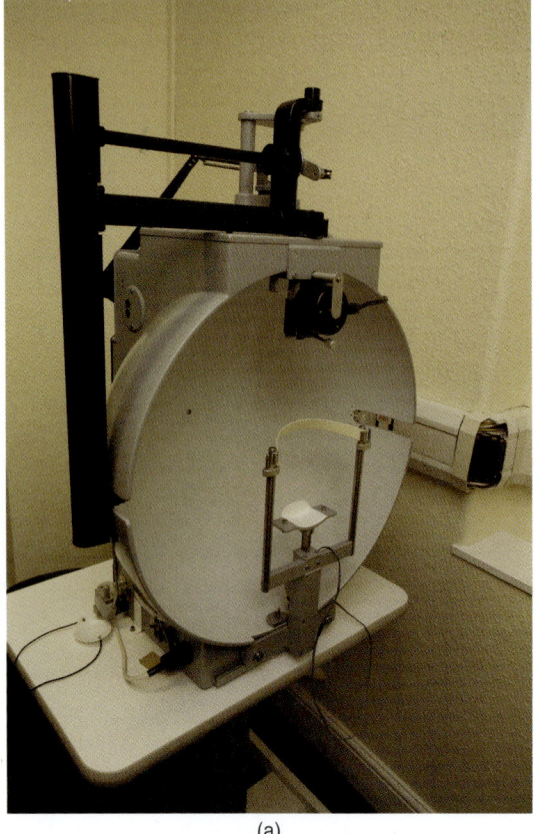 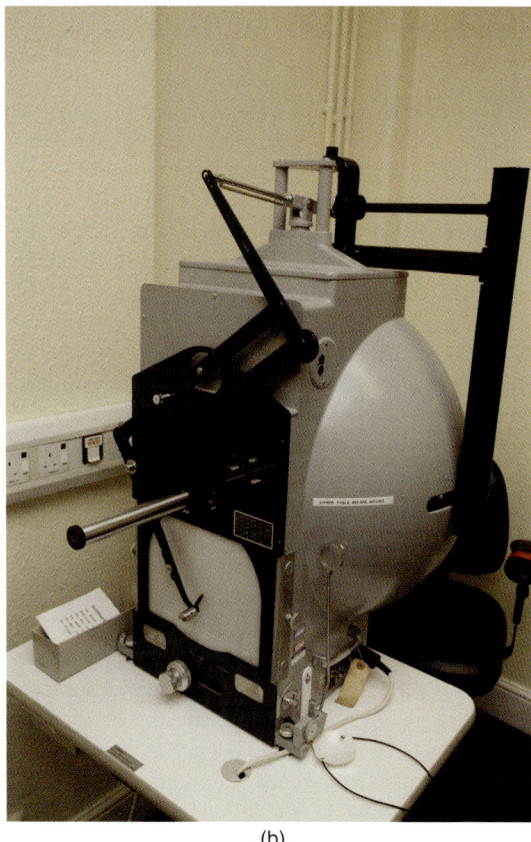

Fig. 1.9 Goldmann Perimeter: (a) patient view and (b) operator view.

independently (Fig. 1.12a and b). One eye is covered while the other maintains accurate, central fixation for the duration of the test. Occasionally, binocular visual field testing is required for patients who have undergone panretinal photocoagulation, resulting in peripheral visual field constriction or defects within the central 20 degrees. This may impact on a person's ability to meet the UK Driver and Vehicle Licensing Agency (DVLA) visual field standard. This requires a binocular assessment to be undertaken, using the Esterman grid testing pattern. A series of 120 points, at a specified light intensity, are presented individually across a rectangular area extending over 150 degrees of the horizontal binocular visual field. Holders of a UK driver's licence are required to meet the standard of a horizontal visual field of at least 120 degrees, with no significant central defect (see Fig. 1.13a and b). (For detailed information on the visual standards required for driving, please refer to the DVLA, www.dvla.gov.uk).

THE APPLICATION OF LASERS IN DIABETIC RETINOPATHY

The acronym laser is defined as light amplification by simulated emission of radiation. Coherence is one of the unique properties of laser light. It arises from the stimulated emission process which provides the amplification, and the emitted photons are 'in step' and have a definite phase relation to each other. Spatial coherence tells us how uniform the phase of the wave front is, which gives us the ability to precisely focus the laser beam to apply very small burns to pathological tissue with minimal disturbance to surrounding tissue. Temporal coherence tells us how monochromatic a source is, and this gives us the ability to select a very narrow bandwidth of light that is preferentially absorbed by the pathological tissue site.

With the improvement of laser technology, different types of laser are used in the diagnosis and treatment of

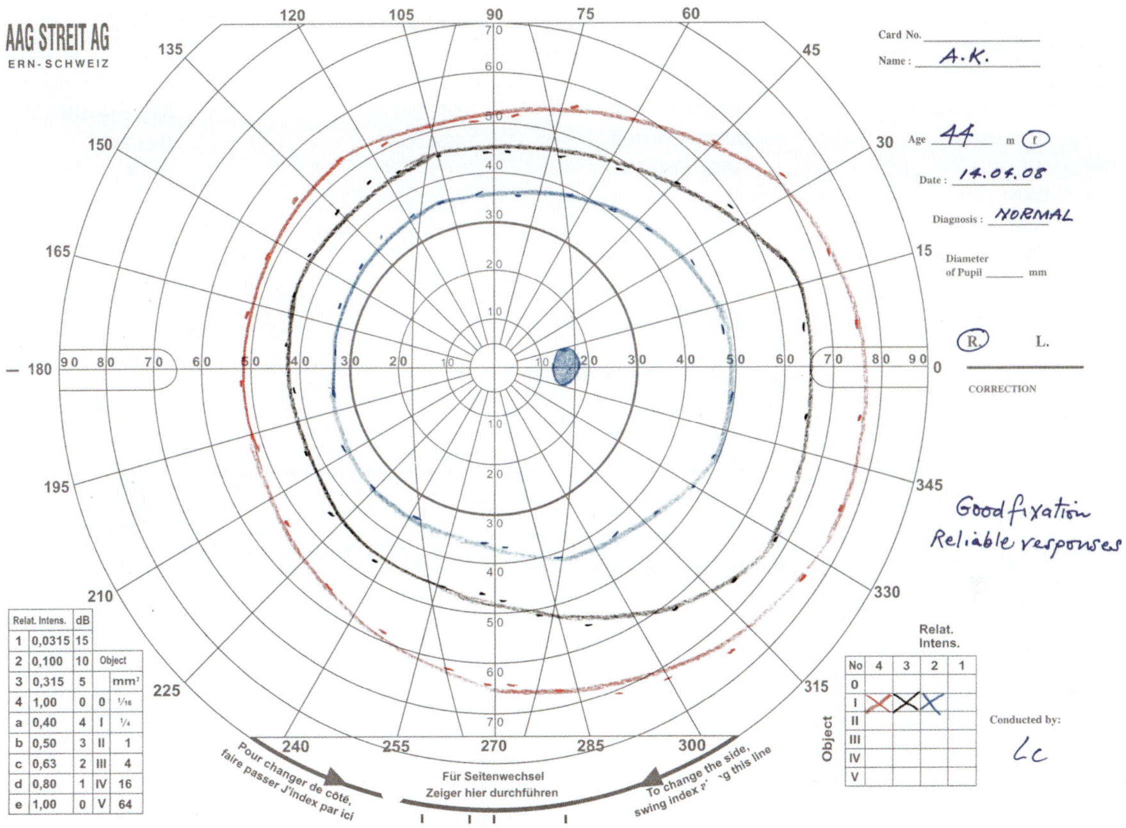

Fig. 1.10 Example of a normal Goldmann visual field.

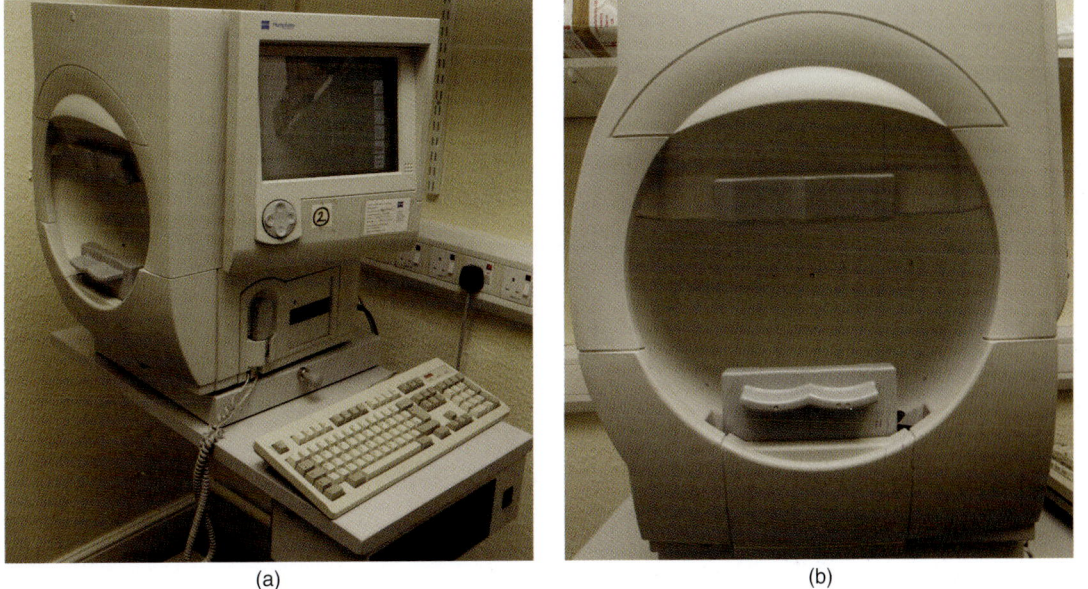

Fig. 1.11 Humphrey visual field analyser: (a) operator's view and (b) subject's view of where the chin and forehead are rested and the view of where individual lights are presented to test the field of vision.

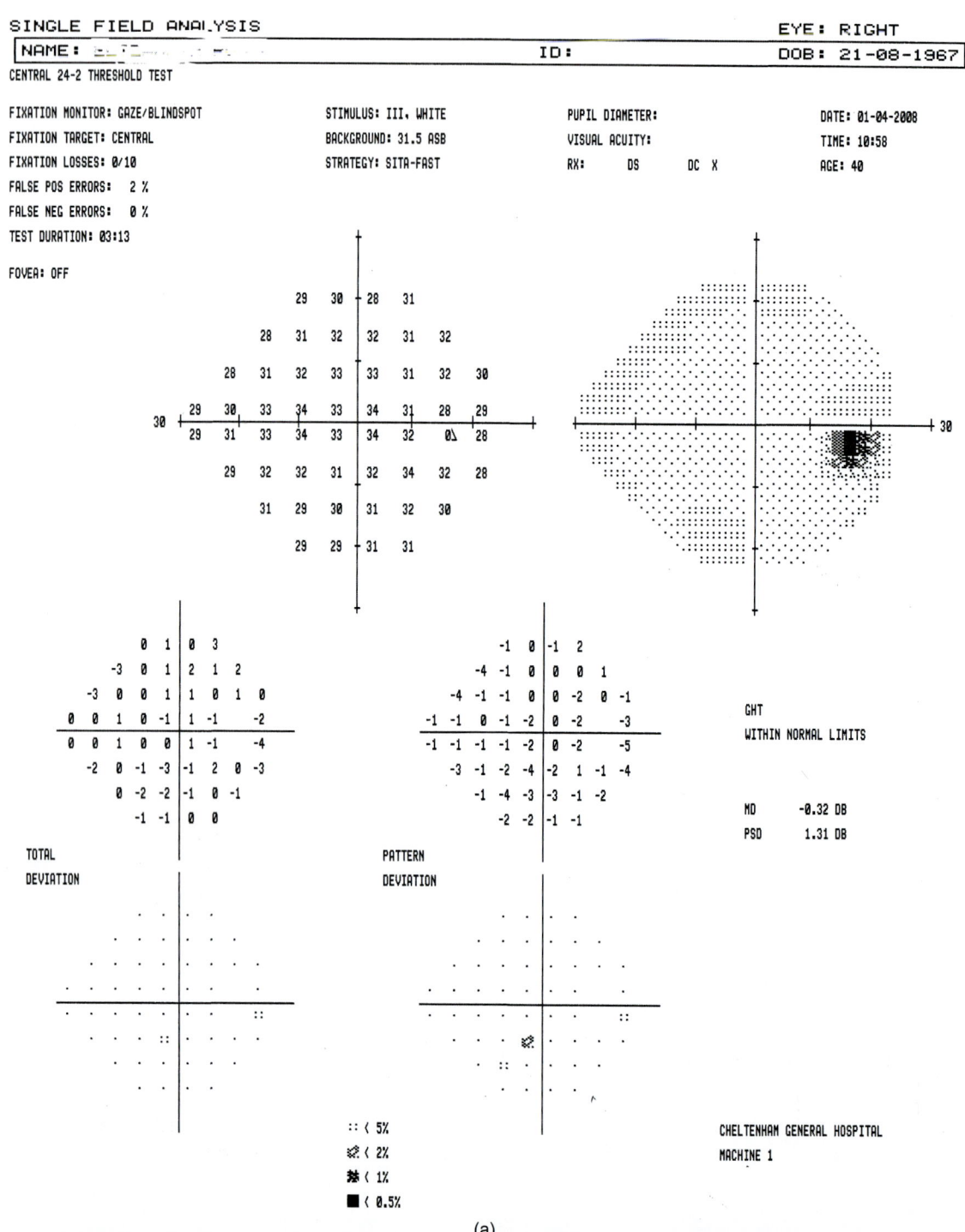

Fig. 1.12 (a, b) Example of a normal Humphrey visual field for right and left eyes.

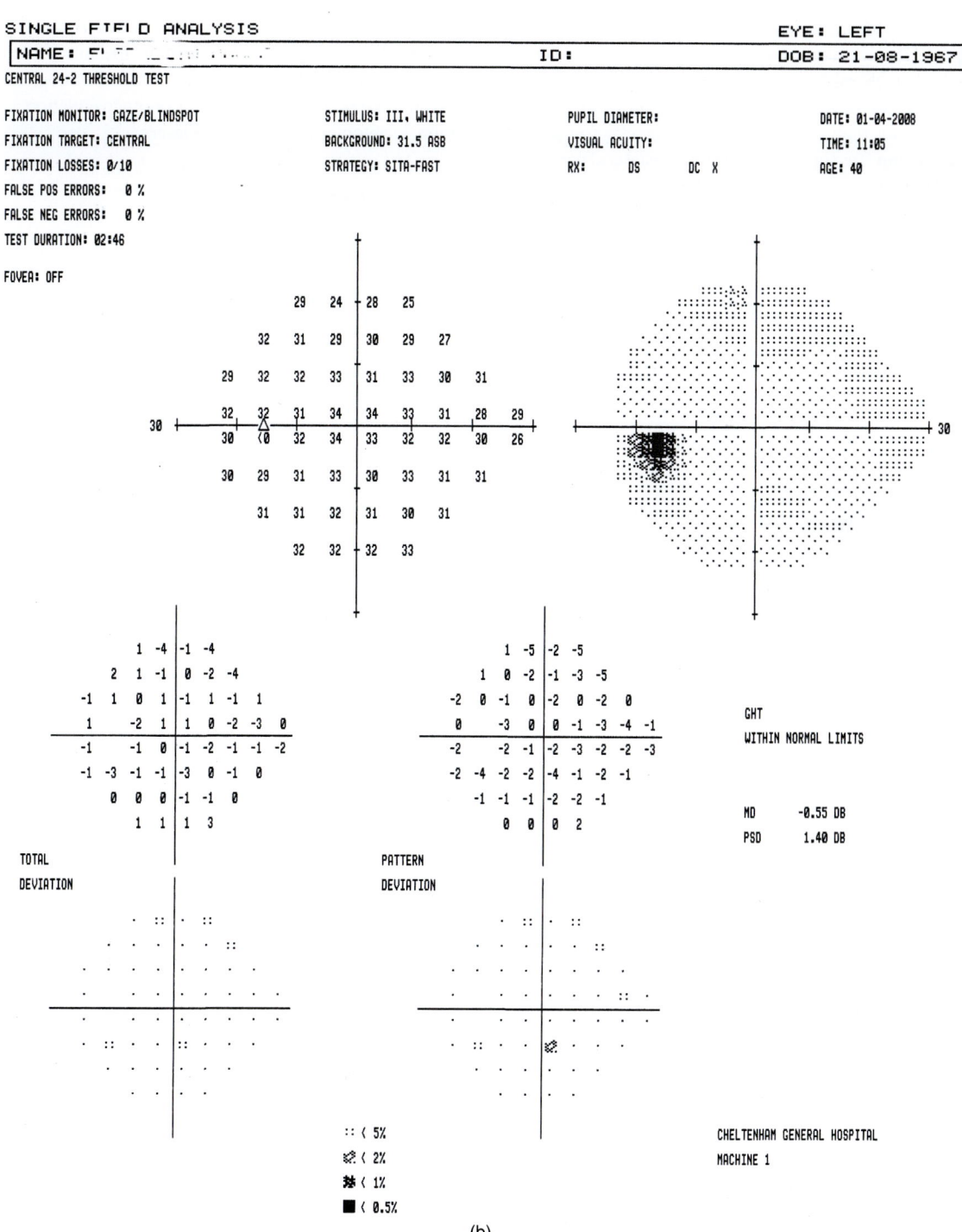

Fig. 1.12 *Continued*

many eye disorders. Laser–tissue interactions can occur in several ways but are broadly grouped under photothermal, photochemical and photoionising effects.

When lasers are used for the treatment of diabetic retinopathy, they rely principally on the effect of photocoagulation. Two other clinical effects of lasers commonly used in ophthalmology are photodisruption and photoablation, all defined in the following.

Photocoagulation

Photocoagulation (photothermal effect) causes denaturation of proteins when temperatures rise sufficiently. The temperature rise in tissues is proportional to the amount of light absorbed by that tissue. The retinal pigment epithelium absorbs light due to the melanin content and blood vessels absorb light due to their haemoglobin content. Lasers commonly used for photocoagulation are argon, krypton or diode Nd:YAG lasers.

Photodisruption

Photodisruption (photoionising effect) is the process by which short-pulsed, high-power lasers disrupt tissues by delivering irradiance to tissue targets such as the peripheral iris, producing a laser iridotomy for the prevention of angle-closure glaucoma using an Nd:YAG Q-switched laser.

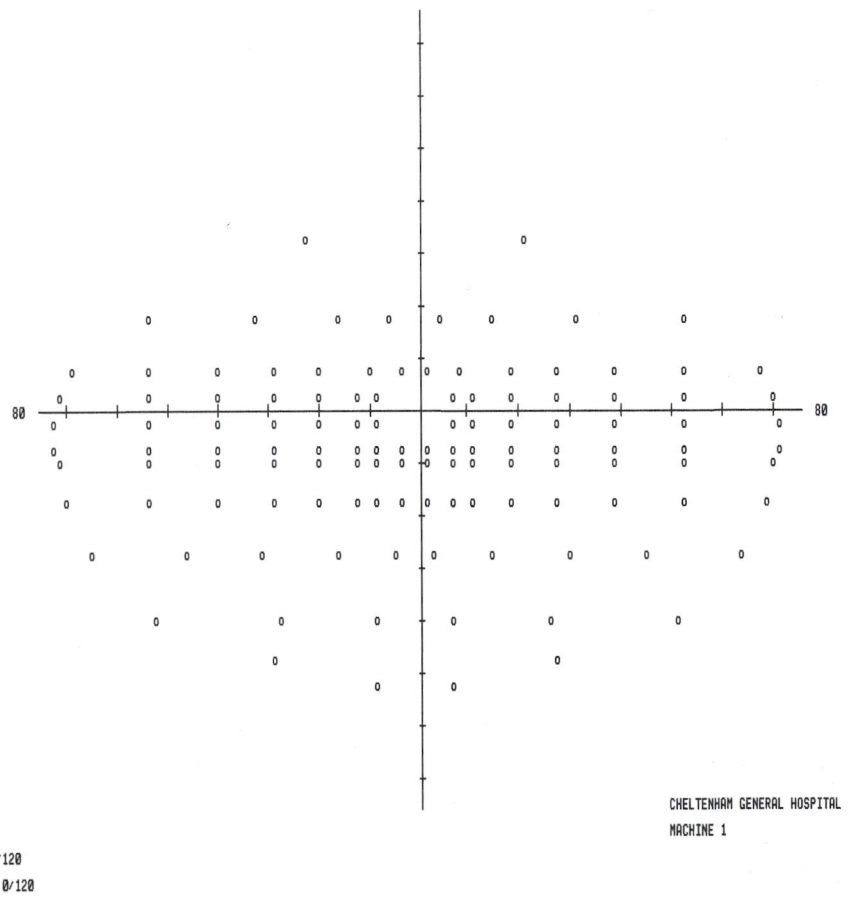

Fig. 1.13 (a) Example of a normal Esterman visual field. (b) Example of a restricted Esterman field in a diabetic patient. The case history of this patient is described in Chapter 9 on proliferative and advanced diabetic retinopathy.

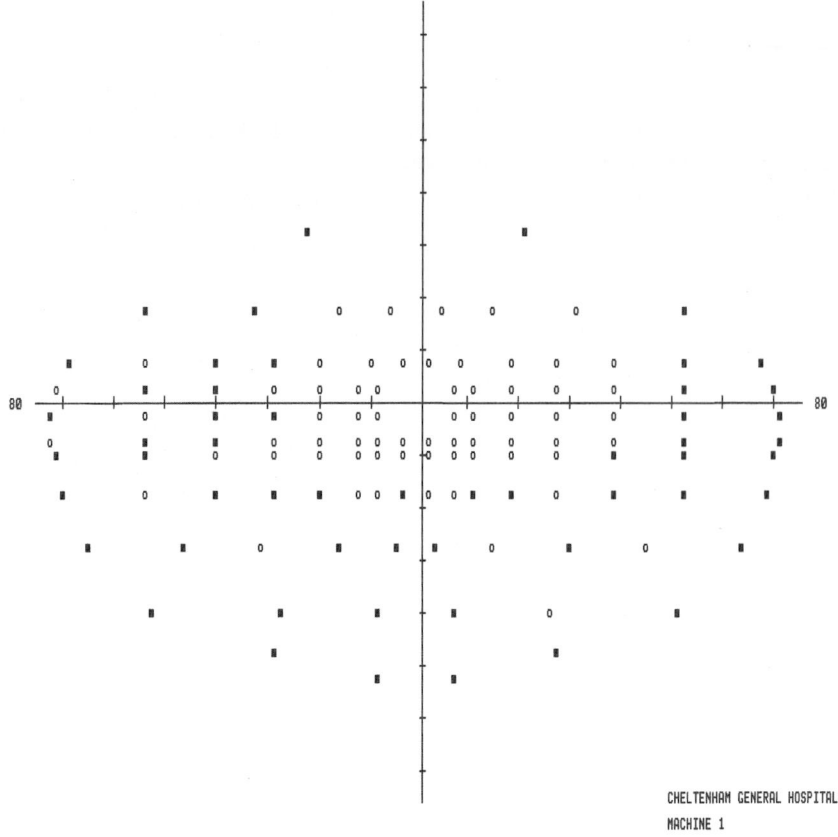

(b)

Fig. 1.13 Continued

Photoablation (photochemical effect)

Photoablation (photochemical effect) describes the process by which tissue is removed in some way by light, such as when intermolecular bands of biological tissues are broken, disintegrating target tissues, and the disintegrated molecules are volatilised. The excimer laser uses photoablation in photorefractive procedures, for example photorefractive keratectomy (PRK) and laser subepithelial keratectomy (LASEK).

Active laser media

Active laser media are available in the following states:
- solid (crystalline or amorphous; e.g. Nd:YAG laser, Rubin laser);
- liquid (e.g. dye laser);
- gaseous (e.g. argon ion laser, CO_2 laser, excimer laser); or
- other (e.g. diode laser).

A laser gain medium is the active medium of the laser which can amplify the power of light. The term gain refers to the amount of amplification. Energy is pumped into the active medium in a very disorganized form and is partially transformed into radiation energy, which is highly ordered.

Light wavelengths produced by different lasers

Argon blue-green lasers produce light over a narrow bandwidth, the main peaks being at 488 and 514 nm.

This laser is the most common laser that is used in diabetic retinopathy treatment for both panretinal laser and macular laser treatment.

The Pascal pattern scan laser is a frequency-doubled Nd:YAG diode-pumped solid-state laser producing light of wavelength 532 nm. This laser was introduced in June 2006 and it is unique in that it allows the operator to apply multiple spots almost simultaneously in pre-chosen patterns of up to 25 spots.

Diode lasers were introduced in 1993 with reports of laser-emitting diodes of gallium-aluminium-arsenide which were portable, and their wavelength of emission was 810 nm. Most of the laser energy from the diode laser is absorbed by the pigment in the melanocytes in the choroid, which made it more difficult for the operator to define the correct treatment power to use and was more painful for patients.

PRACTICE POINTS

Modern technology has produced major advances in the investigations and treatment that can be undertaken in our diabetic patients over the last 30 years. However, a carefully taken history and high-quality clinical examination is a vital component of the care of any patient with diabetic retinopathy.

2 Diabetes

Jonathan Shaw[1] & Peter H. Scanlon[2]

[1] Baker IDI Heart and Diabetes Institute, Melbourne, Australia
[2] Harris Manchester College, University of Oxford; Medical Ophthalmology, University of Gloucestershire, UK

Diabetes mellitus is a chronic condition in which there is an excess of glucose circulating in the bloodstream. Glucose homeostasis is complex and is the result of the interplay of insulin secretion and insulin sensitivity. Typically the differences between type 1 (T1DM) and type 2 (T2DM) diabetes are characterised by the absolute deficiency of insulin in the former and the relative deficiency of insulin associated with insulin resistance in the latter. This insulin deficiency – either complete or partial – is the basic mechanism behind diabetes, although other factors have an influence and can sometimes be more important when considering treatment. Insulin resistance, defined as the reduced capacity of peripheral tissues and the liver to respond to insulin, is almost always found in diabetes; it is especially important in type 2 diabetes where insulin resistance compounds the insulin secretory defects. Because insulin resistance can be such a feature of T2DM, hyperinsulinaemia may be found although the high concentrations are still insufficient to control the glycaemia.

The body normally regulates glucose very precisely in the fasting state between about 4.0 and 5.5 mmol/L in the plasma. Blood glucose concentrations above the normal limits lead to numerous biochemical changes, including excessive glycosylation of proteins, which collectively lead to long-term complications of diabetes. In addition to the direct biochemical effects of hyperglycaemia, other associated conditions, such as hypertension, contribute to the risks of microvascular disease, of which the most common is diabetic retinopathy.

CLASSIFICATION OF DIABETES

Diabetes mellitus is generally divided into the categories type 1 and type 2, with much rarer additional categories of maturity-onset diabetes of the young (MODY) and secondary diabetes. The two major forms differ in the cause and urgency of treatment necessary. It has even been suggested that the dichotomy is false as there is a grey area between the two types[1]. As a broad generalisation, type 1 diabetes occurs in those who are generally younger (so teenagers are more likely to have type 1 and those in middle age type 2) and thinner (being overweight is a risk for type 2 diabetes but not for type 1). Nevertheless, type 2 diabetes can develop in young adults and teenagers, while type 1 diabetes can develop in middle-aged and older adults. Type 1 diabetes typically has a rapid onset and symptoms can be severe; this is especially so in children. Prompt medical intervention is almost always necessary because of the risk of diabetic ketoacidosis, which is potentially fatal. Type 2 diabetes is quite strongly genetic (being found in families from one generation to the next, and in brothers and sisters as they get to middle age or older) and is also related to being overweight and sedentary and consuming unhealthy, energy-dense diets. Type 2 diabetes can have a very slow and insidious onset; the diagnosis may be missed for many years or be found by chance during routine medical screening or in health-check medical investigations. In the UK Prospective Diabetes Study (UKPDS) it was observed that up to 50% of patients had some detectable form of tissue damage at diagnosis, the most common type of which was background diabetic retinopathy.

Case History 2.1: Type 1 diabetes with retinopathy

A 5-year-old girl presented with thirst, polyuria and weight loss. Her father had type 1 diabetes mellitus. She had an elevated blood glucose of 23 mmol/L and a slightly elevated urea, but no signs of diabetic ketoacidosis. She was started on a standard mixture of 30% soluble insulin and 70% isophane insulin with a guesstimated dose of 0.6 units per kg of body weight per day (total). This was

A Practical Manual of Diabetic Retinopathy Management, Second Edition.
Edited by Peter Scanlon, Ahmed Sallam, and Peter van Wijngaarden.
© 2017 John Wiley & Sons Ltd. Published 2017 by John Wiley & Sons Ltd.
Companion Website: www.wiley.com/go/scanlon/diabetic_retinopathy

split into 2/3 in the morning and 1/3 at night (i.e. 0.4 unit/kg in the morning and 0.2 unit/kg in the afternoon). Stabilisation occurred over the next few weeks and 2 years later was requiring 1 unit/kg of body weight/day and a small increase was required during puberty. The diabetes was reasonably well controlled with regular attendance at the paediatric diabetic clinic until the age of 14 years.

Her parents then divorced, and control deteriorated as clinic visits became irregular. At the age of 16 a hospital admission occurred due to diabetic ketoacidosis, but she discharged herself 2 days later when she felt that she could manage again at home. During her teenage years she found that whenever she controlled her diabetes well, she had a tendency to put on weight. She therefore tended to run her blood sugars on the high side in order to stay slim. She had been discharged from the paediatric clinic at the age of 16 years and, following her episode of diabetic ketoacidosis, she was supposed to attend the adult clinic but failed to do so. Her family doctor prescribed her insulin, checked her blood pressure (BP) and looked in her fundi once a year with a direct ophthalmoscope.

At the age of 21 years she had a sudden onset of a floater in her right eye and presented as an emergency to the eye department. The photographs shown in Figure 2.1a and b were taken 2 days after the initial presentation. The photographs show proliferative diabetic retinopathy in her right eye which was also present in her left, and laser treatment was commenced to both eyes. She had one laser treatment to each eye, but failed to attend follow-up appointments. Four months later she presented with a further extensive floaters and some blurring of vision in her right eye, as shown in Figure 2.1c and d.

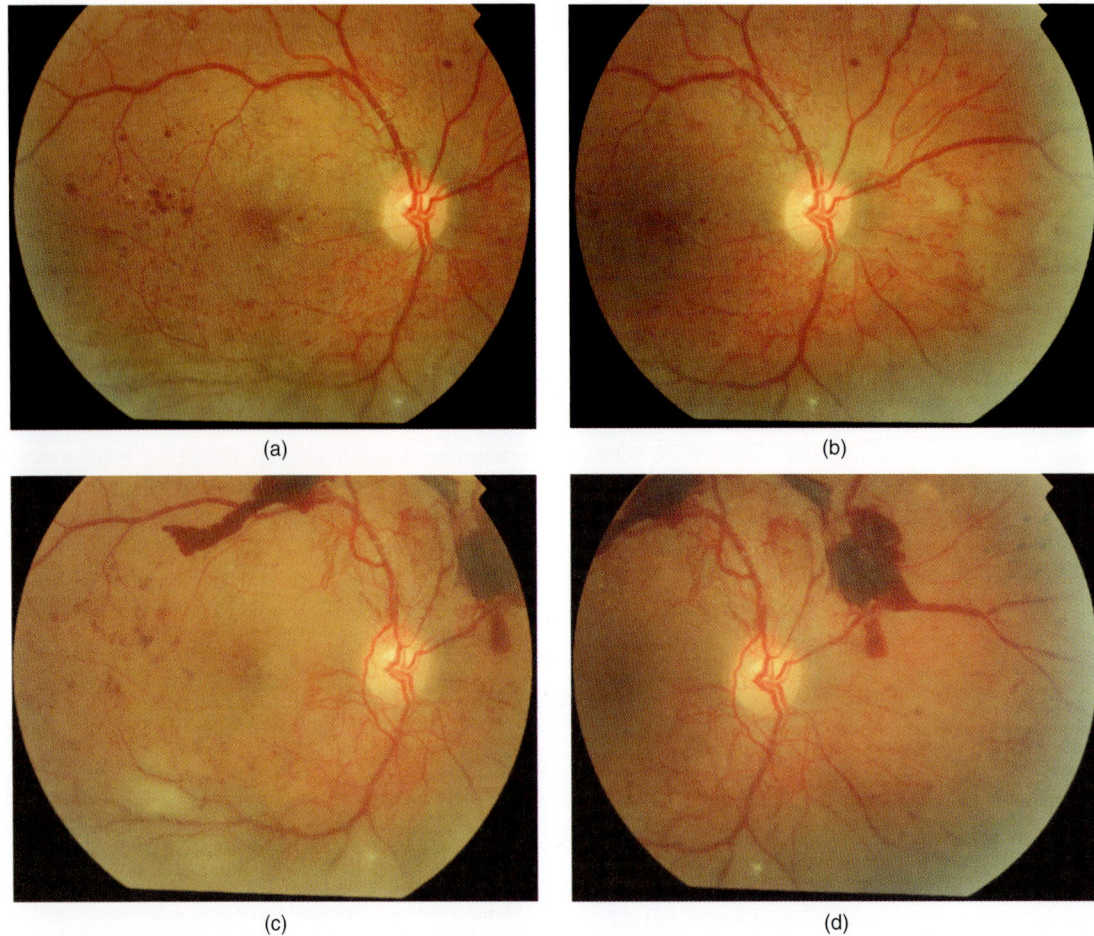

Fig. 2.1 (a) Right macular colour photograph at presentation. (b) Right nasal colour photograph at presentation. (c) Right macular colour photograph 4 months after presentation. (d) Right nasal colour photograph 4 months after presentation.

She needed a vitrectomy in her right eye and laser under general anaesthetic to her left eye. She has subsequently had a vitrectomy to her left eye.

She has attended most of her follow-up visits after the vitrectomy, but has now developed renal problems and is under the care of renal physician.

Case History 2.2: Type 2 diabetes presenting with neuropathy and retinopathy

A 53-year-old man presented to his GP with a year's history of tingling and soreness in his feet. On examination he was hypertensive with a BP of 180/94, his random blood glucose was 15.4 mmol/L and glycated haemoglobin (HbA1c) result 11.4%. He was not obese with a body mass index (BMI) of 24.8. His cholesterol was raised at 8.6 with a high-density lipoprotein (HDL) of 1.6 and low-density lipoprotein (LDL) of 5.2. His renal function was normal with an albumin creatinine ratio of 0.8. He was referred to diabetic eye screening when he showed extensive diabetic maculopathy in both eyes (see Fig. 2.2a–d).

His family doctor has treated him with Metformin 2 g daily, Aspirin 75 mg daily, Simvastatin 40 mg daily, Gliclazide 80 mg daily and Ramipril 2.5 mg daily, and his HbA1c gradually improved over a 3 month period to 8.6%.

He received three treatments of focal laser to each eye (this was before vascular endothelial growth factor or VEGF inhibitors were available) with improvement in macular appearance. He subsequently developed new vessels in the temporal retina of each eye, requiring panretinal photocoagulation to each eye. His vision has been preserved at a level of right 0.3 left 0.28 LogMAR. His macular photographs 5 years after his initial presentation are shown in Figure 2.2e and f.

AETIOPATHOLOGY OF DIABETES

Type 1 diabetes

Type 1 diabetes (Table 2.1) is autoimmune in its aetiology usually with the generation of detectable islet cell antibodies (ICA) or glutamic acid decarboxylase antibodies (GADA). Detection of such antibodies helps to confirm the autoimmune nature of the process, but the presence of the antibodies is neither necessary nor sufficient in the process. Some classical type 1 diabetes occurs without such antibodies being detectable, and

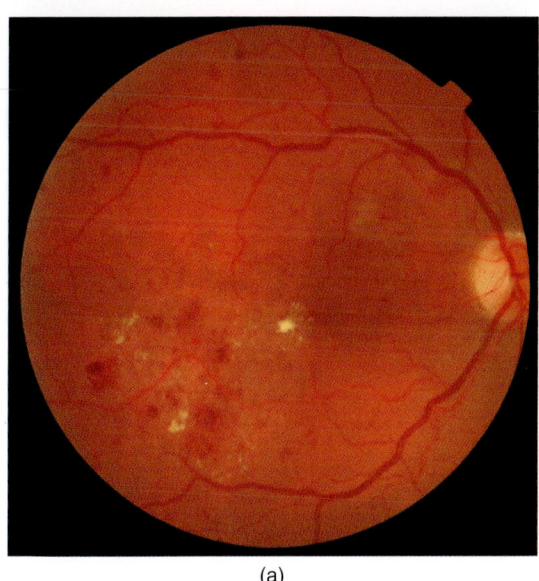

(a)

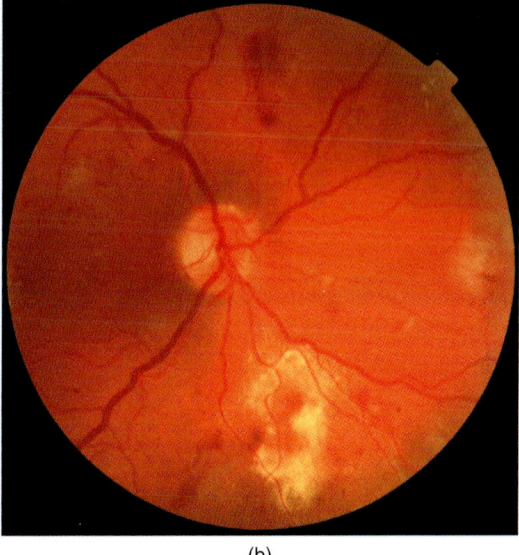

(b)

Fig. 2.2 (a) Right macular colour photo in patient presenting with type 2 diabetes. (b) Right nasal colour photo in patient presenting with type 2 diabetes. (c) Left nasal colour photo in patient presenting with type 2 diabetes. (d) Left macular colour photo in patient presenting with type 2 diabetes. (e) Right macular colour photo 5 years after presentation. (f) Left macular colour photo 5 years after presentation.

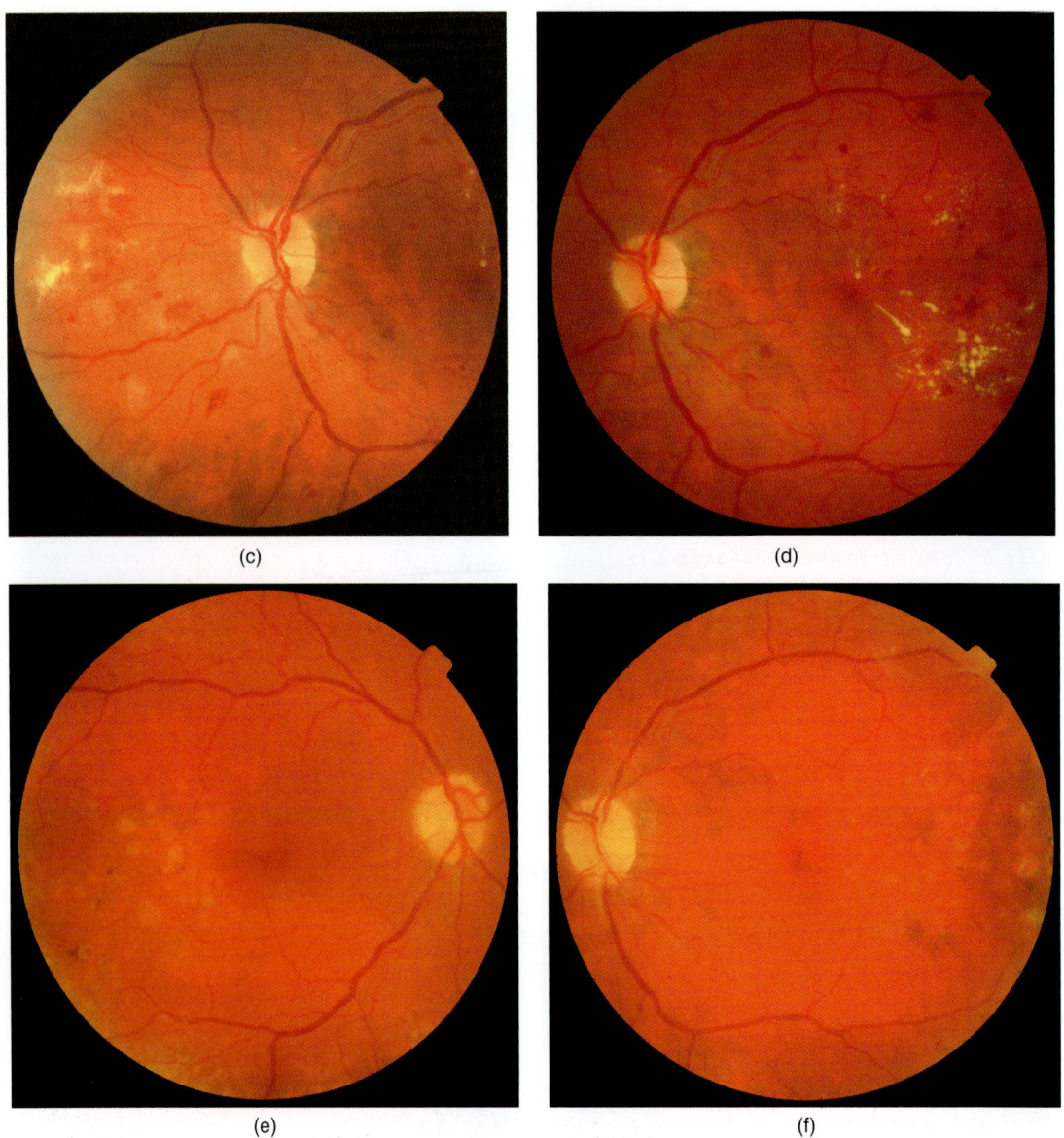

Fig. 2.2 (*Continued*)

some people will have antibodies for many years without developing the clinical condition. There is continuing debate about the triggering effects of other proteins or of infections in sensitising the autoimmune system. Some associations – such as those with milk proteins and cytomegalovirus – are recurrent in the literature, but again the exposure seems neither necessary nor sufficient.

There are genetic propensities, but even identical twins have a discordance rate of 70%.

Type 2 diabetes

Type 2 diabetes (Table 2.1) is common – and 20 times as common as type 1 diabetes – and has an obscure

Table 2.1 Differences between type 1 and type 2 diabetes.

Nomenclature	Type 1 diabetes	Type 2 diabetes
Older and alternative names	Juvenile-onset diabetes; insulin-dependent diabetes mellitus (IDDM)	Maturity-onset diabetes; non-insulin-dependent diabetes mellitus (NIDDM)
Onset	Any time in life, but teenagers and children are most likely to have this type	Generally diagnosed over the age of 40, but can occur in the overweight or in some genetic conditions in younger people
Symptoms at onset	Thirst, tiredness, weight loss, polyuria, ketoacidosis	Tiredness, nocturia, thrush and skin infections; often asymptomatic.
Body type	Generally normal weight or thin	Generally overweight
Speed of onset	Usually becomes critical and needs urgent attention within a few weeks (or even days) of the first symptoms	May not be noticed as a problem; onset can be insidious; diagnosis made often incidental to other pathology
Genetics	Some genetic propensity to run in families, but not caused by a single gene	Quite a strong genetic propensity to run in families, but not caused by a single gene
Triggered by	Autoimmunity; GAD antibody and ICA positive	Relative insulin deficiency where the beta-cells have insufficient function in an internal environment characterised by insulin resistance
Treated by	Insulin from diagnosis	Optimising lifestyle, which may initially be enough; will generally need oral agents initially; progress onto insulin is common.
How common	About 0.2% of the population (2 cases per 1000 people)	Up to 4% UK adult population, up to 8% USA, up to 20% in parts of Asia and up to 50% in Pima Indians and Pacific Islanders
Retinopathy	Rare in the first 5 years if the diabetes is treated adequately; some background retinopathy usual by 15 years duration.	Background retinopathy may be present at diagnosis

pathophysiology. The risks of the disease are related to obesity; with a BMI of >35 the risk is 37 times that of those with a BMI of <22. The condition seems to be genetically coded and concordance between twins over time converges towards about 90%. Many theories have been propounded; lipotoxicity, glucose toxicity, amyloidosis secondary to islet-associated polypeptide beta-pleating and insulin resistance are all currently under close scrutiny. What has become clear, however, is that there is always some element of beta-cell failure whenever type 2 diabetes is diagnosed. Because the pathophysiology tends to be indolent, symptoms can sometimes be slight or so slow in onset that they are not recognised as being pathological; nocturia is the classic example of this. The consequence is that the body may have been exposed to several years of hyperglycaemia and the result is the finding of tissue damage at diagnosis. Retinopathy is the most common finding with up to 30% of all those with newly diagnosed diabetes having detectable retinal lesions. This percentage tends to be lower in settings where active screening or case-finding programs are in place for the early detection of diabetes.

MODY

There are some important monogenic forms of diabetes that have been recognised. About 2% of all diabetes appears similar to type 2 diabetes but is diagnosed in the teenage years and early 20s; this is referred to by the acronym MODY for 'maturity-onset diabetes of the young' or MODY. MODY-1–6 are recognised as having specific monogenic aetiologies (Table 2.2) and they have markedly different outcomes in terms of progression and complications. The most common type (MODY-3) is caused by hepatic nuclear factor (HNF1α) abnormalities, and responds well to low dose sulphonylureas. MODY-2 (c. 20% of all MODY) is important to diagnose because it is a well-regulated hyperglycaemic state with a norm set at about 6 mmol/L rather than 4 mmol/L fasting. Because sustained hyperglycaemia is not a feature, those

Table 2.2 Monogenic aetiologies of maturity-onset diabetes of the young (MODY).

MODY type	Monogenic cause	Complications and features
MODY-1	HNF-4α	Diabetes deteriorates; complications as common as with T2DM
MODY-2	Glucokinase defect (heterozygotic)	c. 20% of all MODY; mild hyperglycaemia; non-progressive form of diabetes; complications mild or none
MODY-3	HNF-1α	c. 60%; most common of the MODY gene defects; responds well to low dose sulphonylurea.
MODY-4	IPF-1	Very rare
MODY-5	HNF-1β	May present with renal disease
MODY-x	Monogenic, but target unidentified	Not known

with MODY-2 rarely have macrovascular complications or significant retinopathy.

Recent discoveries[2,3] of ABCC8 (SUR1) and INS (insulin) gene mutations presenting in patients clinically defined as having MODY will have implications for clinical management.

Case History 2.3: HNF-1α MODY diabetes

A 46-year-old gentleman who attends the eye clinic for monitoring of moderate non-proliferative diabetic retinopathy (pre-proliferative R2; Fig. 2.3) was diagnosed with type 1 diabetes at the age of 18, having presented with a 4-month history of tiredness, polydipsia and polyurea. A random blood glucose at diagnosis was 16.0 mmol/L and he had a BMI of 24 kg/m². He has a positive family history of diabetes, with his sister, father and paternal grandfather having been diagnosed with type 1 diabetes in their late teens, although his father has relatively good glycaemic control despite not being fully compliant with his insulin therapy (Fig. 2.4).

M.F. was initially treated with basal bolus insulin regimen and responded well with good glycaemic control and an HbA1c of 6.7% one month after diagnosis.

At one follow-up appointment 14 years later, he mentioned forgetting to take his insulin for 4 days while on a camping trip. He remained well, and monitored his CBG which never rose above 12.0 mmol/L. He was also noted to be requiring small doses of insulin and have persistent glycosuria despite blood glucose levels in the normal range. A C-peptide level was checked and was found to be positive. Following this, a glutamic acid decarboxylase (GAD) antibody level was checked and found to be negative. At this point he was investigated for a genetic aetiology and found to have the P291fsinsC mutation of HNF1A. He commenced a low dose of gliclazide 40 mg once daily and his insulin therapy was stopped. He responded very well to this dosage with excellent glycaemic control. He has continued on this medication since, although requiring increased dosage, and his HbA1c remains at 6.5%. His family members that have diabetes have undergone a genetic test for the specific HNF1A mutation and are all mutation positive. All except his grandfather have been switched to gliclazide therapy and their insulin stopped.

Secondary diabetes

Secondary diabetes occurs as a result of trauma to the pancreas (surgery, pancreatitis, obstruction) or from the exposure of the body to agents that may affect beta-cell function (major tranquillisers, beta-blockers, thiazide diuretics) or induce insulin resistance (steroids). There are hormonal diseases associated with secondary

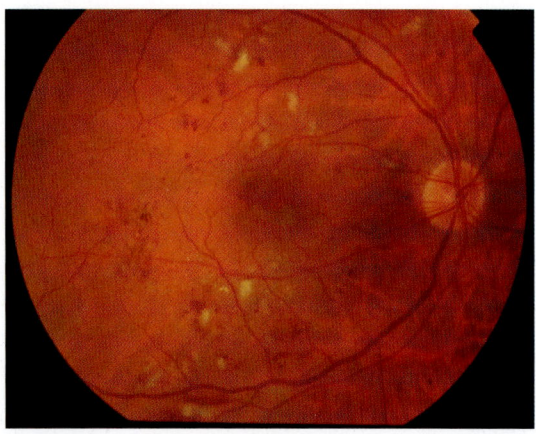

Fig. 2.3 Retinopathy in patient with MODY.

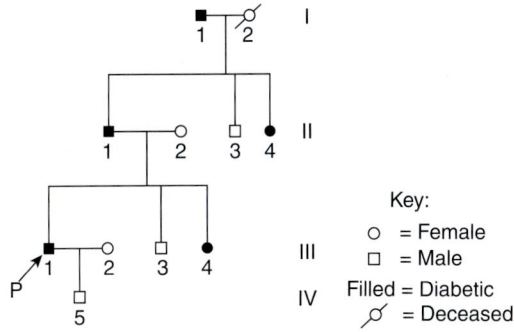

Fig. 2.4 Family history of a person (P) with HNF-1α MODY diabetes.

diabetes – Cushing's disease, acromegaly, phaeochromocytoma – where the secretory product induces insulin resistance. Beta-cell failure can be caused by haemochromatosis and by tropical calcific disease. Secondary diabetes may often need insulin treatment, and the incidence of complications is essentially the same as that of type 1 and type 2 diabetes.

Tissue complications of diabetes

The tissue complications of diabetes are divided into macrovascular (cardiac, cerebrovascular and peripheral vascular) and microvascular (retinopathy, neuropathy and nephropathy). The complications tend to cluster for the obvious reason that processes affecting small vessels

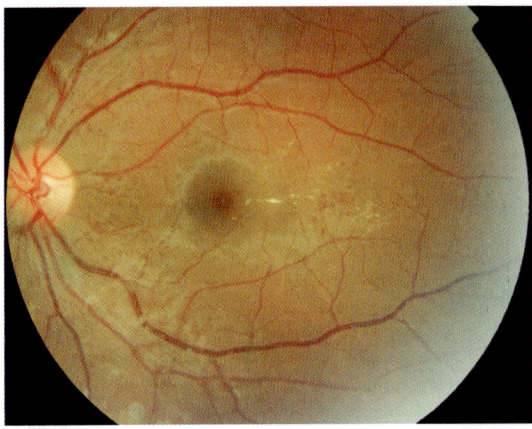

Fig. 2.5 A young woman showing signs of maculopathy with exudate encroaching on the central fovea. There are also some reflections from the flash, especially around the infero-temporal arcade which one sees in young people.

in the eye are likely to be affecting small vessels in the nerves and kidney as well. Retinopathy is often the easiest complication to detect because the smallest of lesions (microaneurysms) can be visualised long before any change to subjective function of the eye would be apparent. Retinopathy tracks closely with nephropathy, and so careful screening of renal function needs to be carried out in those who have retinopathy and vice versa.

Pregnancy can sometimes accelerate retinopathy for reasons that are unclear. Because there is no clear way of distinguishing those who may have fast-developing changes, it is recommended that careful initial and subsequent screening is carried out (Fig. 2.5).

RISK FACTORS FOR DIABETIC RETINOPATHY

Modifiable risk factors

Blood glucose

In 1976, Cahill et al.[4] wrote that the weight of evidence strongly supports the concept that the microvascular complications of diabetes are decreased by a reduction of glucose concentrations. In 1981, Hyman[5] recommended a nationally co-ordinated clinical study of sufficient duration to resolve the issue. Evidence for the link between poor glucose control and greater progression of diabetic retinopathy (DR) was provided by Frank et al.[6], Dahl-Jorgensen et al.[7], Brinchmann-Hansen et al.[8], Joner et al.[9], Klein et al.[10–12], Goldstein et al.[13], Danne et al.[14], Davis et al.[15] and Fong et al.[16].

The study that changed opinion and confirmed that intensive blood glucose control reduces the risk of new-onset DR and slows the progression of existing DR for patients with type 1 diabetes was the Diabetes Control and Complications Trial (DCCT)[17–21]. The trial included 1441 people with type 1 diabetes, 726 with no DR at base line (the primary-prevention cohort) and 715 with mild retinopathy (the secondary-intervention cohort), with mean follow-up of 6.5 years. For the primary-prevention cohort, intensive therapy reduced the risk for the development of DR by 76% (confidence interval or CI 62–85%) compared with conventional therapy. For the secondary-intervention cohort, intensive therapy slowed the progression of DR by 54% (CI 39–66%) and reduced the development of proliferative diabetic retinopathy (PDR) or severe non-proliferative diabetic retinopathy (NPDR) by 47% (CI 14–67%).

The study that changed opinion and confirmed that intensive blood glucose control reduces the risk of new-onset DR and slows the progression of existing DR for patients with type 2 diabetes was the UKPDS[22 25]. This study recruited 3867 adults with type 2 diabetes and the effect of intensive blood glucose control with sulphonylureas or insulin was compared with conventional treatment. Compared with the conventional group, there was a 25% risk reduction (7–40, $P = 0.0099$) in the intensive group in microvascular endpoints, including the need for retinal photocoagulation. Compared to the conventional group, patients allocated metformin had risk reductions of 32% (95% CI 13–47, $P=0.002$) for any diabetes-related endpoint.

> **Case History 2.4: Improvement in retinopathy in a person with improved glucose control**
>
> A 43-year-old lady with type 1 diabetes since the age of 26 years, when she was started on insulin during her third pregnancy, was commenced on insulin pump therapy. Prior to the pump therapy her two previous HbA1c results had been 9.3 and 8.6%, BMI 26.8 and BP 164/98. Figure 2.6a was taken 6 months after starting insulin pump therapy.
>
> Over the next 3 years her HbA1c improved gradually to readings of 6.9 and 7.1% and her BP improved to 145/75 with increased anti-hypertensive medication.
>
> She is currently on approximately 50 units Humalog per day. The pump delivers 30 units automatically over 24 hours and the rest is given as a bolus dependent on carbohydrate intake or exercise. She determines the bolus amount herself, calculating one unit for every 8 g of carbohydrate.
>
> Subsequent photographs (Fig. 2.6b and c) show a clearing of the exudates in her macular area.

Blood pressure

Control of systemic hypertension has been shown to reduce the risk of new-onset DR and slow the progression of existing DR in studies reported by Chase et al.[26], Joner et al.[9], Klein et al.[10], UKPDS[25], Stratton et al.[27], Estacio et al.[28] and Matthews et al.[29]. In young subjects with type 1 diabetes, Chase et al.[26] and Joner et al.[9] demonstrated in the early 1990s that elevation in diastolic blood pressure alone and in combination with elevated systolic blood pressure and higher mean arterial blood pressure correlated with the presence of retinopathy and of progression of pre-existing retinopathy. The UKPDS[25,29] described the effect of tight blood pressure control and risk of microvascular complications in type 2 diabetes. After 9 years of follow-up, the group assigned to tight blood pressure control had a 34% reduction in risk in the proportion of patients with deterioration of retinopathy by two steps (99%; confidence interval 11–50%; $P=0.0004$) and a 47% reduced risk (7–70%; $P=0.004$) of deterioration in visual acuity by three lines of the early treatment of diabetic retinopathy study (ETDRS) chart. However, more recent trials undertaken in an environment of better overall blood pressure have failed to confirm these findings. Neither the ACCORD[30] nor the ADVANCE[31] trials showed benefits for retinopathy of more intensive blood pressure lowering, perhaps because the blood pressure in the control arms was already moderately good (Fig 2.7).

Lipid levels

Evidence that elevated serum lipids are associated with macular exudates, and moderate visual loss, and that partial regression of hard exudates may be possible by reducing elevated lipid levels, comes from studies reported by Chew et al.[32], Fong et al.[16], Klein et al.[33], Sen et al.[34], Cusick et al.[35] and Lyons et al.[36].

In 1996 Chew et al.[32] reported an association of elevated serum lipid levels with retinal hard exudates in diabetic patients from the ETDRS, and Fong et al.[16] later reported that patients with persistent severe visual loss in the ETDRS had higher levels of cholesterol (244.1 v. 228.5 mg/dL; $P=0.0081$) at baseline. Sen et al.[34] and Cusick et al.[35] described the regression of retinal hard exudates in patients with diabetic maculopathy after correction of dyslipidemia (Fig. 2.8). As part of the Diabetes Control and Complications Trial/Epidemiology of Diabetes Interventions and Complications Study cohort in 2004, Lyons et al.[36] demonstrated new associations between serum lipoproteins and severity of retinopathy in type 1 diabetes. Two recent large trials have suggested that fenofibrate, a fibric acid derivative, may have marked beneficial effects on preventing and slowing progression of retinopathy[30,37], although the mechanism does not appear to operate through modification of lipid levels.

Smoking

There is some evidence that smoking may be a risk factor in progression of diabetic retinopathy in type 1 diabetes, as described by Muhlhauser et al.[38,39] and Karamanos et al.[40] However, in type 2 diabetes the evidence is controversial and it may protect[21] against the progression of retinopathy in some patients, despite the fact that it is an independent risk factor for cardiovascular disease in all patients with diabetes.

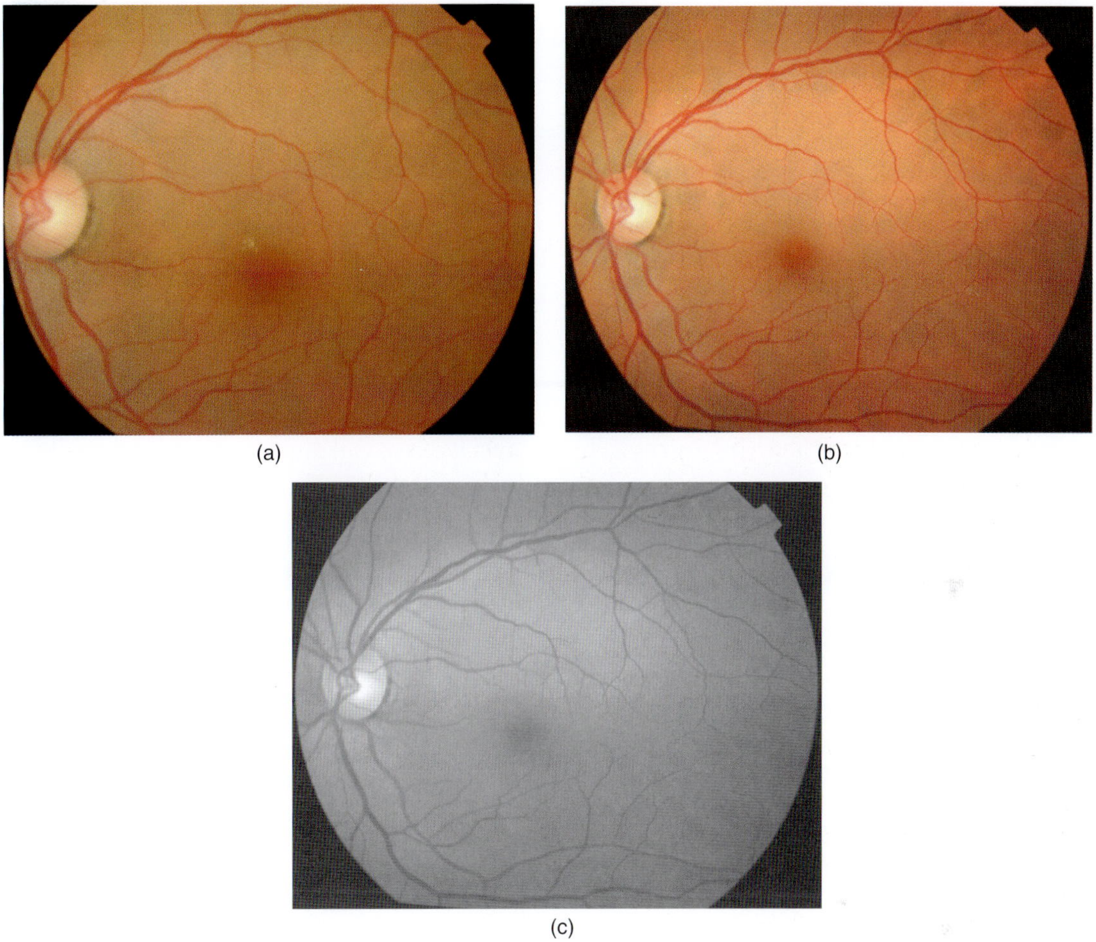

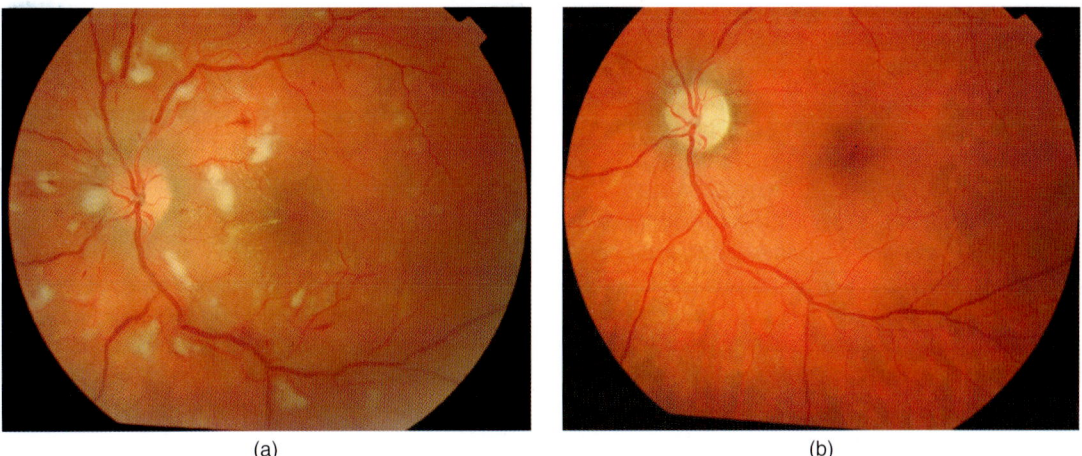

Fig. 2.6 (a) Photograph taken 6 months after starting insulin pump therapy. (b) Colour and (c) red-free photograph taken 3 years after starting insulin pump therapy, showing clearing of the exudates in her macular area.

Fig. 2.7 Uncontrolled hypertension in a person with diabetes. (a) Left macular colour photo showing flame haemorrhages and cotton wool spots and exudates. (b) Improvement in appearance following treatment of the hypertension.

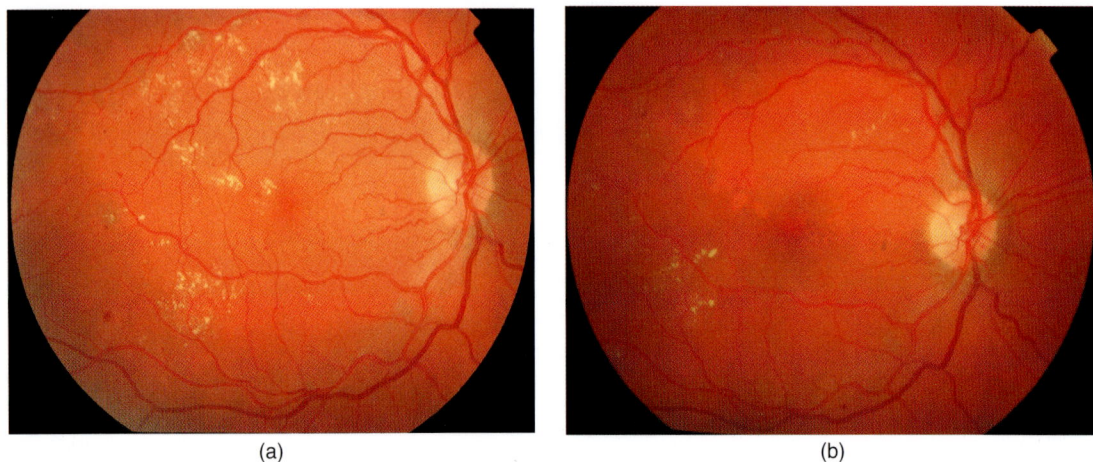

Fig. 2.8 (a) Macular exudates in diabetic retinopathy (a) pre–treatment and (b) post-treatment with laser treatment and a statin.

Non-modifiable risk factors for DR

Duration

Among the non-modifiable risk factors, the major determinant of progression of diabetic retinopathy is duration of diabetes. This has been demonstrated in studies by Palmberg et al.[41], Frank et al.[6], Klein et al.[12,42–48], Burger et al.[49], Kohner and Sleightholm[50], Orchard et al.[51], ETDRS[52,53], Goldstein[13], McNally et al.[54], UKPDS[27,55], Vitale et al.[56], d'Annunzio et al.[57], Donaghue et al.[58,59], Kernell et al.[60], Vitale et al.[61], Danne et al.[62], Davis et al.[15], Henricsson et al.[63], Ling et al.[64], Liu et al.[65] and Younis et al.[66,67]

Palmberg et al.[41] demonstrated in 1981 in a group of 461 juvenile-onset persons with type 1 diabetes, in which no DR had been identified at diagnosis, 50% were found to have DR 7 years after diagnosis and 90% were found to have DR 17–50 years after diagnosis. PDR was first seen 13 years after diagnosis, and 26% were found to have PDR 26–50 years after diagnosis. In the Wisconsin Epidemiological Study of Diabetic Retinopathy (WESDR), Klein et al.[42,43] demonstrated in 1984 that in 996 subjects with younger-onset type 1 diabetes any DR was found in 17% when their diabetes was of less than 5 years duration, while those with diabetes for ≥15 years duration had a prevalence of 97.5%. Proliferative DR was found in 1.2% of those with less than 10 years duration and in 67% of those with ≥35 years duration.

In 1986, Burger et al.[49] studied 231 juvenile-onset insulin-dependent diabetes mellitus (IDDM) in the Berlin retinopathy study who had 1–6 examinations with fluorescein angiography over 5 years. A total of 47% developed retinal changes, half of which were classified as minimal (<5 microaneurysms). The median diabetes duration at the time of development of early DR was 9.1 years.

In 1989 Klein et al.[46,47] reported that of 271 persons with type 1 diabetes diagnosed aged ≤30 years with no DR at first visit in WESDR, 59% developed DR after 4 years. Of 713 persons with no proliferative DR at first visit, 11% developed proliferative DR after 4 years. Worsening of DR occurred in 41% and improvement in only 7%. The incidence of proliferative DR rose to 14% after 13 years of diabetes.

Of 154 persons with type 1 diabetes diagnosed at ≥30 years with no DR at first visit, 47% developed DR after 4 years. Of 418 with no proliferative DR at first visit, 7% developed proliferative DR after 4 years and worsening of DR in 34%.

Of 320 persons with type 2 diabetes diagnosed at 30 years or older with no DR at first visit, 34% developed DR after 4 years. Of 486 with no proliferative DR at first visit, 2% developed proliferative DR after 4 years and worsening of DR occurred in 25%.

Age

The Wisconsin Epidemiological Study[42,43,68] demonstrated that in those whose age of diagnosis was less than 30 years and who had diabetes of 10 years duration or less, the severity of retinopathy was related to older age at examination. When the age at diagnosis was 30 or more years, the severity of retinopathy was related to younger age at diagnosis. In those taking insulin divided by age groups diagnosed before and after age 30 years, the 10-year incidence of retinopathy was 89% and 79%, progression of retinopathy 76% and 69%, and progression to proliferative retinopathy 30% and 24%, respectively. This was in contrast to those not requiring insulin, where there was a lower incidence, general progression and progression to proliferative retinopathy of 67%, 53% and 10% respectively. In the UKPDS[27], in those who already had retinopathy progression was associated with older age.

Genetic predisposition

Diabetic retinopathy (DR) progresses from mild non-proliferative DR to proliferative DR and is considered to develop as a consequence of long duration of diabetes, poor glycaemic control, high blood pressure and several genetic factors. Early studies of identical twins with diabetes mellitus suggest familial clustering of diabetic retinopathy. An association between severity of diabetic retinopathy and human lymphocytic antigens (HLA) has been suggested in a number of studies[69–71], although this has not been uniformly accepted[72]. The Diabetes Control and Complications Trial (DCCT) suggested that, as well as environmental factors, the severity of diabetic retinopathy is influenced by familial factors, probably of genetic origin. Researchers have been searching for many years for the genes responsible for retinopathy. Generally, genes which encode factors involved in the pathogenesis of diabetic retinopathy are considered as candidates. For example, angiotensin I-converting enzyme[73], nitric oxide synthase[74] (NOS2A and NOS3), vascular endothelial growth factor[75–78] (VEGF), pigmented epithelium-derived factor (PEDF), protein kinase C-beta (PKC-beta) and receptor for advanced glycation end products[79–82] (RAGE) have been implicated in the pathogenesis of DR. The majority of candidate genes studied exhibit weak or no association with retinopathy status and, where associations have been detected, these results have not been replicated in multiple populations.

Ethnicity

Emanuele et al.[83] reported ethnicity, race and baseline retinopathy correlates in the veterans affairs diabetes trial, which has a cohort enriched with approximately 20% Hispanics and 20% African Americans. The prevalence of diabetic retinopathy scores of >40 was higher for Hispanics (36%) and African Americans (29%) than for non-Hispanic whites (22%). The difference between Hispanics and non-Hispanic whites was significant ($P<0.05$). Similarly, the prevalence of diabetic retinopathy scores of >40 was significantly higher in African Americans than in non-Hispanic whites ($P<0.05$). These differences could not be accounted for by an imbalance in traditional risk factors such as age, duration of diagnosed diabetes, HbA1c and blood pressure. Simmons et al.[84] compared ethnic differences in the prevalence of diabetic retinopathy in European, Maori and Pacific peoples with diabetes in Auckland, New Zealand. They demonstrated that that moderate or more severe retinopathy is more common in Polynesians than Europeans, and this difference could not be explained by differences in diabetes duration, insulin therapy, the extent of renal disease, blood pressure or glycaemic control. A recent review[85] of diabetic retinopathy prevalence studies around the world showed marked variation in diagnostic criteria and study design, but indicated that the prevalence of DR appeared to be much higher in developing than in developed countries.

PRACTICE POINTS

Diabetic retinopathy is integrally linked to glycaemic control, blood pressure control, lipid levels, smoking and non-modifiable risk factors such as age and duration of diabetes.

It is very important to have good communication between the ophthalmologist, diabetologist and any other health professional looking after someone with diabetic microvascular complications.

Some patients are diagnosed with type 2 diabetes when they present with sight-threatening diabetic retinopathy and have clearly had diabetes for many years without their knowledge.

REFERENCE

Please visit www.wiley.com/go/scanlon/diabetic_retinopathy

3 Lesions and classifications of diabetic retinopathy

Peter H. Scanlon

Harris Manchester College, University of Oxford; Medical Ophthalmology, University of Gloucestershire, UK

Diabetic retinopathy refers to pathology of the capillaries, arterioles and venules in the retina and the subsequent effects of leakage from or occlusion of the small vessels. Diabetes can affect larger blood vessels of the head and neck and of the retina, but pathology of the larger blood vessels does not come under the classification of diabetic retinopathy. Changes that occur within the retinal capillary wall include: (1) thickening of the basement membrane; (2) pericyte loss; (3) epithelial cell dysfunction (loss of epithelial tight junctions); and (4) loss of endothelial cells.

ETDRS CLASSIFICATION

The Early Treatment Diabetic Retinopathy Study[1,2] (ETDRS) classified a number of lesions of diabetic retinopathy and described the progression of diabetic retinopathy in relation to the development of these lesions (Tables 3.1 and 3.2). The lesions that the ETDRS described as critical to the stages of progression of diabetic retinopathy are described in the following sections.

Microaneurysm

A microaneurysm is defined as a red spot <125 microns (approximate width of vein at disc margin) with sharp margins.

Haemorrhage

A haemorrhage is defined as a red spot which has irregular margins and/or uneven density, particularly when surrounding a smaller central lesion considered to be a microaneurysm. If a red lesion is >125 microns in its longest dimension, it is usually a haemorrhage unless features such as round shape, smooth margins and a central light reflex suggest it is possibly a microaneurysm.

HMa

Because the ETDRS recognised that it was very difficult to differentiate between microaneurysms and small haemorrhages (Fig. 3.1) the concept of HMa was introduced, which is a small haemorrhage or microaneurysm.

Other larger retinal haemorrhages

Flame haemorrhages

Flame haemorrhages (Fig. 3.2) are superficial haemorrhages just under the nerve fibre layer that can be seen in relatively mild forms of diabetic retinopathy and also in systemic hypertension.

Blot haemorrhages

Blot haemorrhages (Fig. 3.3) are deeper haemorrhages which are a sign of retinal ischaemia in the area of the retina in which they occur. Large numbers of blot haemorrhages are associated with significant retinal ischaemia.

Hard exudates

The ETDRS defined hard exudates (sometimes now just referred to as exudates; Fig. 3.4) as small white or yellowish-white deposits with sharp margins. Although located typically in the outer layers of the retina, they may be more superficial particularly when retinal oedema is present. Hard exudates rings were defined in the ETDRS by whether 10%, 50% or 90% or more HE present were part of a ring.

A Practical Manual of Diabetic Retinopathy Management, Second Edition.
Edited by Peter Scanlon, Ahmed Sallam, and Peter van Wijngaarden.
© 2017 John Wiley & Sons Ltd. Published 2017 by John Wiley & Sons Ltd.
Companion Website: www.wiley.com/go/scanlon/diabetic_retinopathy

Table 3.1 ETDRS diabetic retinopathy classification of progression to proliferative DR based on 7 × 30 degree field stereo photographs of each eye.

ETDRS final retinopathy severity scale[3]	ETDRS (Final) Grade	Lesions	Risk of progression to PDR in 1 year (ETDRS interim)	Practical clinic follow up intervals (not ETDRS)
No apparent retinopathy	10	DR absent		1 year
	14, 15	DR questionable		
Mild NPDR	20	Microaneurysms only		1 year
	35	One or more of the following:	Level 30 = 6.2%	6–12 months
	a	Venous loops $\geq$ definite in 1 field		
	b	SE, IRMA, or VB questionable		
	c	Retinal haemorrhages present		
	d	HE $\geq$ definite in 1 field		
	e	SE $\geq$ definite in 1 field		
Moderate NPDR	43a	H/Ma moderate in 4–5 fields or severe in 1 field	Level 41 = 11.3%	6 months
	b	IRMA definite in 1–3 fields		
Moderately severe NPDR	47	Both level 43 characteristics:	Level 45 = 20.7%	4 months
	a	H/Ma moderate in 4–5 fields or severe in 1 field and IRMA definite in 1–3 fields. Or any one of the following:		
	b	IRMA in 4–5 fields		
	c	HMA severe in 2–3 fields		
	d	VB definite in 1 field		
Severe NPDR	53	One or more of the following:	Level 51 = 44.2%	3 months
	a	≥ 2 of the 3 level 47 characteristics		
	b	H/Ma severe in 4–5 fields		
	c	IRMA $\geq$ moderate in 1 field	Level 55 = 54.8%	
	d	VB $\geq$ definite in 2–3 fields		
Mild PDR	61a	FPD or FPE present with NVD absent or	1976. Diabetic Retinopathy Study[4] Protocol changed to treat untreated eyes with high risk characteristics	
	b	NVE = definite		
Moderate PDR	65a	NVE $\geq$ moderate in 1 field or definite NVD with VH and PRH absent or questionable, or	1981. Diabetic Retinopathy Study[5] recommendation to treat eyes with new vessels on or within one disc diameter of the optic disc (NVD) $\geq$0.2–0.33 disc area, even in the absence of preretinal or vitreous haemorrhage. Photocoagulation, as used in the study, reduced the risk of severe visual loss by 50% or more.	
	b	VH or PRH definite and NVE < moderate in 1 field and NVD absent		
High-risk PDR	71	Any of the following:		
	a	VH or PRH $\geq$ moderate in 1 field		
	b	NVE $\geq$ moderate in 1 field and VH or PRH definite in 1 field		
	c	NVD = 2 and VH or PRH definite in 1 field		
	d	NVD $\geq$ moderate		
High-risk PDR	75	NVD $\geq$ moderate and definite VH or PRH		
Advanced PDR	81	Retina obscured due to VH or PRH		

Table 3.2 ETDRS maculopathy classification.

ETDRS: clinically significant macular oedema[6] as defined by:	Outcome
A zone or zones of retinal thickening one disc area or larger, any part of which is within one disc diameter of the centre of the macula.	Consider laser
Retinal thickening at or within 500 microns of the centre of the macula	Consider laser
Hard exudates at or within 500 microns of the centre of the macula, if associated with thickening of the adjacent retina (not residual hard exudates remaining after disappearance of retinal thickening)	Consider laser

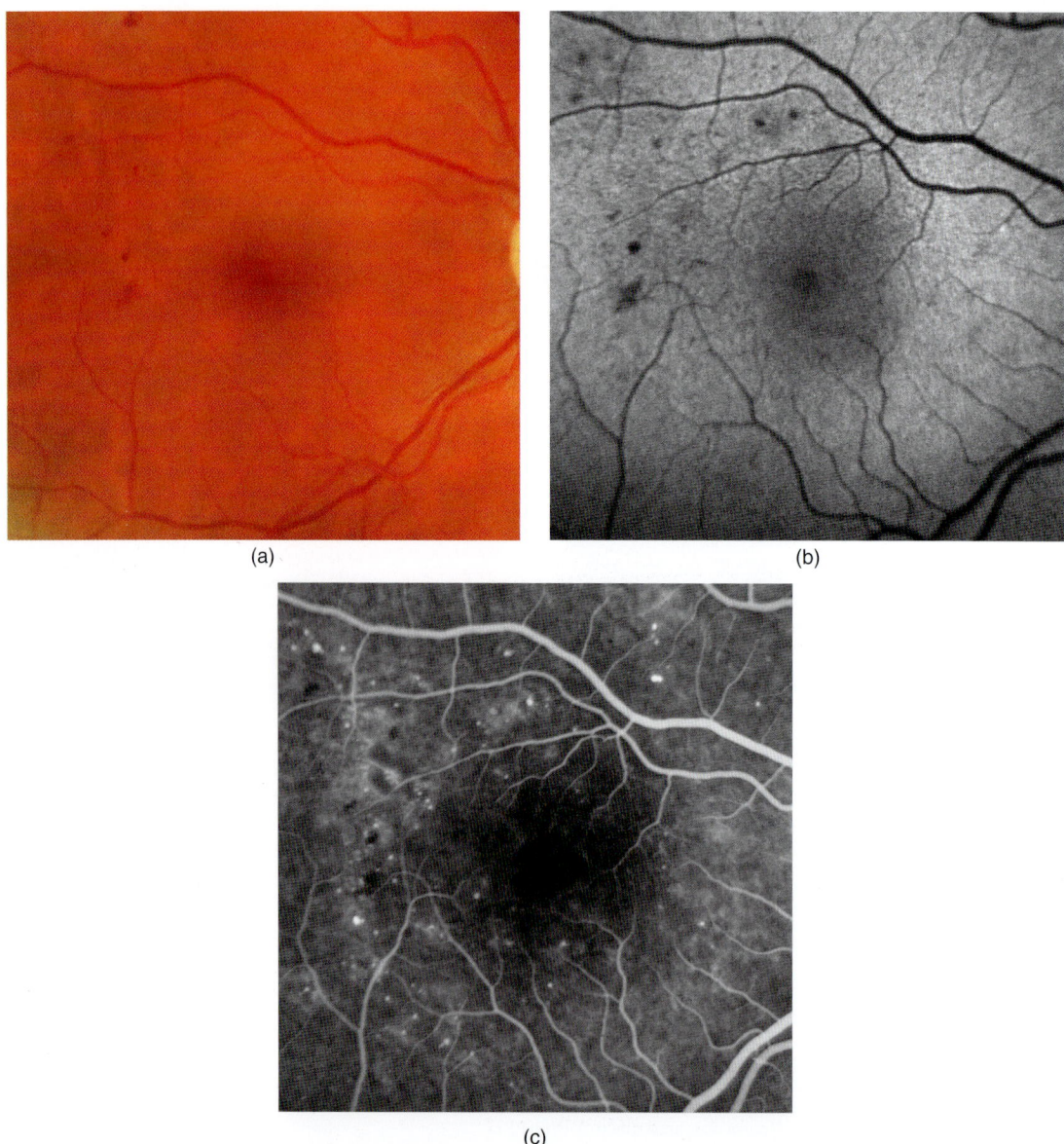

Fig. 3.1 (a) An example of microaneurysms and small haemorrhages in the right macular area. (b) Figure (a) autofluorescence image. (c) Figure (a) fluorescein at 2 min 17 s, showing leakage from some of the microaneurysms as shown by a fluffy fluorescence appearing around the microaneurysm.

Lesions and classifications of diabetic retinopathy 29

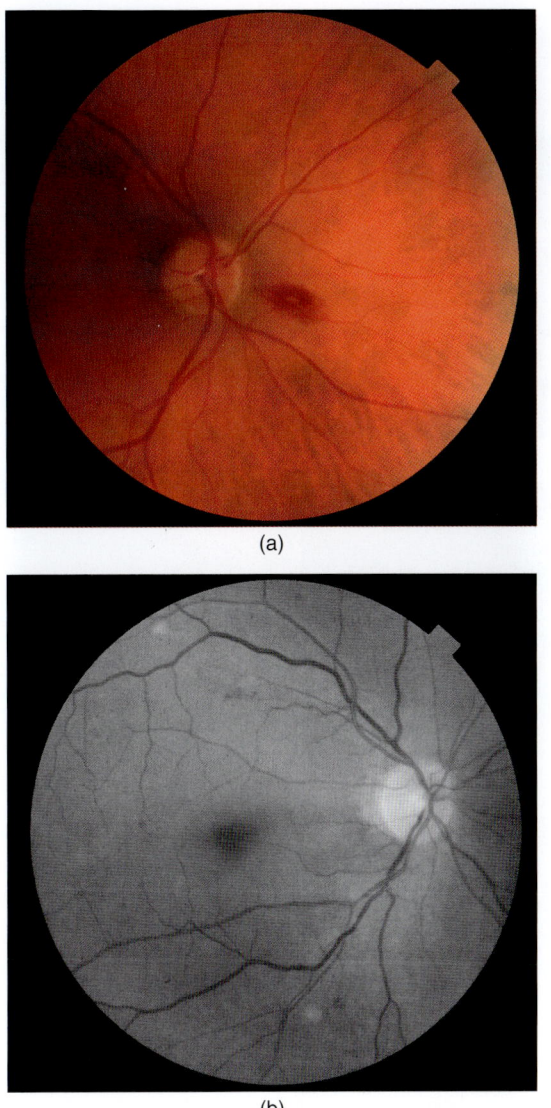

Fig. 3.2 An example of (a) a flame haemorrhage and (b) a superficial haemorrhage in the nerve fibre layer with Hmas and CWS.

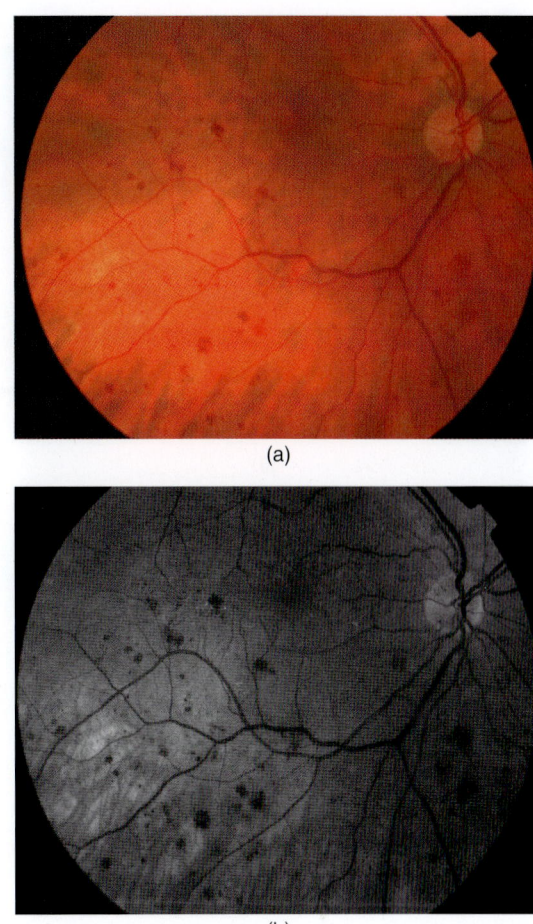

Fig. 3.3 (a) An example of blot haemorrhages in the right infero-temporal retina and a small patch of NVE. (b) Red-free photo of patient (a) with blot haemorrhages and small NVE.

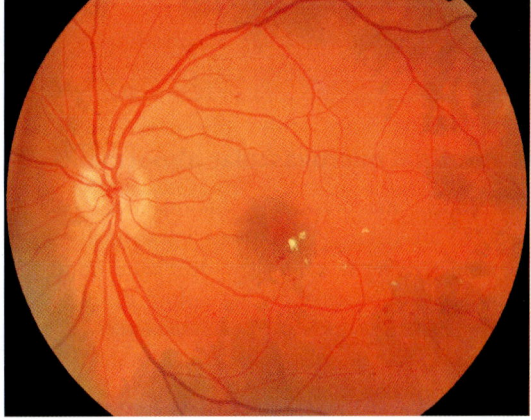

Fig. 3.4 An example of (hard) exudates encroaching on the central fovea.

Cotton wool spots

Cotton wool spots (referred to as soft exudates in the ETDRS, but this term is now rarely used; Fig. 3.5) are fluffy white opaque areas caused by an accumulation of axoplasm in the nerve fibre layer of the retina. They are caused by an arteriolar occlusion in that area of the retina, which is apparent on a fluorescein angiogram. Haemorrhages

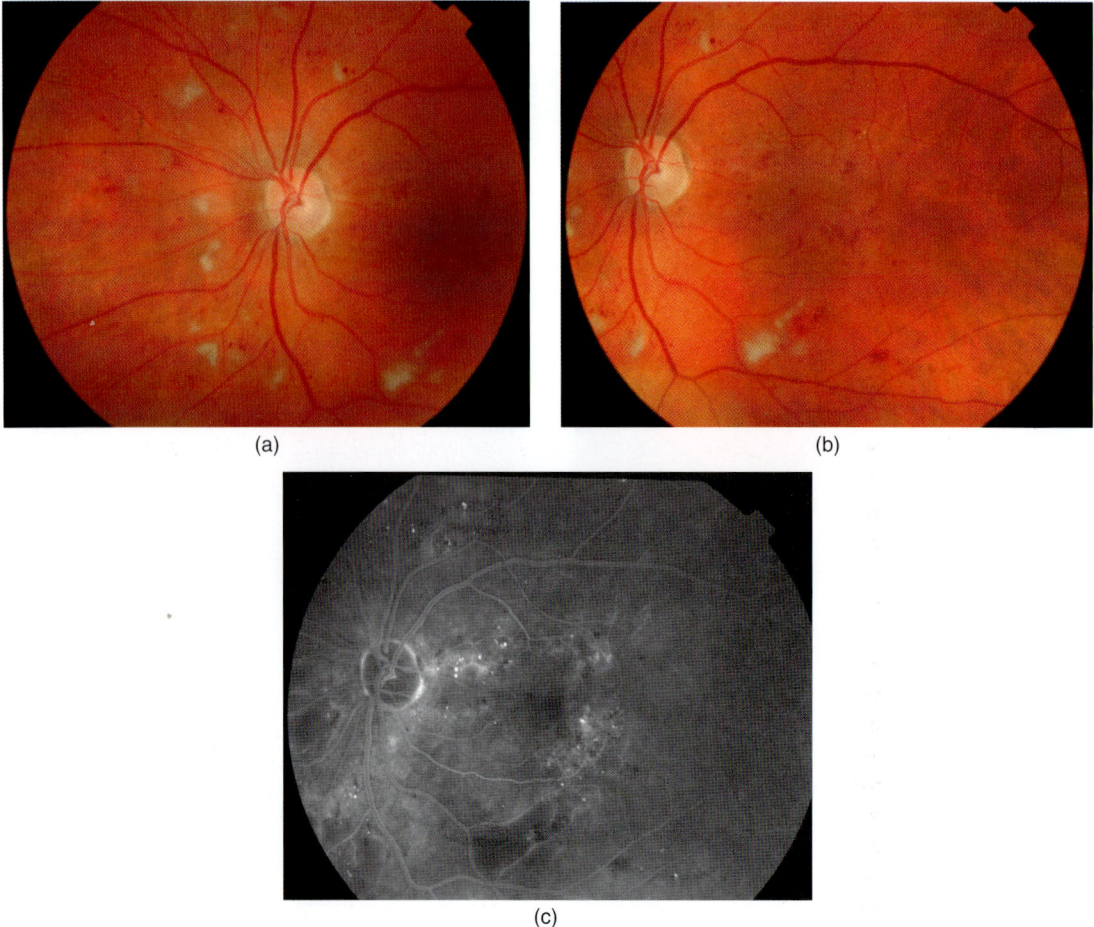

Fig. 3.5 An example of cotton wool spots (CWS) in (a) the nasal view and (b) the macular view of the same patient. (c) Fluorescein of patient (a)'s macular view showing ischaemia in the areas of CWS.

and intraretinal microvascular abnormalities are often seen in the retina adjacent to a cotton wool spot.

Intraretinal microvascular abnormality

Intraretinal microvascular abnormalities (IRMAs; Fig. 3.6) are defined as tortuous intraretinal vascular segments varying in calibre. By definition, intraretinal microvascular abnormalities are not on the surface of the retina and do not break through the internal limiting membrane. Intraretinal microvascular abnormalities are derived from remodelling of the retinal capillaries and small collateral vessels in areas of microvascular occlusion. They are usually found on the borders of areas of non-perfused retina, and are therefore a sign of retinal ischaemia.

Venous abnormalities

Venous loops and/or reduplication

A venous loop is defined by the ETDRS as an abrupt curving deviation of a vein from its normal path. There are mild forms that can be present in mild non-proliferative DR (Fig. 3.7a) and larger loops that develop in more ischaemic retinae (Fig. 3.7b).

Reduplication is dilation (Fig. 3.8) of a pre-existing channel or proliferation of a new channel adjacent to and approximately the same calibre as the original vein.

Lesions and classifications of diabetic retinopathy 31

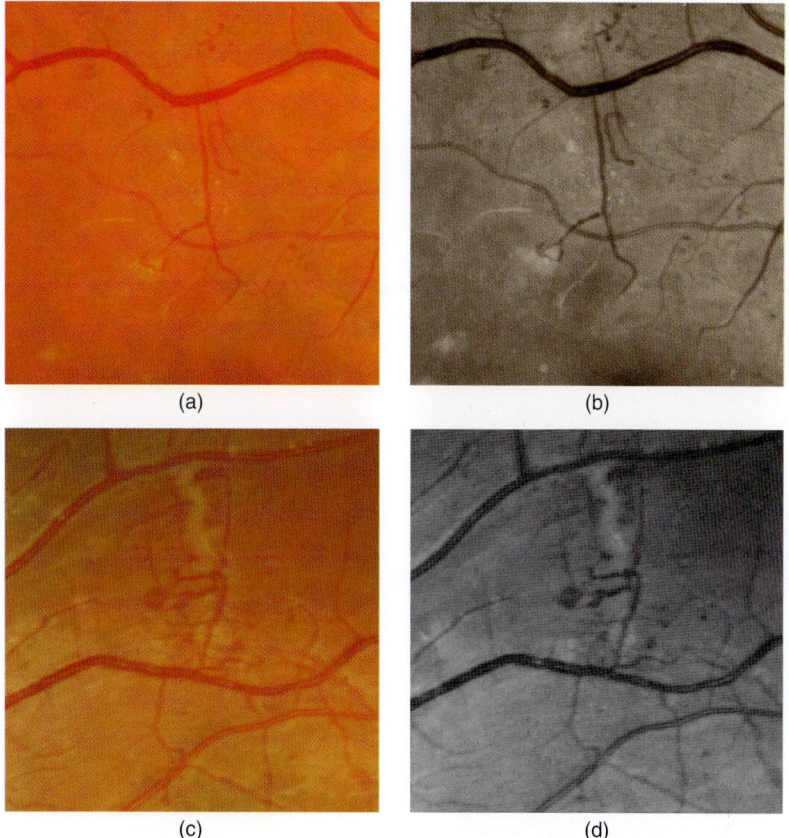

Fig. 3.6 Example of IRMA: (a, c) colour photograph and (b, d) red-free photograph.

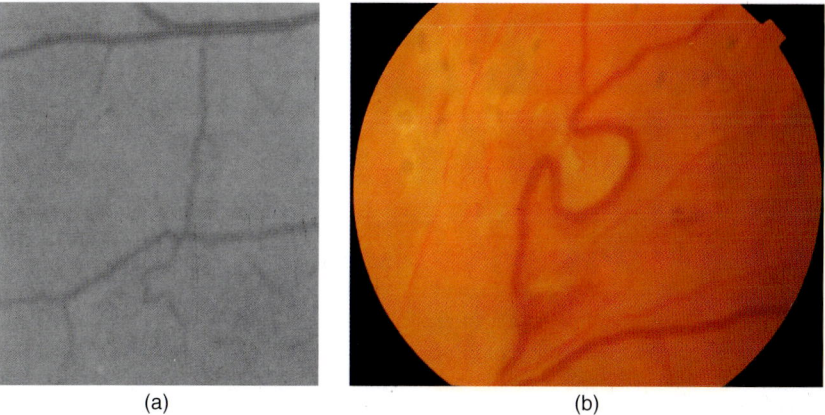

Fig. 3.7 An example of a venous loop (a) in the temporal retina of a patient with mild NPDR and (b) in a more ischaemic retina (colour photograph superior retina).

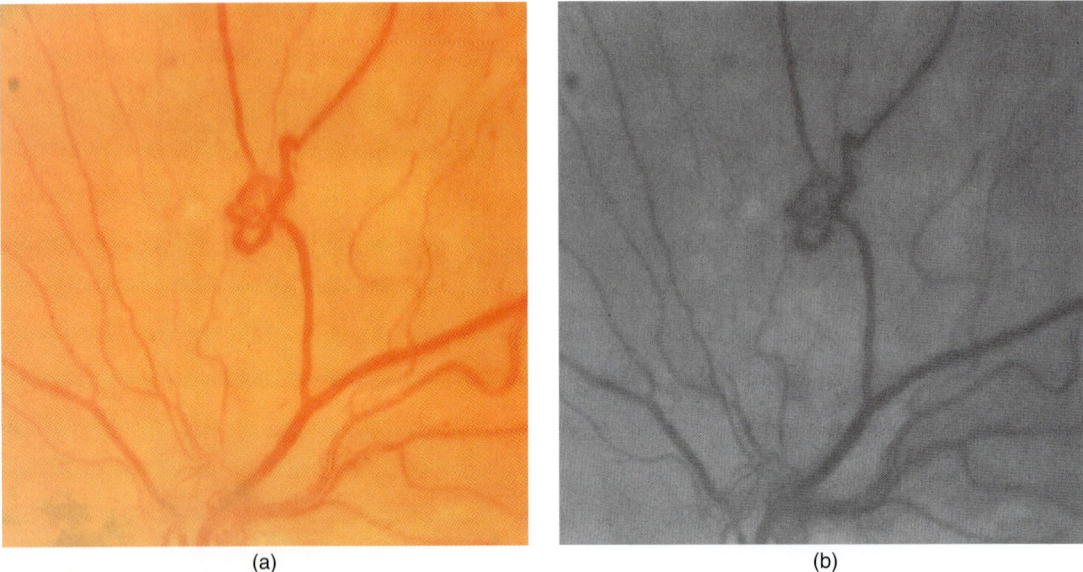

Fig. 3.8 An example of a venous reduplication: (a) colour photograph and (b) red-free photograph.

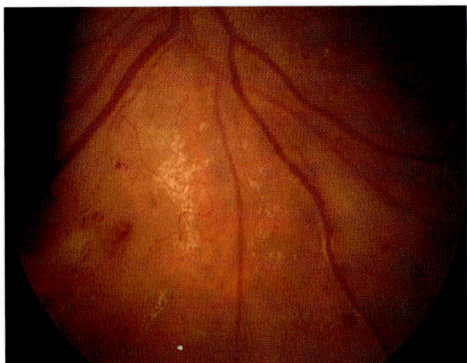

Fig. 3.9 An example of venous dilation, venous beading and IRMA in an area of ischaemic retina.

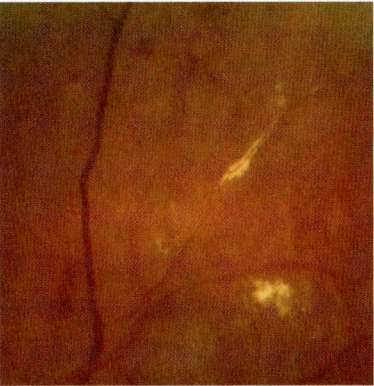

Fig. 3.10 An example of venous narrowing and perivenous exudates.

Venous beading

In the ETDRS venous beading was described as a localised increase in calibre of the vein, the severity of which was dependent on the increase in calibre and the length of vein involved. Venous beading was found to be associated with retinal ischaemia. It is used for assessment of severity of diabetic retinopathy and response to laser treatment, as venous dilation and beading do respond to scatter laser treatment. Other venous changes that also occur in diabetic retinopathy are: (1) venous dilation (Fig. 3.9); this is common in diabetic retinopathy and an obvious return to normal calibre is often apparent following panretinal photocoagulation for retinal neovascularisation; (2) venous narrowing (Fig. 3.10); (3) opacification of the venous wall (venous sheathing or 'white threads'; Fig. 3.11); and (4) perivenous exudate (Fig. 3.12).

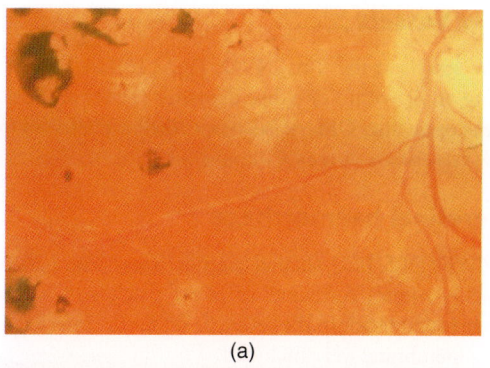

(a)

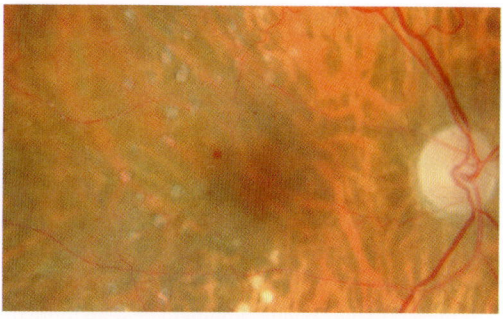

Fig. 3.13 An example of arteriolar narrowing.

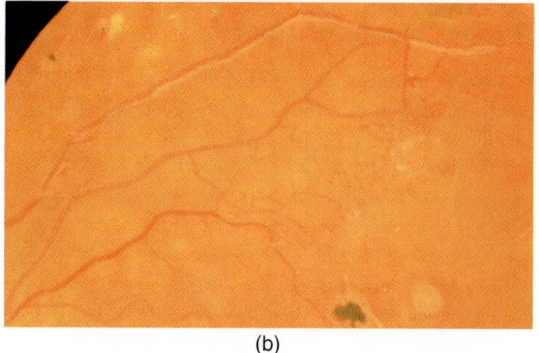

(b)

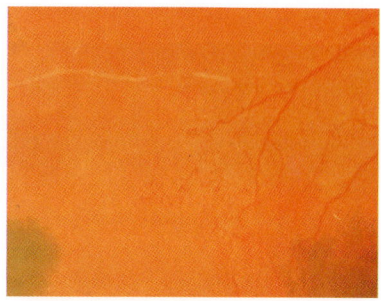

Fig. 3.14 An example of opacification of arteriolar walls.

Fig. 3.11 An example of venous sheathing: (a) nasal view left eye and (b) macular view left eye.

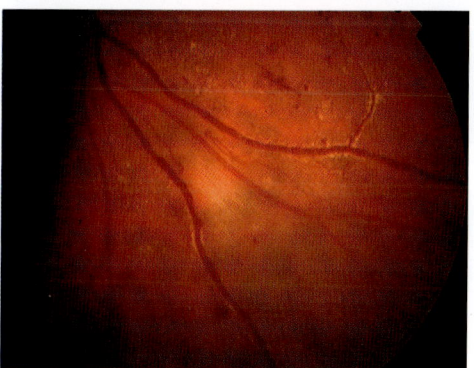

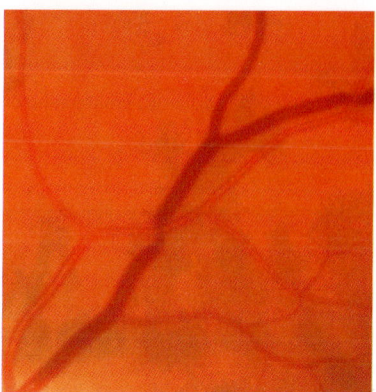

Fig. 3.15 An example of arterio-venous nipping.

Fig. 3.12 An example of perivenous exudates.

Arteriolar abnormalities

Other arteriolar changes that occur in diabetic retinopathy are: (1) arteriolar narrowing (Fig. 3.13); (2) opacification of arteriolar walls (sheathing or 'white threads'; Fig. 3.14); and (3) arterio-venous nipping (Fig. 3.15), narrowing of the venous diameter where it is crossed by a branch artery. The latter is often a feature of hypertension.

Fibrous proliferations

On or within the disc
Fibrous proliferation on or within one disc diameter (1DD) of the disc margin (FPD; Fig. 3.16) is fibrous tissue opaque enough to be seen at the disc or less than 1DD from the disc margin with or without accompanying new vessels.

Elsewhere
FPE is fibrous tissue opaque enough to be seen more than 1DD from the disc margin, with or without accompanying new vessels (Fig. 3.17).

New Vessels
New vessels at the disc (NVD; Fig. 3.18) are defined as being on or within one disc diameter (1DD) of the edge of the optic disc. Otherwise, new vessels are referred to as new vessels elsewhere (NVE; Fig. 3.19).

Preretinal haemorrhage
In the ETDRS, boat-shaped haemorrhages (Fig. 3.20) and roughly round, confluent or linear patches of haemorrhage just anterior to the retina or under the internal limiting membrane were included.

Vitreous haemorrhage
A vitreous haemorrhage (VH; Figs 3.21 and 3.22) is a haemorrhage that is in the vitreous gel, having penetrated through the internal limiting membrane.

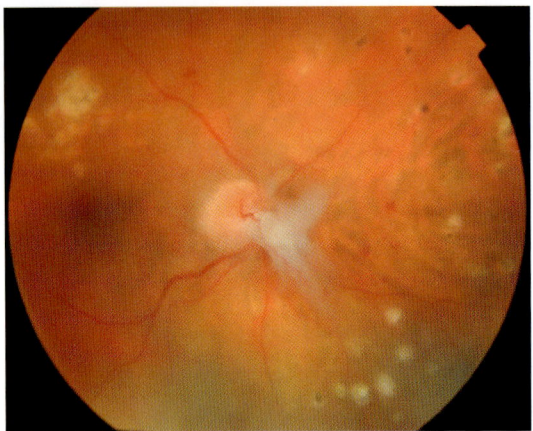

Fig. 3.16 An example of FPD (fibrous proliferation on the disc).

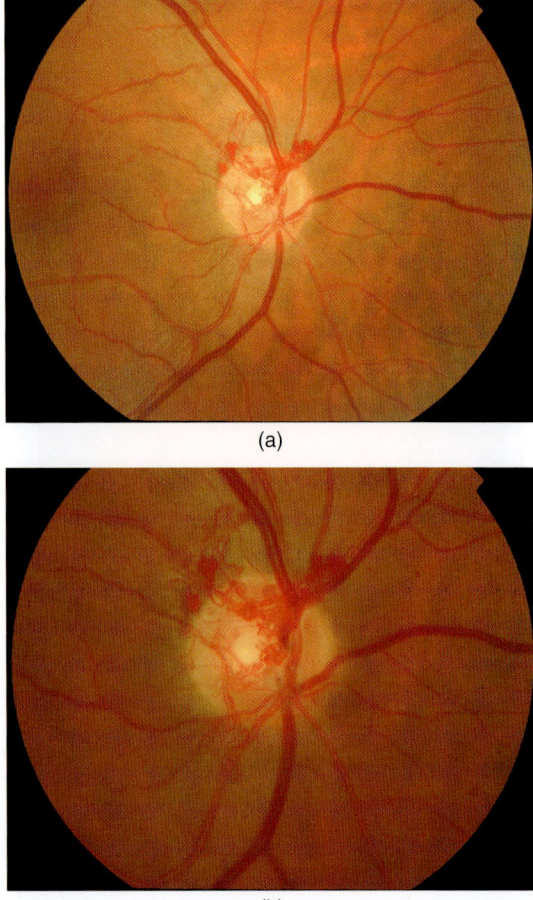

Fig. 3.18 (a) An example of NVD and (b) magnified view.

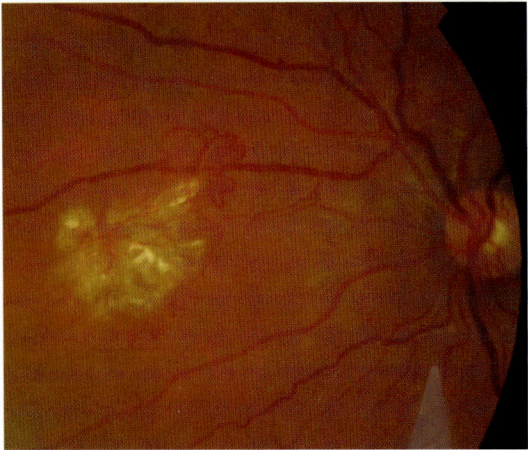

Fig. 3.17 An example of FPE (fibrous proliferation elsewhere), showing partial fibrosis of NVE in nasal retina.

Lesions and classifications of diabetic retinopathy 35

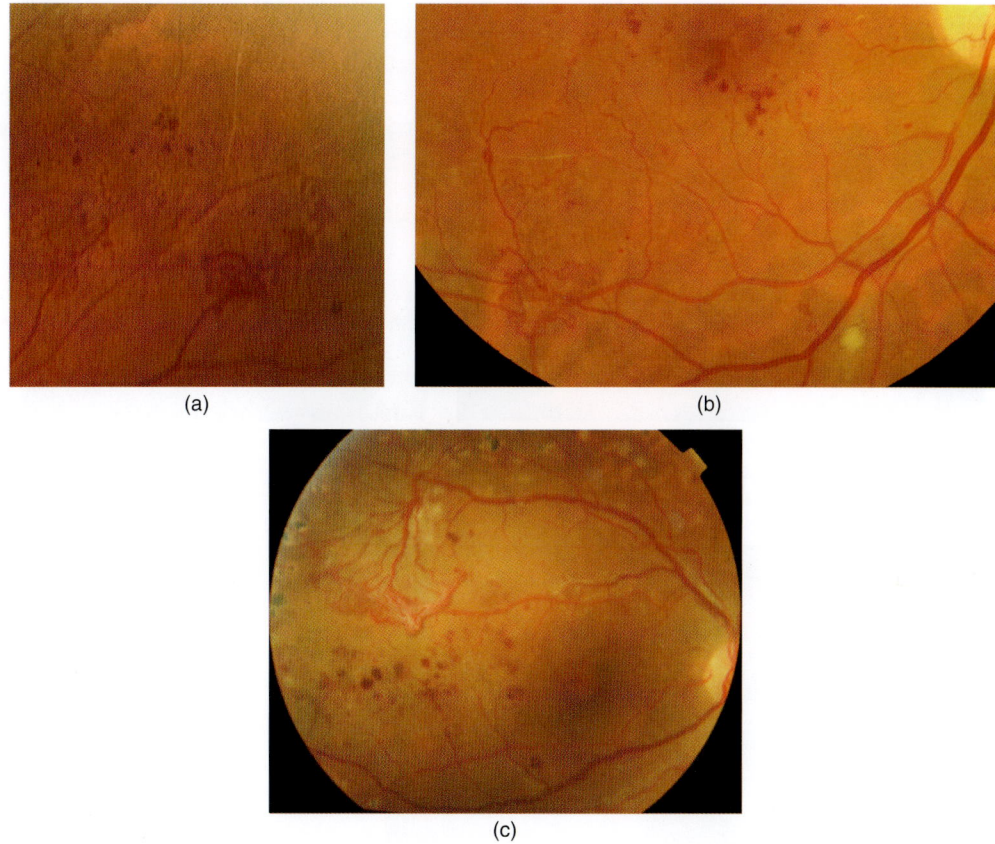

Fig. 3.19 An example of NVE forming (a) on the edge of an ischaemic area due to an occluded arteriole and (b) in the right infero-temporal retina. (c) An example of large NVE forming in the right temporal retina.

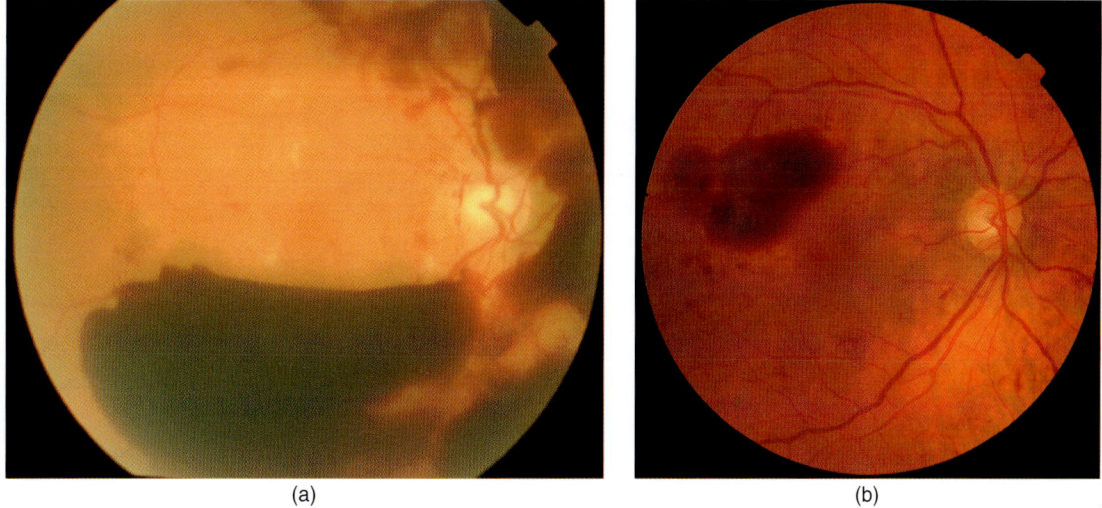

Fig. 3.20 (a, b) Examples of a preretinal haemorrhage (PRH): large boat-shaped with flat top and extension to nasal retina.

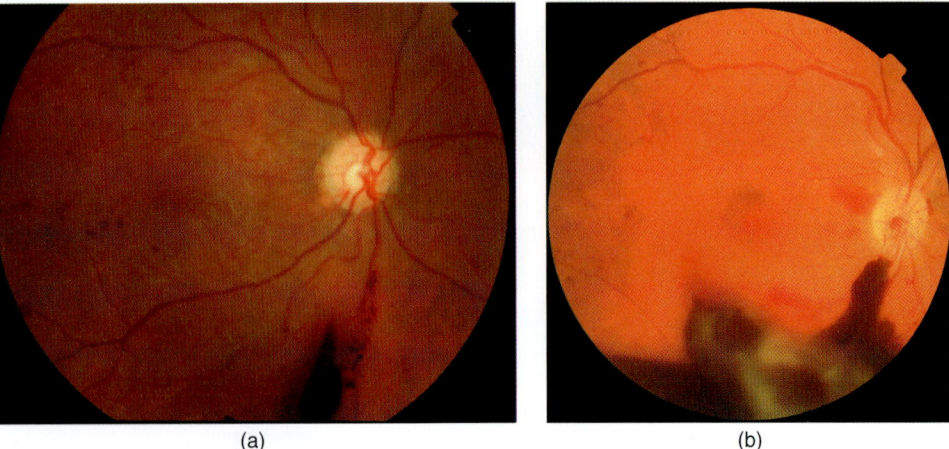

Fig. 3.21 An example of (a) a small VH and (b) a larger VH.

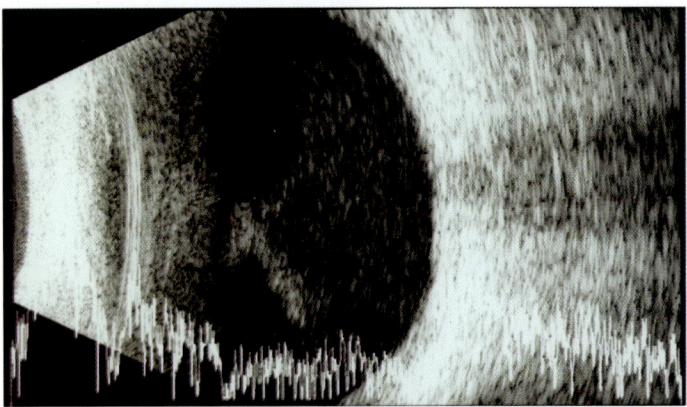

Fig. 3.22 An example of a B-scan of a more pronounced vitreous haemorrhage.

Post-maculopathy laser treatment

Photocoagulation scars may be present after macular laser treatment (Fig. 3.23). The best result would be clearing of clinically significant macular oedema and all hard exudates. Assessment of residual retinal oedema to decide whether further laser treatment is required will depend on an assessment of the amount of residual oedema, its location and the likely source and location of the leakage.

Post-scatter laser treatment for proliferative diabetic retinopathy

Photocoagulation scars are usually visible following scatter laser treatment (Fig. 3.24). The best result would be complete regression of the new vessels. However, one is often left with partial regression of new vessels and

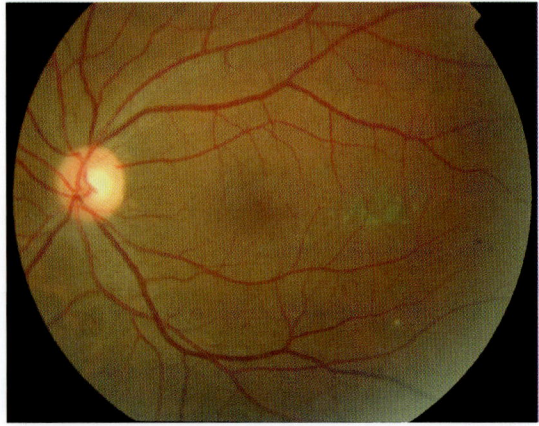

Fig. 3.23 An example of laser scars resulting from maculopathy treatment.

Lesions and classifications of diabetic retinopathy 37

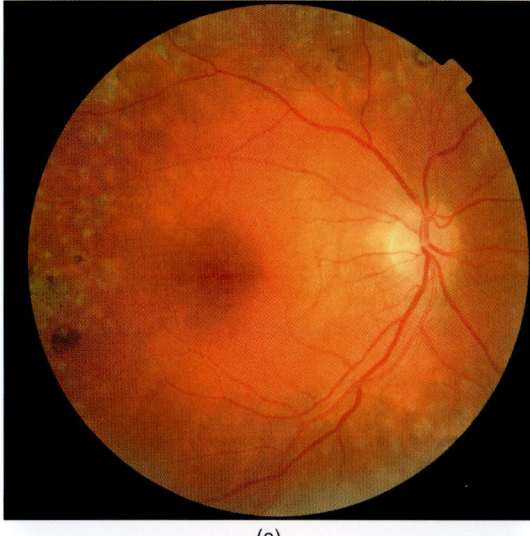

(a)

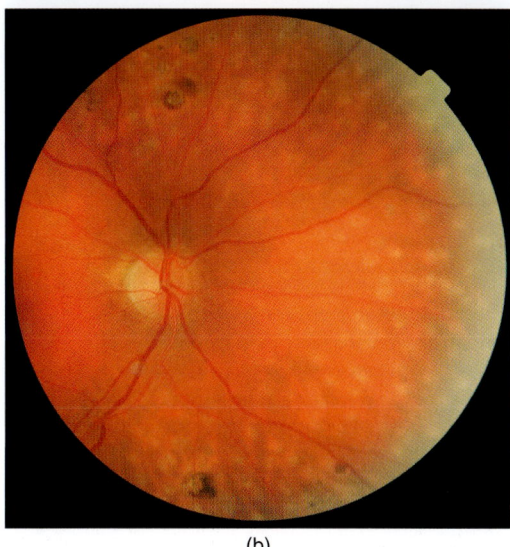

(b)

Fig. 3.24 Examples of laser scars post-scatter (panretinal) laser treatment: (a) right macular view and (b) right nasal view.

a decision needs to be made on the merits of further laser treatment. This decision will be based on the areas of retina that show laser photocoagulation scars, the appearance of the new vessels themselves, whether the frond-like tips still show circulation of red blood cells suggesting activity, whether the new vessels continue to grow or have shrunk and finally the appearance of areas of retina. In an area of retina that has been adequately treated the venous calibre returns to normal, having very

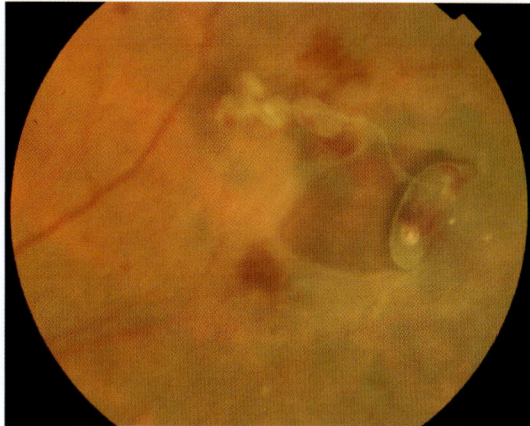

Fig. 3.25 Avulsion of NVE, leaving horseshoe tear.

often shown signs of venous dilation and sometimes beading. There may also be areas of retina that show obvious signs of inadequate treatment as well as areas that show good treatment results, evident by the presence of photocoagulation scars and changes in venous calibre.

Posterior vitreous detachment

A posterior vitreous detachment (PVD) is a common condition of the eye in which the vitreous humour separates from the retina. The vitreous is attached to the retina, more strongly in some places than others, particularly around the optic nerve head and around the peripheral retina. In people with proliferative diabetic retinopathy, where new vessels have penetrated the internal limiting membrane, vitreous haemorrhage is the usual result. Once a complete posterior vitreous detachment has occurred, this removes the structure that new vessels rely on to proliferate anteriorly and a posterior vitreous detachment can therefore be helpful in preventing further anterior neovascularisation. This is, of course, one of the rationales behind vitrectomy surgery. Rarely, a posterior vitreous detachment can result in a retinal tear when the new vessel complex is pulled away from the retina (Fig. 3.25).

ENGLISH AND INTERNATIONAL CLASSIFICATION

Because of the difficulty in correlating seven-field stereo-photography to the clinical setting, particularly in the screening environment where the level of referral

Table 3.3 International and English retinopathy classifications.

International clinical classification of diabetic retinopathy severity or diabetic macular oedema[7]		English Screening Programme levels[8]
	Optimise medical therapy, screen at least annually	R0 Currently screen annually
Microaneurysms only		R1
More than just microaneurysms but less severe than severe NPDR	Refer to ophthalmologist	Screen annually **Background** microaneurysm(s) or HMa retinal haemorrhage(s) venous loop any exudate or cotton wool spots (CWS) in the presence of other non-referable features of DR R2
Severe NPDR Any of the following: a) Extensive intraretinal haem (>20) in 4 quadrants b) Definite venous beading in 2+ quadrants c) Prominent IRMA in 1+ quadrant And no signs of PDR	Consider scatter photocoagulation for type 2 diabetes	Refer to ophthalmologist **Pre-proliferative** venous beading venous reduplication intraretinal microvascular abnormality (IRMA) multiple deep, round or blot haemorrhages
Neovascularisation Vitreous/preretinal haemorrhage	Scatter photocoagulation without delay for patients with vitreous haemorrhage or neovascularisation within 1DD of the optic nerve head	R3A Urgent referral to ophthalmologist **R3A. Proliferative** new vessels on disc (NVD) new vessels elsewhere (NVE) preretinal or vitreous haemorrhage preretinal fibrosis ± tractional retinal detachment **R3S.** Follow up annually within screening or at appropriate interval in surveillance. **R3S. Stable treated proliferative** Evidence of peripheral retinal laser treatment AND Stable retina from photograph taken at or shortly after discharge from the Hospital Eye service (HES)

to an ophthalmologist needed to be clearly defined, two further simplified classifications have been developed (Tables 3.3 and 3.4). The international classification has been developed for healthcare settings in countries such as the USA where there are an adequate number of ophthalmologists to undertake the slit-lamp biomicroscopy examinations on patients with microaneurysms only. In England, the referral level has been defined to refer patients with retinopathy to an ophthalmologist at a later stage in the disease process.

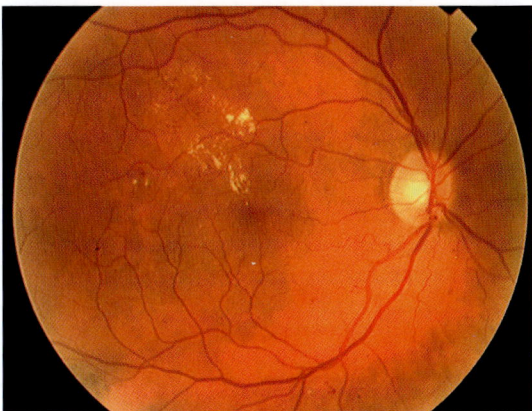

Fig. 4.2 Macular exudates before argon laser photocoagulation.

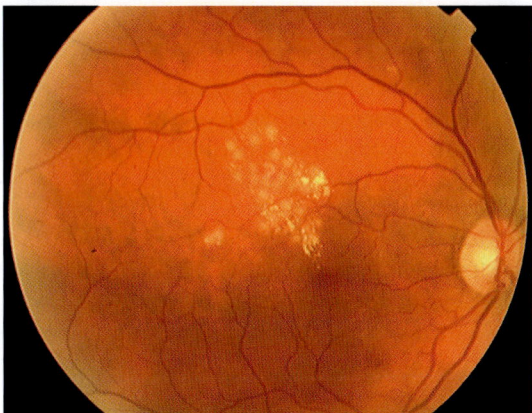

Fig. 4.3 Macular exudates immediately after laser photocoagulation.

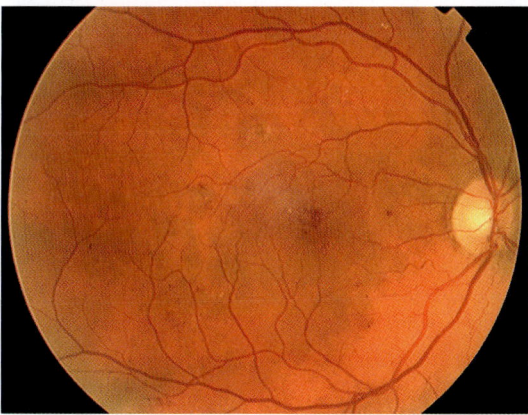

Fig. 4.4 Macular exudates 6 months after laser photocoagulation.

shown favourable long-term visual results of photocoagulation.

More recent studies[21–24] have shown beneficial effects from VEGF inhibitor treatments in centre-involving diabetic macular oedema.

Prevention/deterioration reduction by improved control of blood glucose, blood pressure and lipid levels

The evidence that intensive blood glucose control reduces the risk of new-onset DR and slows the progression of existing DR comes from the Diabetes Control and Complications Trial (DCCT)[25] and UKPDS[26]. Evidence that control of systemic hypertension reduces the risk of new-onset DR and slows the progression of existing DR has been provided by the UKPDS[27,28] and other studies[29,30]. There is evidence that elevated serum lipids are associated with macular exudate[31], and that prevention of moderate visual loss and partial regression of hard exudates may be possible by reducing elevated lipid levels[32].

Is there a suitable, reliable and acceptable screening test available?

There is widespread agreement that digital photography is the best method of screening for sight-threatening DR. The use of selective mydriasis and the number of fields captured have been more controversial. The reasons for digital photography being the preferred method are described in the following sections.

Direct ophthalmoscopy

Studies of direct ophthalmoscopy against a recognised reference standard of seven-field stereo photography, an ophthalmologist using slit-lamp biomicroscopy or fluorescein angiography showed variable results in studies by Palmberg et al.[33], Sussman et al.[34], Foulds et al.[35], Moss et al.[36], Kleinstein et al.[37], Awh et al.[38], Nathan et al.[39], Pugh et al.[40] and Harding et al.[41]. The results are considered too variable between different professional groups; even in the hands of a specialist registrar in ophthalmology[41] the sensitivity achieved for the detection of sight-threatening retinopathy was only 65% (CI 51–79%).

Optometrist's slit-lamp biomicroscopy

A number of studies have assessed the performance of optometrist's slit-lamp biomicroscopy including those by been overtaken by inherited retinal disorders. This may relate in part to the introduction of nationwide diabetic retinopathy screening programmes and improved glycaemic control. Kocur and Resnikoff[6] reported that, in European people of working age, diabetic retinopathy is the most frequently reported causes of serious visual loss. In the middle-income countries of Europe, diabetic retinopathy is the third most common cause (advanced cataract and glaucoma being more frequently observed).

Zheng et al.[7] reported that, globally, the number of people with DR will grow from 126.6 million in 2010 to 191.0 million by 2030, and estimated that the number with vision-threatening diabetic retinopathy (VTDR) will increase from 37.3 million to 56.3 million in that time.

Is it a constant or growing public health problem?

In 1997, Amos et al.[8] estimated that 124 million people worldwide had diabetes, 97% of these having non-insulin-dependent diabetes mellitus (NIDDM). In 2000, Sorensen[9] reported body weight and the prevalence of obesity was rising so rapidly in many countries that the World Health Organisation had recognised that there is a 'global epidemic of obesity'. The prevalence of type 2 diabetes is rising in parallel. The International Diabetes Federation (IDF) forecast[10] a rise from the current level of 387 million people with diabetes worldwide in 2014 to 592 million by 2035.

Is there a recognisable latent or early symptomatic stage?

The Wisconsin Epidemiological Study[11], the Berlin Retinopathy Study[12], the Early Treatment Diabetic Retinopathy Study[13] and the UKPDS[14] have all observed the natural history of diabetic retinopathy. In 2003, Younis et al.[15,16] reported yearly and cumulative incidence of any retinopathy, maculopathy and sight-threatening diabetic retinopathy in patients with type 1 diabetes and type 2 diabetes who underwent 2742 and 20,570 screening events, respectively. There is clear evidence from these studies that sight-threatening diabetic retinopathy has a recognisable latent or early symptomatic stage (Fig. 4.1).

Is treatment effective and agreed universally?

The evidence that laser treatment is effective

There is clear evidence that laser treatment is effective and universally agreed for the treatment of proliferative diabetic retinopathy. The Diabetic Retinopathy Study Research Group[17] study provided evidence that photocoagulation treatment was of benefit in preventing severe visual loss in eyes with proliferative retinopathy. The Early Treatment Diabetic Retinopathy Study[18] (ETDRS) showed that focal photocoagulation (Figs 4.2–4.4) of 'clinically significant' diabetic macular oedema substantially reduced the risk of visual loss. Further reports[19,20] have

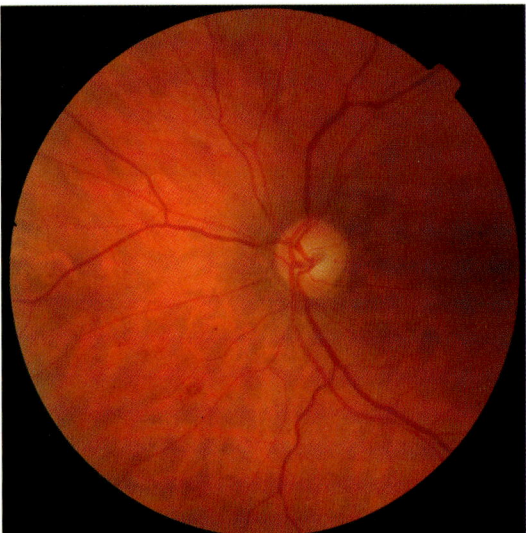
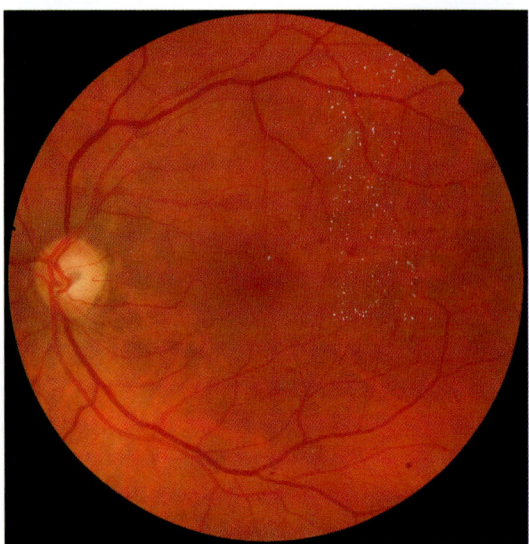

Fig. 4.1 Diabetic retinopathy detected during screening.

4 Screening for diabetic retinopathy

Peter H. Scanlon

Harris Manchester College, University of Oxford; Medical Ophthalmology, University of Gloucestershire, UK

PRINCIPLES OF SCREENING

The definition of screening that was adapted by the World Health Organisation (WHO)[1] in 1968 was 'the presumptive identification of unrecognised disease or defect by the application of tests, examinations or other procedures which can be applied rapidly. Screening tests sort out apparently well persons who probably have a disease from those who probably do not. A screening test is not intended to be diagnostic. Persons with positive or suspicious findings must be referred to their physicians for diagnosis and necessary treatment.'

The principles for screening for human disease that were derived from the public health papers produced by the WHO[1] in 1968 were as follows.

1. The condition sought should be an important problem.
2. There should be an accepted treatment for patients with recognised disease.
3. Facilities for diagnosis and treatment should be available.
4. There should be a recognisable latent or early symptomatic stage.
5. There should be a suitable test or examination.
6. The test should be acceptable to the population.
7. The natural history of the condition, including development from latent to declared disease, should be adequately understood.
8. There should be an agreed policy on whom to treat as patients.
9. The cost of the case-finding programme (including early diagnosis and treatment of patients diagnosed) should be economically balanced in relation to possible expenditure on medical care as a whole.
10. Case-finding should be a continuing process and not a 'one-time' project.

Applying these principles to sight-threatening diabetic retinopathy raises the following questions[2].

1. Is there evidence that sight-threatening diabetic retinopathy is an important public health problem?
2. Is there evidence that the incidence of sight-threatening diabetic retinopathy is going to remain the same or become an even greater public health problem?
3. Is there evidence that sight-threatening diabetic retinopathy has a recognisable latent or early symptomatic stage?
4. Is there evidence that treatment for sight-threatening diabetic retinopathy is effective and agreed universally?
5. Is a suitable and reliable screening test available, acceptable to both healthcare professionals and (more importantly) to the public?
6. Are the costs of screening and effective treatment of sight-threatening diabetic retinopathy balanced economically in relation to total expenditure on healthcare, including the consequences of leaving the disease untreated?

Is it an important public health problem?

The UK Prospective Diabetes Study (UKPDS) reported a baseline prevalence of retinopathy in 39% of diabetic men and 35% of diabetic women. In 2002, Younis et al.[3] reported baseline prevalence in the type 1 group of any diabetic retinopathy (DR), proliferative diabetic retinopathy (PDR) and sight-threatening diabetic retinopathy (STDR) of 45.7%, 3.7% and 16.4%, respectively. Baseline prevalence in the type 2 group of any DR, PDR and STDR was 25.3%, 0.5% and 6.0%, respectively.

In 1995, Evans[4] reported that diabetes was the most important cause of blindness in the working population (13.8%) in England with 11.9% due to diabetic retinopathy. A recent study[5] has shown that, for the first time in at least five decades, diabetic retinopathy/maculopathy is no longer the leading cause of certifiable blindness among working age adults in England and Wales, having

A Practical Manual of Diabetic Retinopathy Management, Second Edition.
Edited by Peter Scanlon, Ahmed Sallam, and Peter van Wijngaarden.
© 2017 John Wiley & Sons Ltd. Published 2017 by John Wiley & Sons Ltd.
Companion Website: www.wiley.com/go/scanlon/diabetic_retinopathy

Table 3.4 International and English maculopathy classification.

International classification[7]	Outcome	English classification[8]	Outcome
Diabetic macular oedema: Present as defined by some retinal thickening or hard exudates in the posterior pole and subclassified into: Mild diabetic macular oedema: Some retinal thickening or hard exudates in the posterior pole but distant from the macula	Referral	Circinate or group of exudates within the macula (The macula is defined as that part of the retina which lies within a circle centred on the centre of the fovea whose radius is the distance between the centre of the fovea and the temporal margin of the disc) (A circinate exudate needs to be at least a ½ disc area which needs to be within the macular area as defined above)	Referral
		Any microaneurysm or haemorrhage within 1DD of the centre of the fovea only if associated with a best VA of $\leq 6/12$ (if no stereo)	Referral
Moderate diabetic macular oedema: Retinal thickening or hard exudates approaching the centre of the macula but not involving the centre	Referral	Exudate within 1DD of the centre of the fovea	Referral
		Retinal thickening within 1DD of the centre of the fovea (if stereo available)	Referral
Severe diabetic macular oedema: Retinal thickening or hard exudates involving the centre of the macula	Referral		

PRACTICE POINTS

There are a number of different classifications of diabetic retinopathy which have been developed to give indications of the risks of progression to proliferative diabetic retinopathy or vision-threatening maculopathy, and the appropriate referral criteria, the latter depending on individual healthcare systems. The key factor in these classifications is accurate identification of the lesions that occur in diabetic retinopathy, as described in this chapter.

REFERENCE

Please visit www.wiley.com/go/scanlon/diabetic_retinopathy

Hammond et al.[42], Burnett et al.[43], Prasad et al.[44], Hulme et al.[45], Olson et al.[46], Sharp et al.[47], Tu et al.[48] and Warburton et al.[49]. The best-designed study is that of Olson et al.[46] and Sharp et al.[47], in which all those patients seen by an optometrist are also examined by a retinal specialist and a comparison with digital photography and 35 mm photography is made. In this study, slit-lamp examination by optometrists for the detection of sight-threatening retinopathy (referable) achieved a sensitivity of 73% (52–88%) and a specificity of 90% (87–93%). No technical failure was reported. However, with two-field imaging, manual grading of red-free digital images achieved a sensitivity of 93% (82–98%) and a specificity of 87% (84–90%). The technical failure rate for digital imaging reported was 4.4% of patients. Two-field digital photography as a method of screening achieved a higher sensitivity and specificity for screening than slit-lamp biomicroscopy by a number of trained optometrists. Slit-lamp biomicroscopy schemes also have the disadvantage that, for quality assurance purposes, a percentage of patients require re-examination as opposed to re-examination of the images in a scheme using digital photography.

Widefield scanning laser ophthalmoscopes

Widefield scanning laser ophthalmoscopes have been proposed for diabetic retinopathy screening but have not as yet demonstrated the same level of resolution as digital cameras. Wilson et al.[50] reported results of a comparative trial of scanning laser ophthalmoscopy against digital photography. The study also reported that images were of lower resolution than conventional digital photographs, limiting the detection of microaneurysms (identifying 79.2% v. 95.9%; $P < 0.001$).

Although there are some advantages of the ultra-widefield technology in angiographic identification[51,52] of areas of ischaemia in the peripheral retina and in detection of peripheral lesions[53], further publications[54–59] have not, in my view, demonstrated that the central resolution detects the required level of detail that digital photography detects in diabetic retinopathy screening.

Mydriatic photography (< seven fields) using 35 mm film or Polaroid

Studies of mydriatic photography with 35 mm film or Polaroid against a recognised reference standard of seven-field stereo photography, an ophthalmologist using slit-lamp biomicroscopy or fluorescein angiography showed consistently good results by Kalm et al.[60], Lee et al.[61], Pugh et al.[40], Schachat et al.[62], Aldington et al.[63], Harding et al.[41], Kiri et al.[64], Taylor et al.[65], Broadbent et al.[66], Moller et al.[67], Stellingwerf et al.[68], Pandit and Taylor[69], Olson et al.[46] and Sharp et al.[47]. These studies have shown that consistently good results can be achieved, with sensitivities of >80% and high levels of specificity, using mydriatic photography with 35 mm film or Polaroid in screening for referable or sight-threatening diabetic retinopathy. In these studies, specificity does vary depending on whether ungradeable images are regarded as test positive, but levels of >85% are consistently achieved.

Non-mydriatic photography

There have been strong proponents of non-mydriatic photography for many years. In 1993, ungradable image rates were reported as low as 4% by Leese et al.[70]. However, it has been recognised in more recent years, following the publication of studies by Scanlon et al.[71] and Murgatroyd et al.[72] that ungradeable image rates for non-mydriatic digital photography in a predominantly white Caucasian population are of the order of 20–26% (19.7% and 26% being reported in the two studies). Age is the strongest correlator to poor-quality images in non-mydriatic digital photography, as shown in the publication by Scanlon et al.[71]. The Health Technology Board for Scotland used data from the Scanlon et al.[71] study in their report[73] and concluded that similar sensitivities and specificities could be achieved by dilating those patients with ungradeable images. This relies on the ability of the screener to accurately determine an ungradeable image at the time of screening and, in the Scottish system, relies on the assumption that the grading of one field will detect referable retinopathy with the same degree of accuracy as the grading of two fields (giving evidence from Olson's study[46]). Other proponents of digital photography have attempted to capture three fields[74–76], five fields[77] and, remarkably, Shiba et al.[78] excluded the over 70 years age group and attempted nine overlapping non-mydriatic 450 fields. Some recent[76,77,79,80] have been based on small numbers of patients, with low mean ages, and they do not report confidence intervals.

Digital camera systems have lower flash intensities than those using Polaroid or 35 mm film. Taylor et al.[65] reported a low flash power (10 W v. 300 W) of one of the earlier digital systems. This has now increased since the modern digital camera backs require more light, but not to the level of 35 mm film or Polaroid cameras.

Mydriatic digital photography

Studies of mydriatic digital photography (Fig. 4.5) against a recognised reference standard of seven-field stereo photography and an ophthalmologist using slit-lamp biomicroscopy have shown showed consistently good results; see Taylor et al.[65], Razvi et al.[81], Rudnisky et al.[82], Olson et al.[46], Sharp et al.[47] and Scanlon et al.[71]. The study by Olson et al.[46] and Sharp et al.[47] demonstrated in 586 patients that, for the detection of sight-threatening retinopathy, manual grading of two-field red-free digital images achieved a sensitivity of 93% (82–98%) and a specificity of 87% (84–90%). The reference standard was slit-lamp biomicrocopy by retinal specialists. Digital imaging had an ungradeable image rate of 4.4% of patients. In 2003, the Gloucestershire Diabetic Eye study[71] demonstrated the effectiveness of mydriatic digital photography against a reference standard of an ophthalmologist's slit-lamp biomicroscopy, which was further validated[83] against seven-field stereo-photography. The same study published results on reasons for poor image quality in digital photographic screening programmes[84] and on the effect of the introduction of the screening programme on the workload of the local ophthalmology department[85]. In 2004, Williams produced a report for the American Academy of Ophthalmology summarising the use of single-field fundus photography for diabetic retinopathy screening.

Two review articles from the USA were written in 2006; the first by Chew[86] concluded that, although screening techniques do not replace the eye examination, in populations with poor access to ophthalmic care screening techniques such as the non-mydriatic camera used in offices of primary care physicians may be useful in identifying lesions of diabetic retinopathy requiring treatment. The second article by Whited[87], which included very few non-US-based studies, concluded that based on existing data teleophthalmology appears to be an accurate

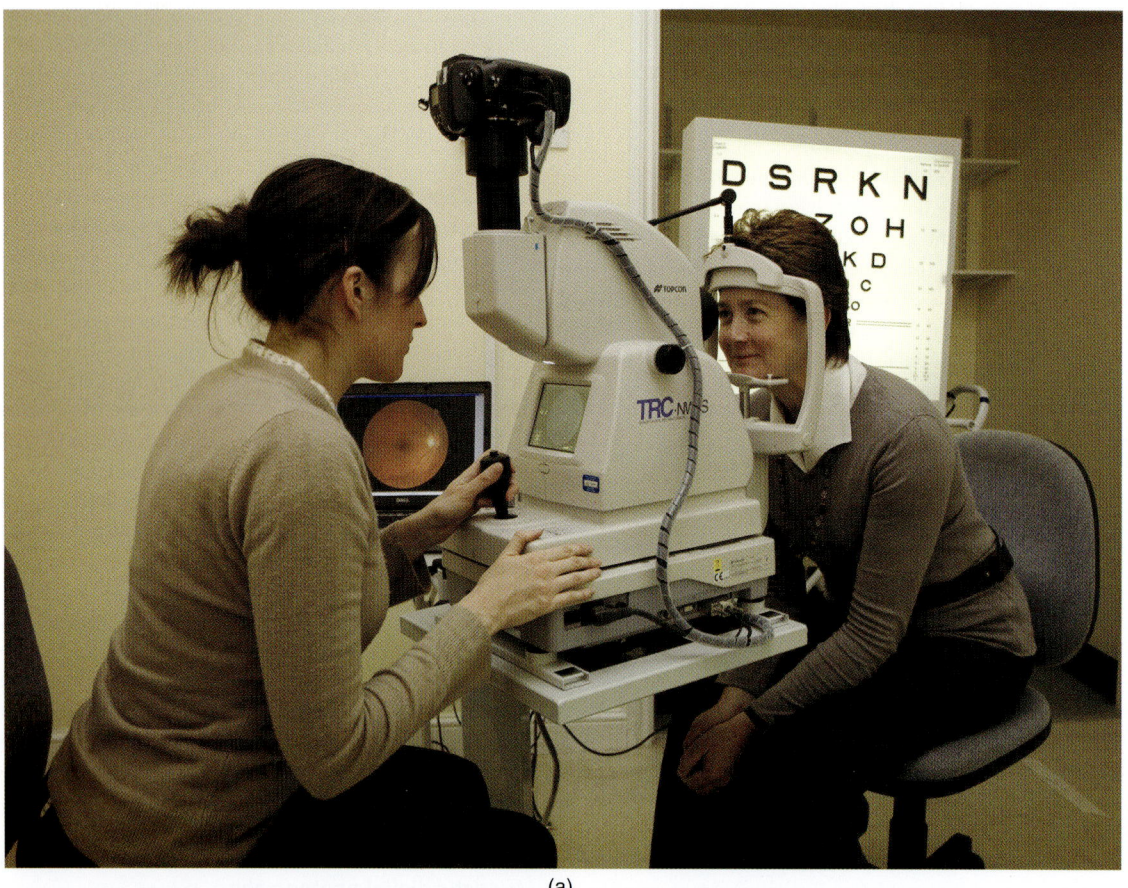

(a)

Fig. 4.5 (a) Screening using two-field mydriatic digital photography as recommended in the English Screening Programme. (b) A screening episode being undertaken.

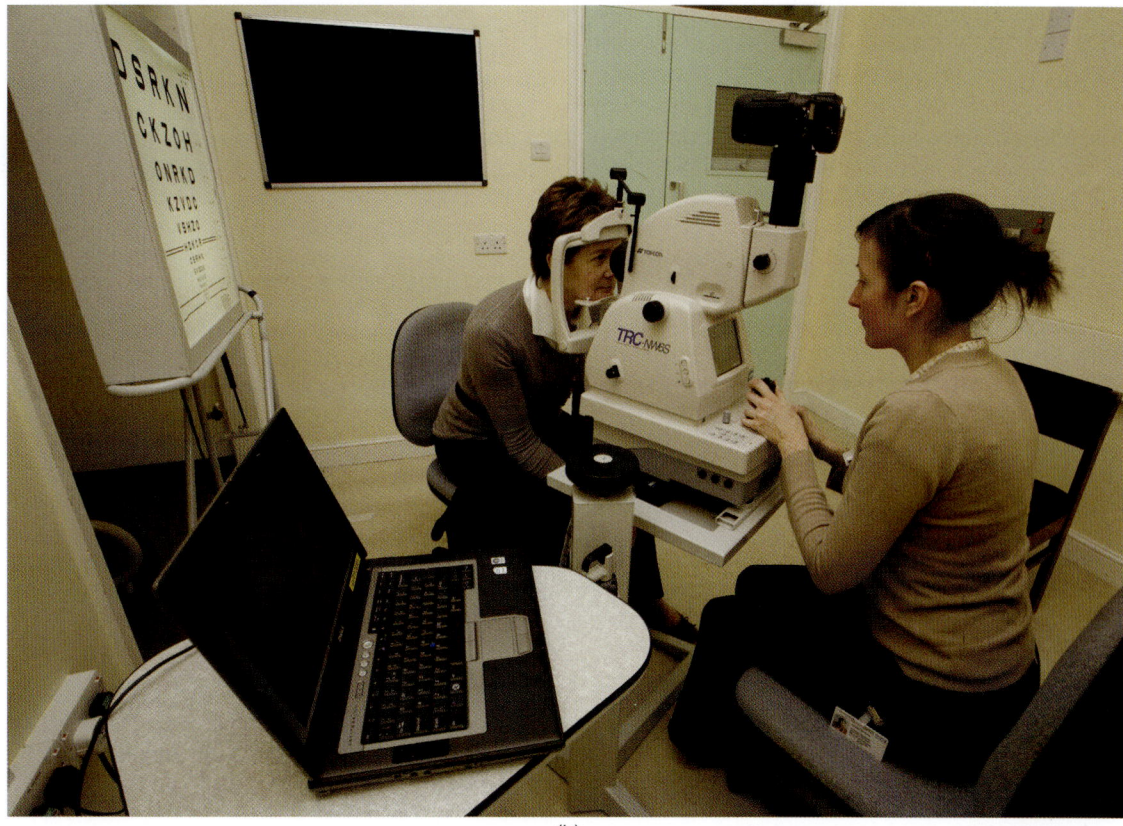

(b)

Fig. 4.5 (*Continued*)

and reliable test for detecting diabetic retinopathy and macular oedema.

Are the costs of screening and effective treatment justified?

In 1982, Savolainen and Lee[88] reported on the cost-effectiveness of photocoagulation for sight-threatening diabetic retinopathy in the UK. There have been reports of computer simulation models by Javitt et al.[89–92], Dasbach et al.[93], Caro et al.[94] and Fendrick et al.[95] based on the health systems in the USA and Sweden[96]. Modelling studies from the Wessex Institute[97] suggested that there is greater benefit in reducing the screening interval when the screening programme retains patients until they require treatment than when the screening programme detects early, background retinopathy, with prompt referral to specialist services. James et al.[98] reported results for an organised screening programme using 35 mm retinal photography, and demonstrated this to be more cost-effective than the previous system of opportunistic screening.

Meads and Hyde[99] reviewed published studies of the costs of blindness and compared the 1983 estimate of Foulds et al.[35] inflated to £7433 in 2002 costs, Dasbach et al.'s 1991 estimate[93] inflated to £5391 in 2002 costs and Wright et al.'s 2000 estimate[100] inflated to £7452 (£4070–11,250) in 2002 costs. He concluded that much of the uncertainty in any sensitivity analysis of the cost of blindness in older people is associated with the cost of residential care and that the excess admission to care homes caused by poor vision is impossible to quantify at the present time.

Only two studies have assessed the costs of screening using digital photography. Bjorvig et al.[101] assessed the costs of telemedicine screening for diabetic retinopathy in a trial conducted in northern Norway. At low workloads, telemedicine was more expensive than conventional examination. However, at higher workloads telemedicine was cheaper. The break-even-point occurred at a patient workload of 110 per annum. Tu et al.[48] calculated the cost of screening each patient as £23.99 per patient for an optometry model and £29.29 per patient for a digital photographic model. However, in this study there were poor compliance rates with the newly introduced screening programme in both models.

The UK National Screening Committee has recommended digital imaging as the preferred method of retinal photography for screening[102,103]. They have used estimates of costs by Garvican[103] for a theoretical population of 500,000. For a mobile photographic screening service, the cost of the initial screen is estimated at approximately £21 per diabetic patient registered, or £24 per attendee at 85–90% uptake.

The Exeter Standards

The Exeter Standards form the basis for an acceptable method for use in a systematic screening programme for DR in the UK. The Exeter Standards recommend that a screening test for sight-threatening DR should achieve a minimum sensitivity of 80% and a minimum specificity of 95%. In the Liverpool Diabetic Eye study[104], 35 mm photography achieved 84% sensitivity and 89% specificity for mydriatic 35 mm film photography and the Gloucestershire Diabetic Eye study[71] achieved 87.8% sensitivity and 86.1% specificity for mydriatic digital photography with an ungradeable image rate of 3.7%. This suggests that 95% specificity may have been set too high and sensitivity too low, but these have not been challenged and the standard has been maintained for guidance. In some studies the specificity is reported as higher than those quoted, but a difference in whether ungradeables are counted as positive test results often explains this difference. If the sensitivity and specificity studies were repeated with modern digital cameras, the results are likely to improve because of the higher resolution of the modern cameras.

Case History 4.1: Screening for sight-threatening diabetic retinopathy

A 20-year-old man with type 1 diabetes diagnosed at the age of 7 years attended his local optician for a sight test and was told that he did not have any significant diabetic retinopathy. Two months later he received an invite for a local photographic screening service, and attended (Fig. 4.6a and b).

Laser treatment was commenced to his left eye with right 30 burns, 100 micron size, 210–230 mW, 0.1 s, Area Centralis lens, argon laser. One year after presentation, the vision deteriorated in the left eye to 6/24 (20/180) and red-free (Fig. 4.6c) and fluorescein photographs (Fig. 4.6d and e) were taken. Further laser treatment was given to the left macular area with left 53 burns, 100 micron size, 180–250 mW, 0.1 s, Area Centralis lens, argon laser.

The following week, panretinal photocoagulation was commenced to the left eye with 1522 burns, 350 micron spot size, power 140–180 mW, Transequator lens, argon laser split over 2 sessions 1 week apart, and a further session of 706 burns, 500 micron spot size, power 170 mW, Karickhoff lens, argon laser. The vision in the left eye remained at the level of 6/24 (20/180), and a retrohyaloid haemorrhage then developed in the left eye as shown in the red-free (Fig. 4.6f) and fluorescein photographs (Fig. 4.6g). Some exudates and leakage were seen in the right macular area (Fig. 4.6h–j).

A B-scan was performed which showed an appearance similar to a detachment but was, in this instance, caused by the retrohyaloid haemorrhage (Fig. 4.6k). A left pars plana vitrectomy was performed. Laser treatment was commenced to his right eye with right 36 burns, 100 micron size, 190 mW, 0.1 s, Area Centralis lens, argon laser.

Three years later (age 25 years), the fluorescein angiogram was repeated. At this stage the visual acuity was right 6/4 (20/14) and the left was 6/9 (20/30) (Fig. 4.6l–o).

At the age of 31 years he developed peripheral neovascularisation in his right eye and required a course of panretinal photocoagulation (1899 burns, 200 micron size, 350–400 mW, 0.02 s over two sessions) with the Pascal laser to his right eye. He is now 35 years old and his vision has remained good at right 6/6 (20/20) and left 6/9 (20/30).

ADVANCES IN SCREENING

Risk-based screening intervals

The current epidemic of diabetes has necessitated further research into extending the screening interval for those at very low risk of sight-threatening retinopathy. There are three possible approaches as described in the following.

1. Risk based on a previous screening result[105–107]. This was originally proposed by a group in Iceland[12] where it was introduced in an area of Sweden[105].
2. Risk based on two consecutive screening results[108]. The Gloucestershire UK Research Group developed a simple risk stratification model for time to development of sight-threatening diabetic retinopathy[108],

Screening for diabetic retinopathy 47

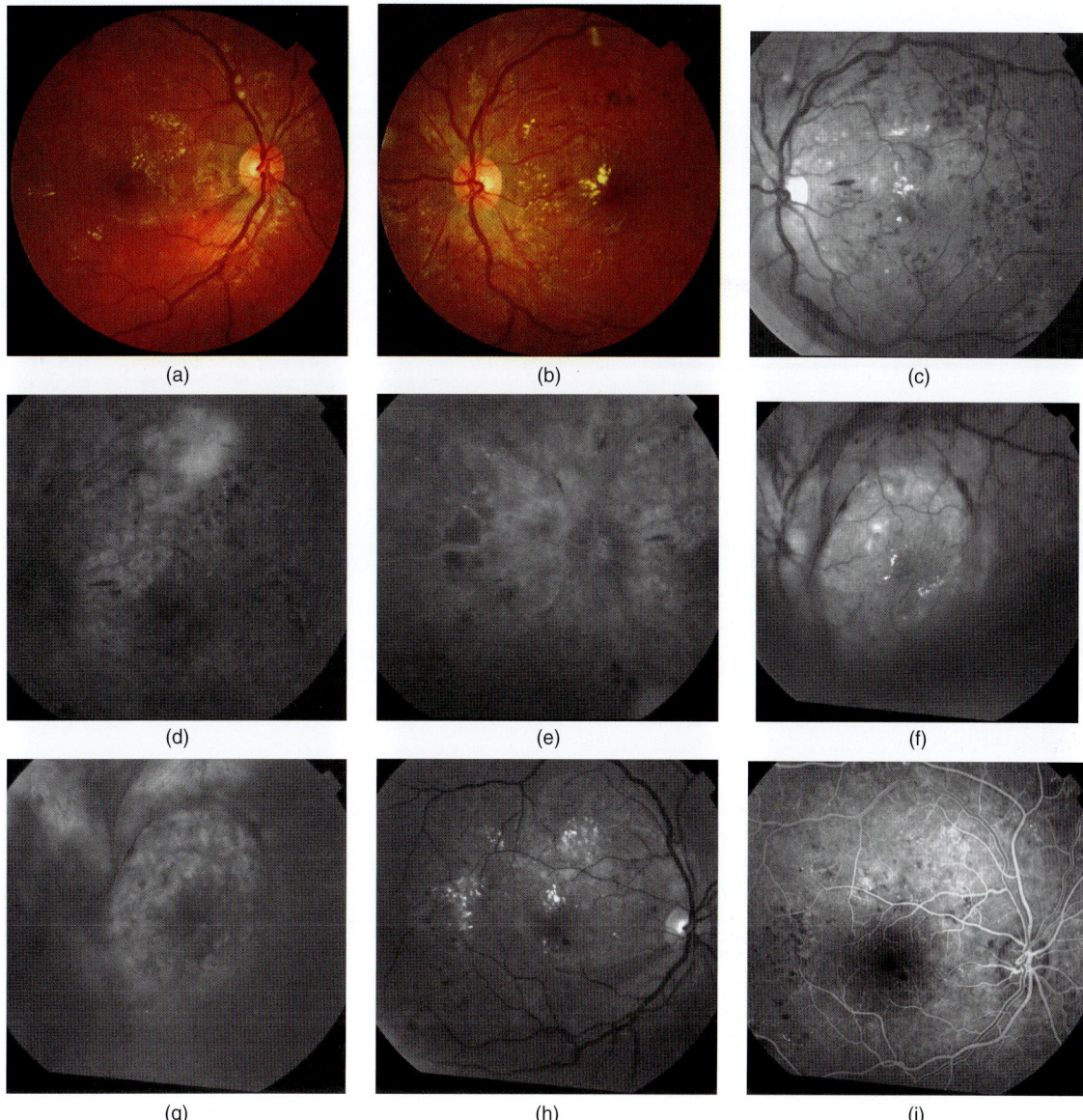

Fig. 4.6 Year 0 macula colour (a) right and (b) left. Year 1 left (c) macula red-free and (d) fluorescein showing left macular oedema and leakage from NVE above the left macula. (e) Year 1 left disc/nasal view fluorescein showing extensive leakage and ischaemic area in left nasal retina. Year 2 left macula (f) red-free, showing retrohayloid haemorrhage with sparing around the fovea, and (g) fluorescein, showing vitreous haemorrhage with sparing around the fovea. Year 2 right macula (h) red-free showing exudates in right macular area, (i) fluorescein of right macular area at 21 s, and (j) fluorescein of right macular area at 2 min 31 s. (k) B-scan appearance caused by retrohyaloid haemorrhage. Year 5 right macula (l) colour and (m) fluorescein at 25 s. Year 5 left macula (n) colour and (o) fluorescein at 2 min 44 s.

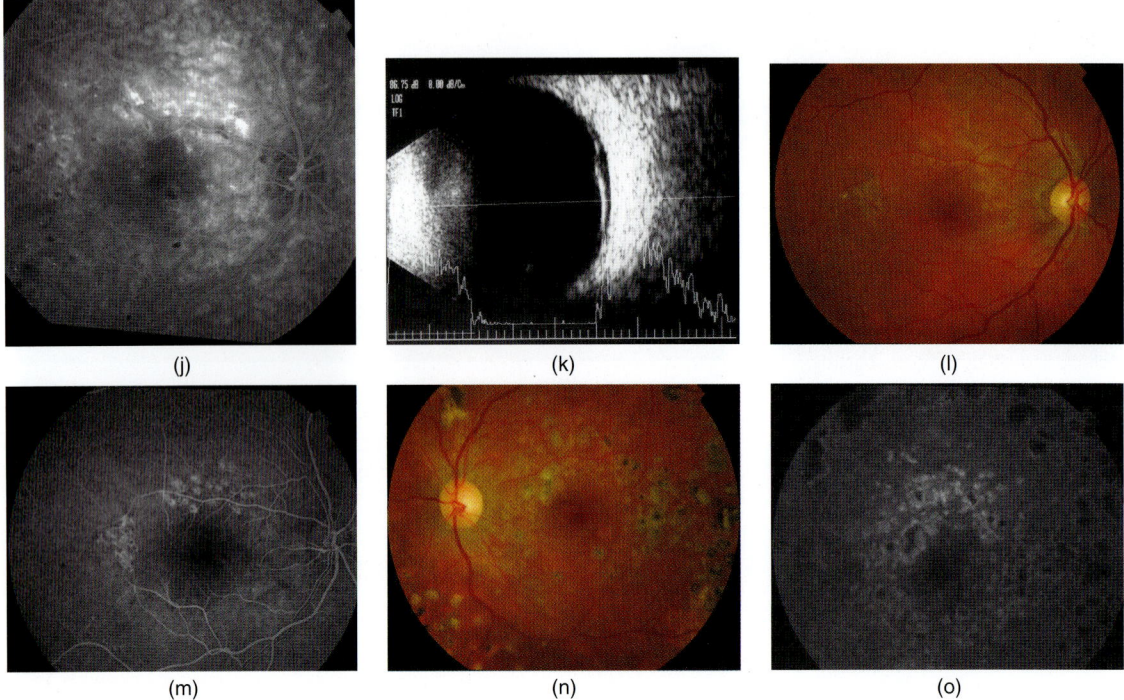

Fig. 4.6 (*Continued*)

which was based on categorising the digital photographic screening results from two consecutive annual digital photographic screenings. This was linked to another study[109] that reported the influence of background diabetic retinopathy in the second eye on rates of progression of diabetic retinopathy in our cohort of patients in Gloucestershire between 2005 and 2010. There has been a further publication[110] from within the UK testing this model on different datasets, and the UK National Screening committee is considering adopting this model in the UK.

3. Risk based on individualised risk factors[111]. The rates of incidence and progression of diabetic retinopathy are greater in people with a longer duration of diabetes and in those with poor glycaemic control (higher HbA1c) and may also vary with other risk factors. A study from Denmark developed a model using data from the UKPDS and other trials to identify those at higher absolute risk of sight-threatening DR[112] in order to identify subgroups of those with diabetes in whom the screening interval can be extended without risk of sight-threatening diabetic retinopathy developing before the next screening visit.

Further work is being undertaken in this area, but the difficulty is the ready availability of the risk factor information on a population level.

Automated analysis

It has been demonstrated[113,114] that computer algorithms can detect microaneurysms and some other features of diabetic retinopathy to a high degree of accuracy. There are scientific, ethical, legal and political issues[115] to be addressed. One of the main areas of concern is that the current screening cameras use digital backs from the general photographic markets with commercially sensitive compression algorithms which are subject to frequent change. Raw images (the original images produced without any compression) from modern digital camera backs are now too large to be realistically used in population-based screening.

Optical coherence tomography/photographic clinics

The introduction of a second level of screening using a combined colour camera and optical coherence tomography (OCT) for those who are screen-positive for diabetic maculopathy using two-dimensional markers has been shown to be effective[116]. Further work to determine how this could be introduced in a cost-effective manner is required before general introduction in the UK screening programmes is recommended. It is unlikely that these machines will be shown to be cost effective as a primary screening tool because of their cost.

PRACTICE POINTS

An effective treatment has been available for most patients with diabetic retinopathy since the first reports from the Diabetic Retinopathy Study[117] were published in 1976. It is therefore a tragedy that so many patients, in healthcare systems where appropriate treatment is readily available, are presenting so late in the course of the disease that treatment is much more difficult and unnecessary blindness is often the result.

Systematic screening programmes with good population coverage do reduce the incidence and prevalence of blindness in the population with diabetes, and many countries are now looking to introduce these programmes.

Case History 4.2: Screening for sight-threatening diabetic retinopathy

A man with type 1 diabetes diagnosed at the age of 28 years was screened at the age of 42 years and referred to the Hospital Eye Service for right maculopathy (Fig. 4.7a).

Laser treatment was commenced to his right eye with right 12 burns, 100 micron size, 150 mW, 0.02 s, Area Centralis lens, Pascal laser. He attended a 3-month follow-up, when there was a reported improvement in the appearance of his right macular area. He did not attend any further follow-up appointments.

He attended for screening at the age of 45 years and bilateral maculopathy and proliferative diabetic retinopathy were observed (Fig. 4.7b–e). He attended the Hospital Eye Service and the OCT photographs (Fig. 4.7f and g) showed thickening in both macular areas.

He received macular laser treatment (35 burns, 100 micron size, 120 mW, 0.05 s) and panretinal photocoagulation (1705 burns, 200 micron size, 300–350 mW,

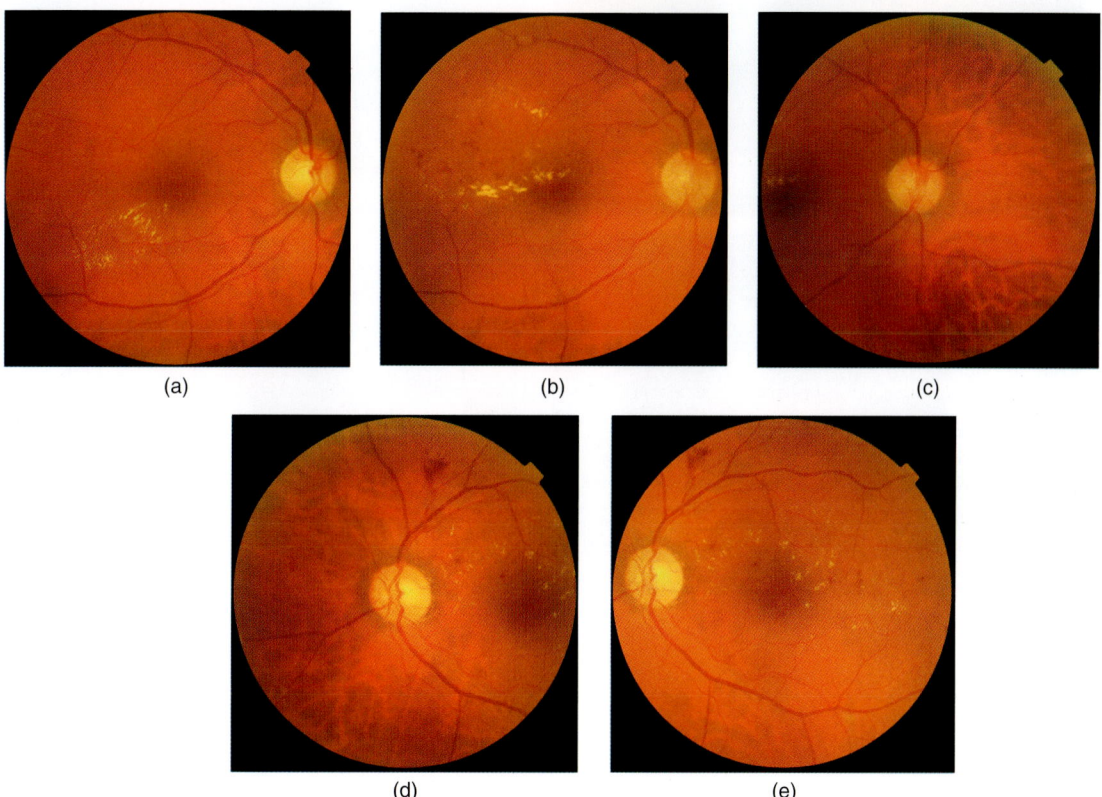

Fig. 4.7 (a) Year 0, first screening episode: right macula colour. (b) Year 3, second screening episode: (b) right macula colour and (c) right and (d) left disc colour. (e) Year 3, second screening episode: left macula colour. OCT (f) right and (g) left macular area. (h) OCT right macular area 2 months after macular and first panretinal laser treatment.

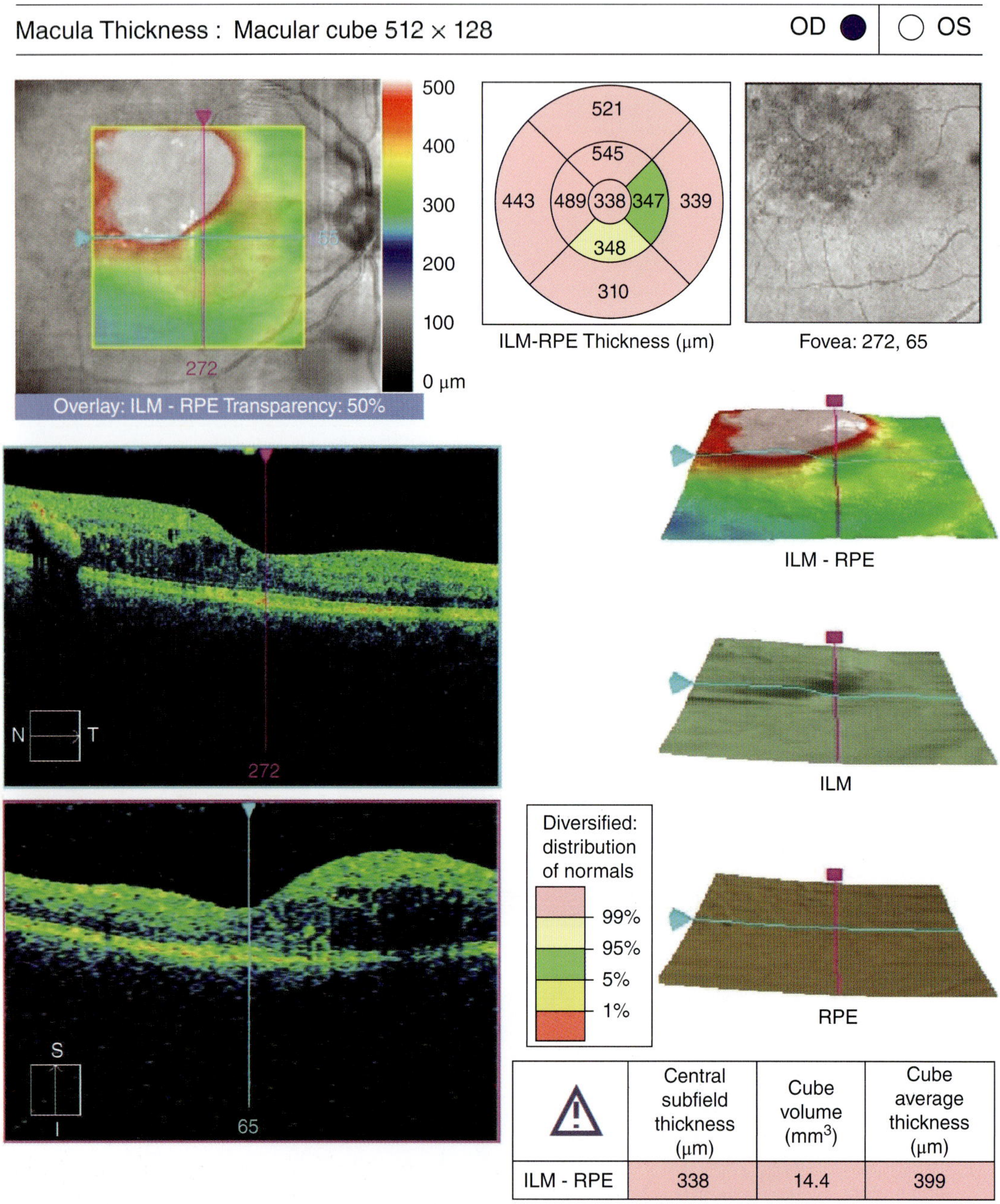

Fig. 4.7 (*Continued*)

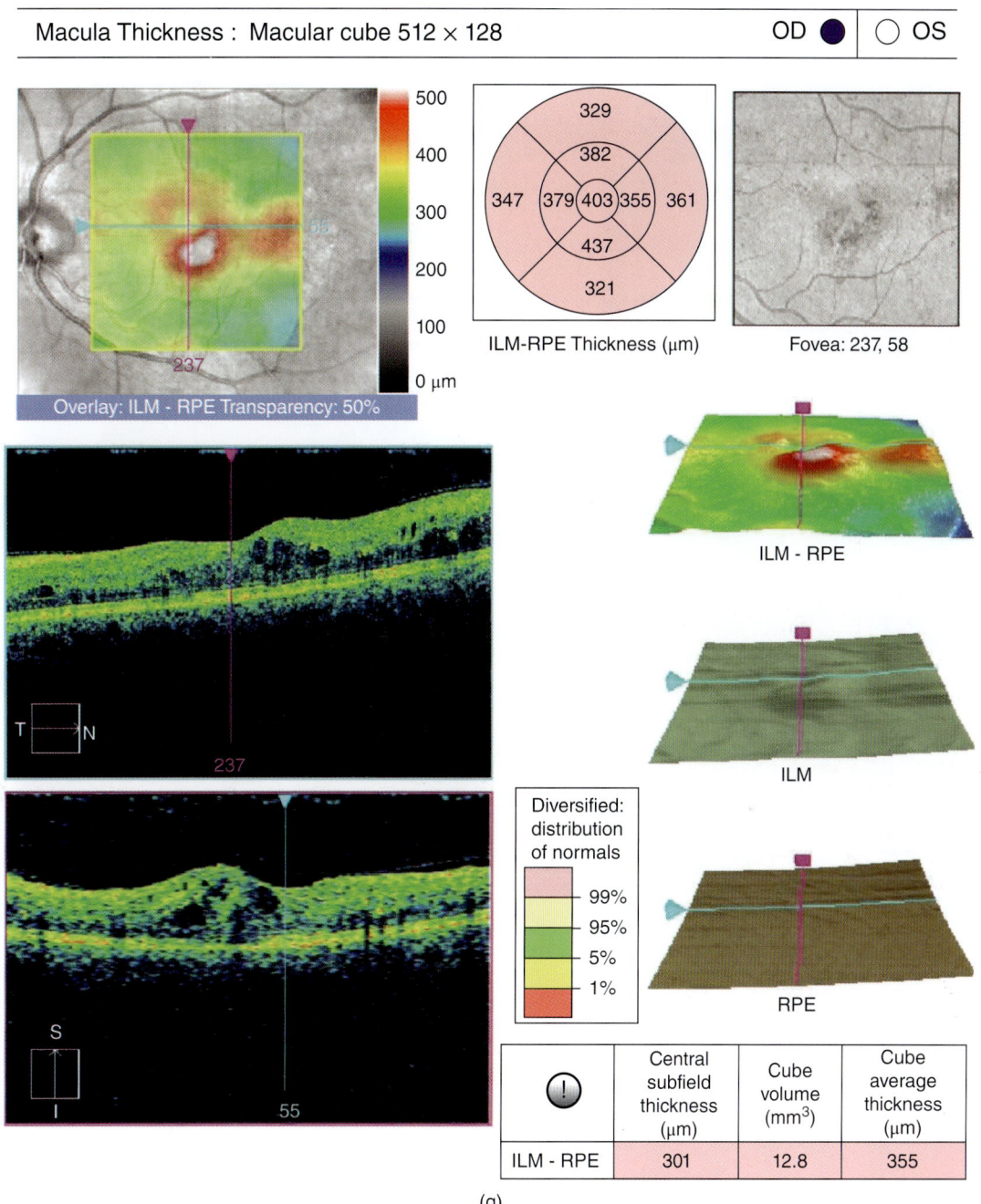

Fig. 4.7 (*Continued*)

52 A practical manual of diabetic retinopathy management

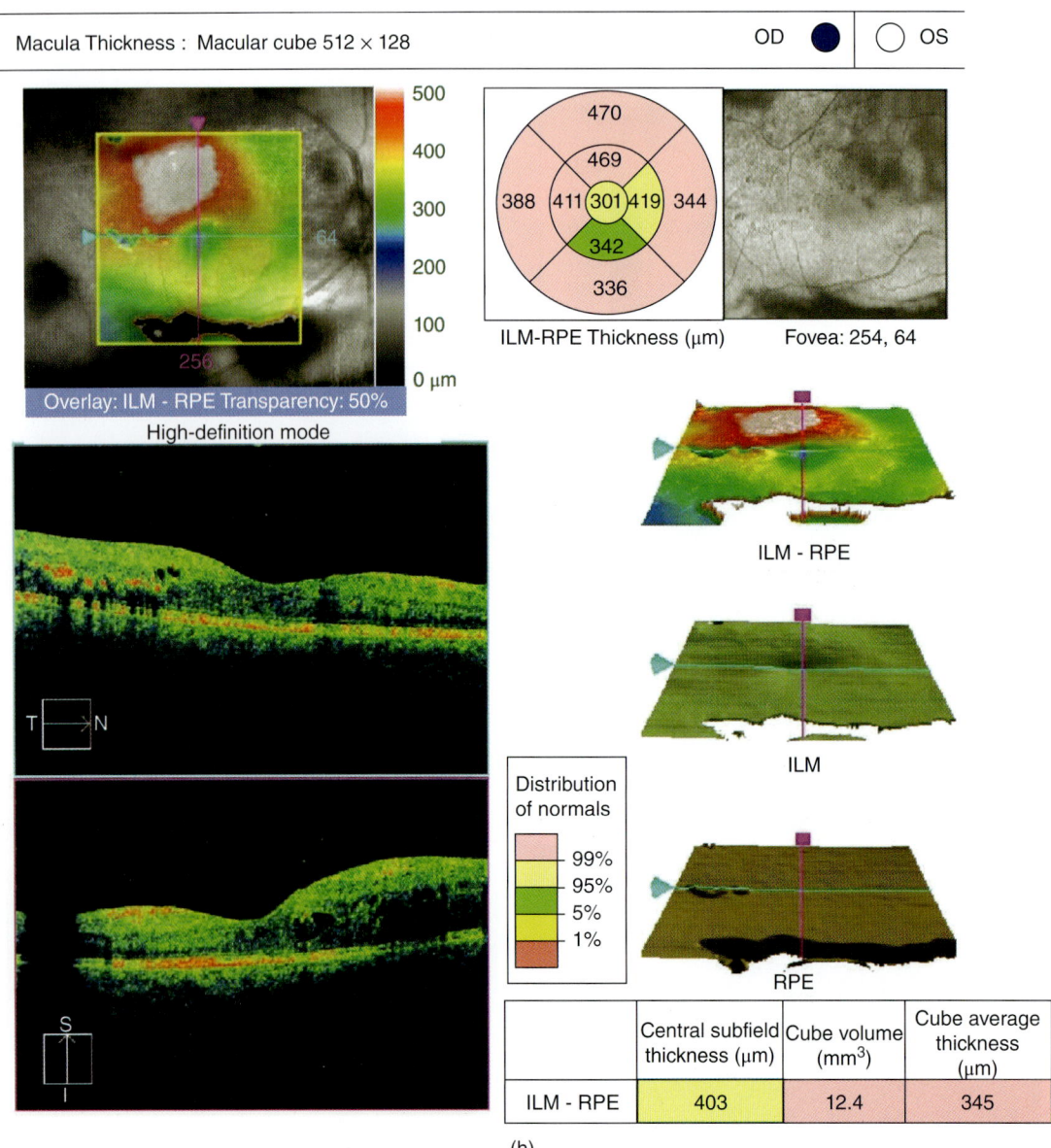

(h)

Fig. 4.7 (*Continued*)

0.02 s over two sessions) with Pascal laser to his right eye. He also received panretinal laser to his left eye (1654 burns, 200 micron size, 275–300 mW, 0.02 s) with the Pascal laser over two sessions. The Superquad lens was used for the panretinal laser and a Mainster lens for the macular laser. The macular laser treatment was applied to areas of leakage outside the foveal avascular zone in the right eye at the first panretinal laser treatment session.

He has subsequently commenced monthly intravitreal injections of ranibizumab for the centre thickening in his left eye and has had two of these treatments so far. The right eye had required one further treatment of panretinal photocoagulation because the new vessels at the right disc were still active and there had been a small amount of improvement in the thickening in the right macular area (Fig. 4.7h).

He is still in the early stages of treatment. His visual acuity is currently LogMAR 0.14 (20/30) right and left.

REFERENCE

Please visit www.wiley.com/go/scanlon/diabetic_retinopathy

5 Imaging techniques in diabetic retinopathy

Peter van Wijngaarden[1] & Peter H. Scanlon[2]

[1]Consultant Ophthalmologist, Centre for Eye Research Australia, Royal Victorian Eye and Ear Hospital, Australia
Ophthalmology, Department of Surgery, University of Melbourne, Australia
[2]Harris Manchester College, University of Oxford; Medical Ophthalmology, University of Gloucestershire, UK

Clinical imaging tools have become an integral part of ophthalmic practice, serving to identify, document and monitor pathology as well as provide useful aids for patient counselling. Of the growing suite of imaging modalities at the disposal of clinicians, retinal photography, optical coherence tomography (OCT), fluorescein fundus angiography and B-scan ultrasonography are central to the management of patients with diabetic retinopathy. Recent advances have seen the emergence of autofluorescence imaging, widefield retinal photography and angiography, as well as OCT angiography. The place of these new imaging modalities in the management of diabetic retinopathy is currently being defined. The development of adaptive optics, non-invasive retinal oximetry and hyperspectral imaging, as well as continual improvements in OCT technology, mean that cellular and metabolic imaging may soon be available in the clinic.

These advances in imaging technologies are informing our understanding of retinal diseases and challenging established diagnostic and treatment paradigms. Moreover, corneal confocal microscopy and retinal OCT have been useful in the detection and monitoring of the neurodegenerative sequelae of diabetes and are increasingly likely to inform the systemic management of diabetes and its complications[1]. Many of these imaging techniques are performed by non-medical staff, and virtual clinics are increasingly used to screen for and monitor retinopathy. In addition, the integration of real-time retinal imaging and image registration technology with laser allows for more precisely targeted delivery of laser photocoagulation therapy, with scope for treatment pre-planning on the basis of angiographic findings[2]. Image registration technology and image analytics will increasingly allow for precise monitoring of retinopathy progression and potentially disease prognostication[3].

RETINAL PHOTOGRAPHY

Retinal photography has long been used as a means of documenting retinopathy status in clinical practice and has served as the principal imaging tool in human clinical studies of diabetic retinopathy. Digital retinal photography has been embraced by eye health professionals, as it does away with the need for film processing and has simplified image storage and retrieval. Electronic transmission of digital retinal images facilitates clinical referral, remote retinal image grading and teleophthalmology. Furthermore, viewing software provides clinicians with tools to manipulate images to optimise lesion detection. Objective longitudinal monitoring of retinopathy is possible with the aid of retinal photographs.

Conventional retinal photographs (Figs 5.1, 5.2) provide monoscopic images, meaning that no direct depth discrimination is possible. Indirect cues, such as changes in retinal vessel angulation and defocus, can be used to infer depth. In practice, reliable detection of diabetic macular oedema is not possible with monoscopic photography in the absence of macular hard exudates. Stereoscopic photography (Fig. 5.3) is a technique that is used to generate a virtual, depth-enhanced image that simulates retinal biomicroscopy. The technique involves capturing two images of the same retinal field from slightly different angles on the horizontal axis and presenting these left and right images to the left and right eyes of the observer using optical stereo-viewing devices. Image fusion by the observer can evoke a perception of depth in the image that can be

A Practical Manual of Diabetic Retinopathy Management, Second Edition.
Edited by Peter Scanlon, Ahmed Sallam, and Peter van Wijngaarden.
© 2017 John Wiley & Sons Ltd. Published 2017 by John Wiley & Sons Ltd.
Companion Website: www.wiley.com/go/scanlon/diabetic_retinopathy

Imaging techniques in diabetic retinopathy   55

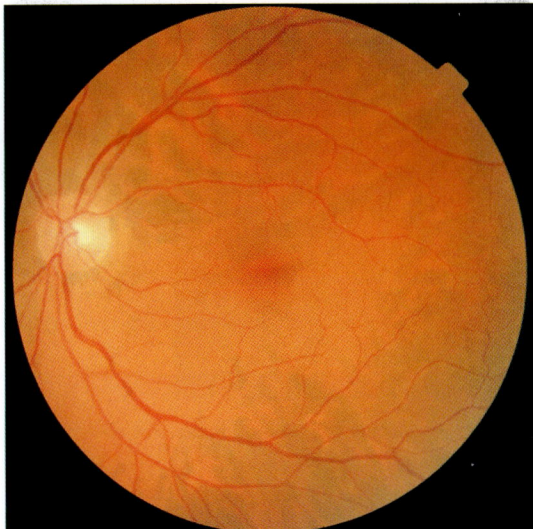

Fig. 5.1 Normal left macular field image.

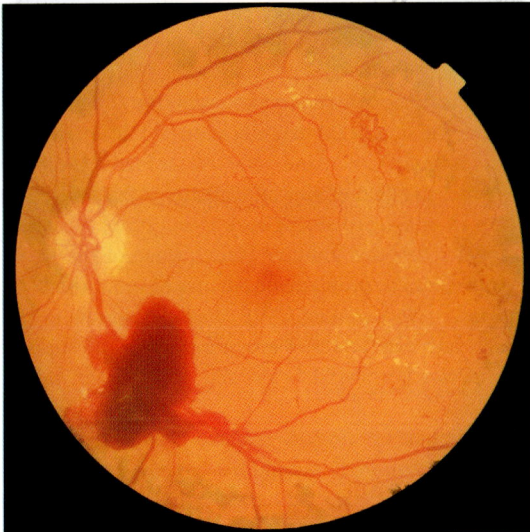

Fig. 5.2 Left macular field image with preretinal haemorrhage, small NVD, NVE, intraretinal haemorrhages and hard exudates.

of value in assessing diabetic macular oedema. In the era of OCT imaging, stereoscopic photography is rarely used.

Standard retinal cameras (Figs 5.4–5.6) capture fields of view ranging from 30° to 50° (based on the external angle), corresponding to 5–14% of the total retinal surface area[4]. While a single macula-centred photograph includes the optic disc, it is conventional to capture at least two images of each eye when documenting diabetic retinopathy (one disc-centred and one macula-centred; Figs 5.7, 5.8) to ensure that pathology in the nasal retina is not missed. A standard mydriatic fundus camera can be used to capture seven fields which, when montaged (Figs 5.9, 5.10), can cover a field of view of up to 90° or approximately 42% of the entire retinal surface. Indeed, our current classification system for diabetic retinopathy, as well as our understanding of the risks of retinopathy progression, vision loss and the likely response to treatment, are based upon early seminal studies the Diabetic Retinopathy Study and Early Treatment of Diabetic Retinopathy Study utilised seven-field stereoscopic photography with 35 mm slide film[5]. While seven-field photography remains the gold standard in clinical studies, it is rarely used in clinical practice as it can be demanding for patients and photographers alike.

Box 5.1: Digital retinal photography

Filters placed in the path of the illuminating light can be used to enhance features of interest. For example, red-free photography (Figs 5.11, 5.12) utilises a green illumination source to highlight retinal vessels and pathology, including haemorrhages and exudates, and is a useful adjunct to colour photography in the assessment of diabetic retinopathy.

ULTRA-WIDEFIELD IMAGING

Cameras with imaging angles that exceed the 30–50° of typical fundus cameras have been referred to as 'widefield' (Figs 5.13, 5.14). The recent development of imaging technologies that allow extensive visualisation of the retinal periphery has led to the adoption of the term 'ultra-widefield' imaging, although the distinction between widefield and ultra-widefield is unclear[6]. Ultra-widefield imaging systems utilise confocal scanning laser ophthalmoscopy (cSLO) to image a significantly greater proportion of the retinal surface than is possible with conventional retinal photography (Fig. 5.15a, b). As its name implies, confocal scanning laser ophthalmoscopy utilises a laser to scan the retina. Images are acquired point-by-point at high speed and reconstructed by computer.

One popular non-contact UWF system (Optos Optomap, Optos) utilises cSLO together with an ellipsoidal mirror that functions as a virtual intraocular scanning

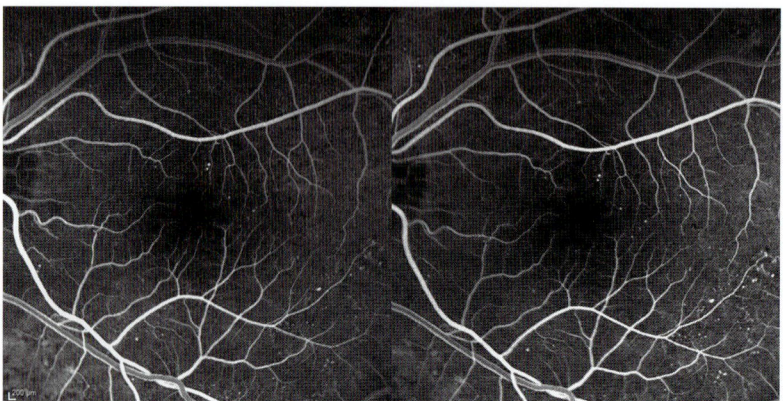

Fig. 5.3 Stereo fluorescein angiogram images of the left eye showing two images of the same retinal location captured at slightly different angles in a patient with microaneurysms.

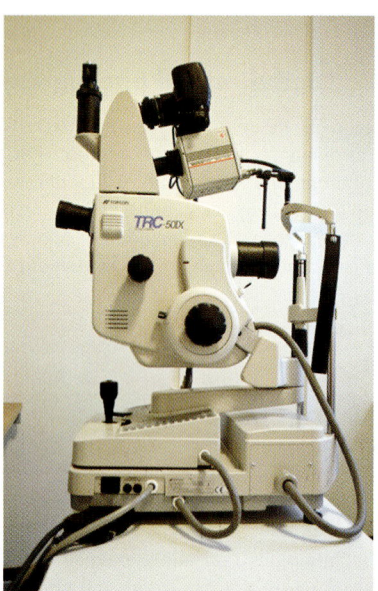

Fig. 5.4 Topcon fundus camera.

point to capture up to 82% of the total retinal surface area (equivalent to an internal angle of 200°) in a single image that is acquired in seconds, without the requirement for mydriasis, and at a resolution of 14 microns[5]. In this system, images are simultaneously acquired with red, green and blue lasers to allow visualisation of all retinal layers and the generation of a composite coloured retinal image (Figs 5.16–5.18). Another leading non-contact UWF system (Heidelberg UWF module, Heidelberg Engineering)

offers a field of view of approximately 102° and the generation of a high-resolution greyscale image (Fig. 5.19).

When ultra-widefield images of a spherical surface are presented on a flat screen, more peripheral parts of the image are subject both to distortion (peripheral non-linearity) and to magnification relative to the centre of the image, a phenomenon known as the Greenland effect after the significant magnification and distortion seen in depictions of Greenland on Mercator map projections. The wider the field of view, the greater is this effect. Advances in image processing seek to minimise this effect. Peripheral defocus, another consequence of the retinal curvature, can be problematic but may be minimised with mydriasis[5]. Non-contact UWF images are prone to eyelid and lash artefacts that obscure parts of the superior and inferior peripheral fields, and can result in missed pathology[7].

A number of clinical studies, chiefly case series, have demonstrated substantial agreement between non-mydriatic UWF imaging and both mydriatic clinical biomicroscopy and seven-field stereophotography for diabetic retinopathy severity grading [5,7–9]. For example, a recent comparison of seven-field photography with non-mydriatic and mydriatic UWF imaging found no major differences in diabetic retinopathy severity grading[7]. Exact agreement with seven-field photography occurred in 76% of cases and agreement within one level of retinopathy in 99% of cases. In more than two-thirds of cases where there was disagreement, the discrepancy was due to the identification of pathology in UWF images that was beyond the field of view of seven-field photography[7].

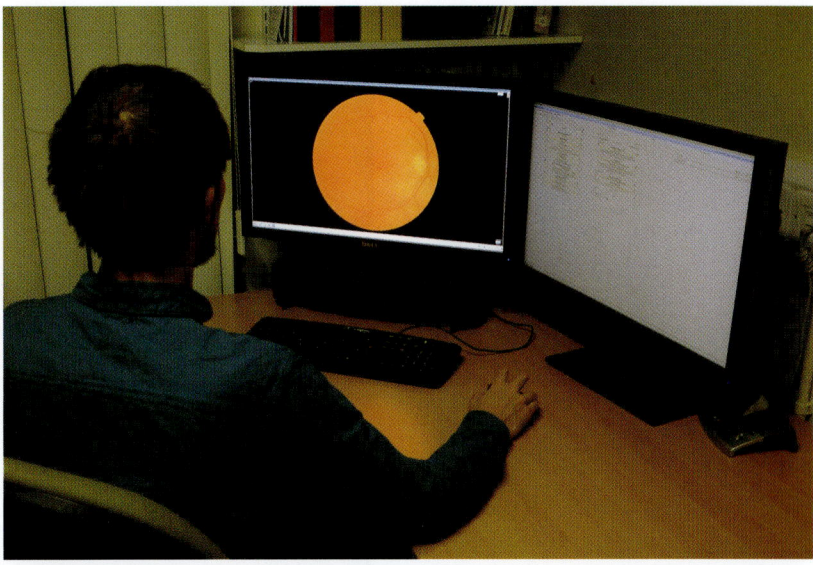

Fig. 5.5 Viewing a digital fundus image.

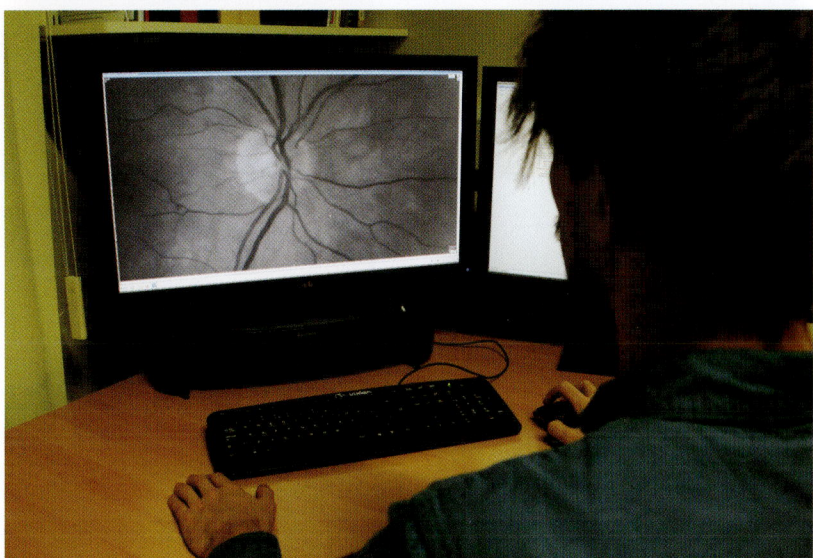

Fig. 5.6 Viewing a magnified red-free digital fundus image.

Similarly, in another study, approximately one-third of all lesions (haemorrhages, microaneurysms, intraretinal microvascular abnormalities and neovascularisation NVE) were located outside of the traditional seven photographic fields, and their identification suggested more severe retinopathy than was assigned by seven-field photography in 10% of cases[8].

Data from large, multi-centre comparative cohort studies with retinopathy at all levels of the severity spectrum are required to provide definitive answers regarding the place of UWF imaging systems in the grading of diabetic retinopathy. In the absence of such studies, the existing evidence suggests that UWF imaging is at least comparable to seven-field photography for the detection of referable

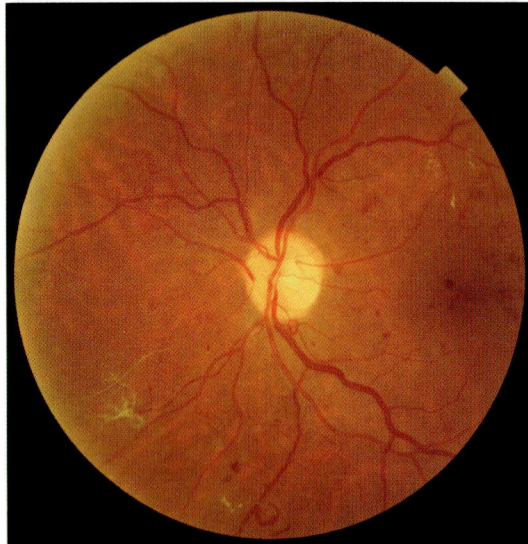

Fig. 5.7 Disc-centred image of a left eye showing IRMA, venous loops, NVD, NVE and preretinal haemorrhage. A large tuft of NVE is seen in the superonasal quadrant.

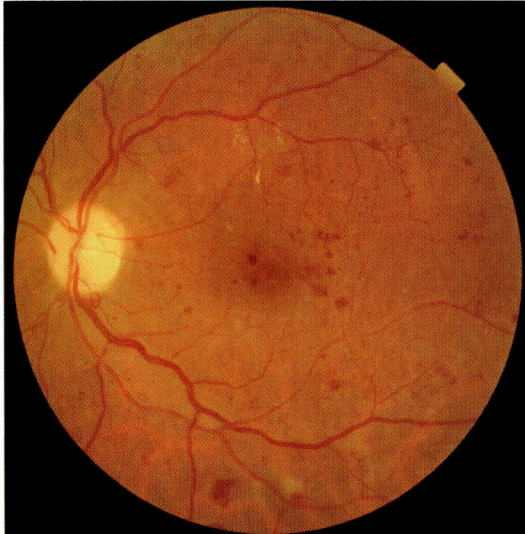

Fig. 5.8 Macular centred image of the same eye showing NVD, NVE and preretinal haemorrhage.

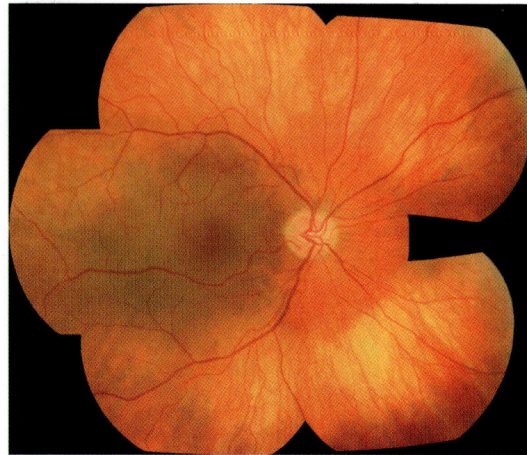

Fig. 5.9 Seven-field montage of a right eye: normal fundus.

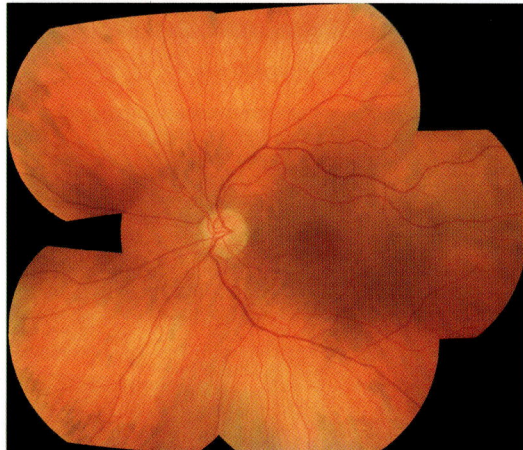

Fig. 5.10 Seven-field montage of a left eye: normal fundus.

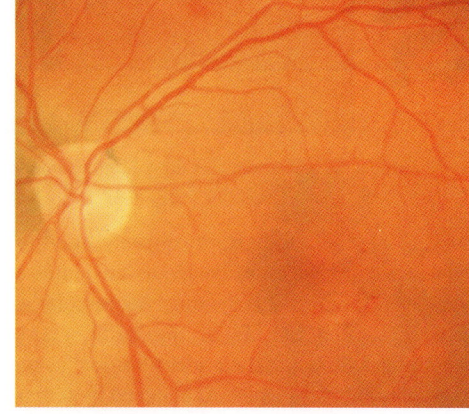

Fig. 5.11 Colour fundus image showing HMas below the left fovea.

disease. While it is not yet clear how the detection of more peripheral retinopathy with UWF imaging will influence clinical risk stratification for progression, evidence suggests that the impact may be significant. In a recently reported study, retinopathy lesions that were located predominantly outside the conventional seven photographic

Imaging techniques in diabetic retinopathy 59

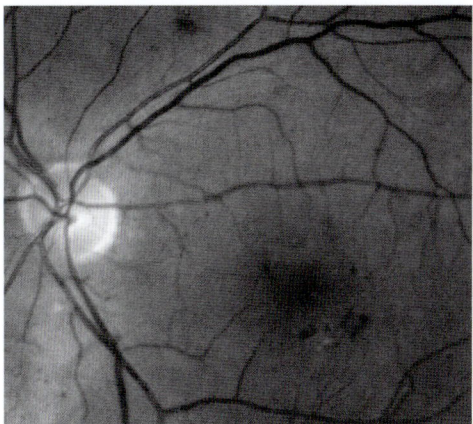

Fig. 5.12 Red-free image of the same eye showing HMas below the left fovea.

fields were found at baseline in half of those patients without proliferative diabetic retinopathy[10]. The presence of these peripheral lesions significantly increased the risk of retinopathy progression and the development of PDR at 4 years (3.2-fold, $P<0.004$; and 4.7-fold, $P<0.009$, respectively), even when adjustments were made for traditional risk factors[10]. Interestingly, no association was found between peripheral lesions and the risk of diabetic macular oedema development or progression.

FUNDUS AUTOFLOURESCENCE

In vivo retinal autofluorescence imaging (Fig. 5.20) has become a standard technique to evaluate macular disease and may have a prognostic role in diabetic macular oedema. Largely due to lipofuscin in the retinal pigment epithelium (RPE), retinal autofluorescence is ordinarily reduced in the fovea due to the absorption of short-wavelength light by photopigments, chiefly lutein and zeaxanthin, which are concentrated in the axons of cone photoreceptors. Fundus autofluorescence can be detected with confocal scanning laser ophthalmoscopy or by fundus photography with the use of specialised excitation and barrier filters that optimise the excitation lipofuscin fluorescence, without eliciting significant fluorescence from the crystalline lens.

The loss of normal foveal hypoautofluorescence (Fig. 5.21) has been identified as a marker of diabetic macular oedema and has been considered by some to be due to the displacement of macular photopigments and thus an unmasking of RPE fluorescence[11,12]. Others have demonstrated that increased foveal autofluorescence

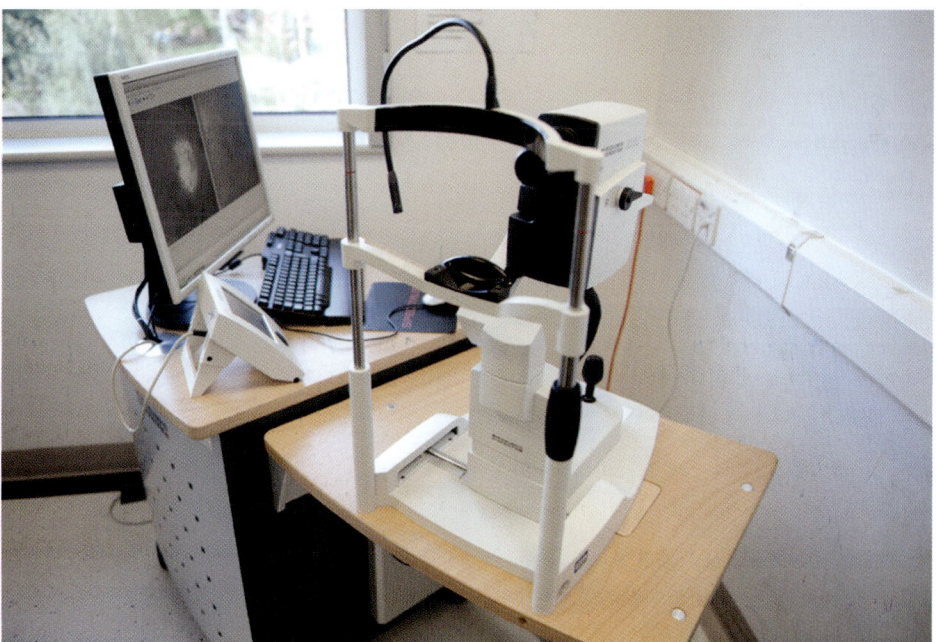

Fig. 5.13 Heidelberg UWF imaging system.

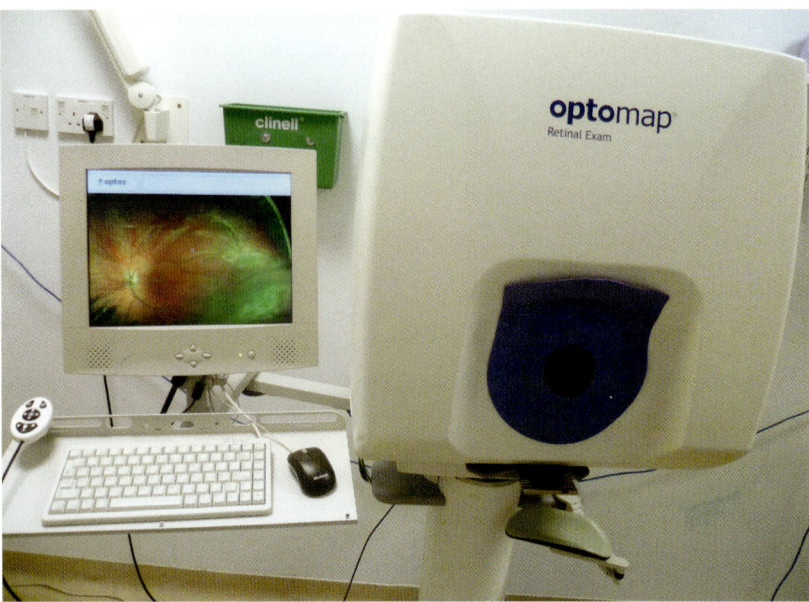

Fig. 5.14 Optos UWF imaging system.

is more closely associated with inner segment/outer segment photoreceptor disruption than the degree of oedema and may portend poorer visual acuity and lower likelihood of improvements in vision with resolution of oedema[13]. The place of retinal autofluorescence in the assessment of diabetic macular oedema is still being defined.

ULTRASONOGRAPHY

Ultrasonography plays an important role in the assessment of diabetic retinopathy when opacification of the ocular media precludes a satisfactory view of the retina. Ultrasound can enable clinicians to evaluate the extent of vitreous haemorrhage, vitreoretinal traction, fibrovascular membranes or retinal detachment. Serial scanning can be used to monitor the resolution of vitreous haemorrhage, as indicated by a reduction in the extent and density of vitreous hyperreflectivity over time.

Ophthalmic ultrasonography quite literally employs sound waves beyond the range of human hearing (beyond 20 kHz), and typically in the range of 8–15 MHz, to generate images of the eye. Ultrasound is produced in an ultrasonography probe via the oscillation of a piezoelectric crystal. When a probe is applied to the eye, the emitted ultrasound passes through the tissues in a series of advancing wavefronts and is differentially absorbed by the ocular media and variably scattered, refracted and reflected at interfaces between tissues of differing densities (acoustic interfaces). Ultrasound that is reflected from acoustic interfaces (echoes) is detected by the probe and converted into a visual representation of the acoustic densities of the ocular structures. The intensity of the reflected ultrasound signal is greatest when the probe is positioned perpendicular to the interface of interest. Highly reflective surfaces, such as the posterior lens and inner scleral surfaces, are those at the interface between tissues with significant acoustic density differences and appear smooth. The interfaces between tissues with similar acoustic densities reflect ultrasound relatively weakly and appear less regular and less bright.

Two distinct ultrasound modes are used to image the eye: so-called A-scan and B-scan modes. A-scan ultrasonography (Fig. 5.22) is predominantly used for ocular biometry and employs a parallel, non-focused beam emitted from a stationary piezoelectric crystal (typically 8 MHz). Ultrasound is emitted in a single direction and echoes detected by the probe are displayed as a function of time (delay between emission and detection) and intensity (reflectivity). Ocular structures are identified by their characteristic reflectivity profiles on the A-scan image and distance is represented by time.

In contrast, B-scan ultrasonography (Figs 5.23–5.27) uses a focused piezoelectric crystal (typically 10 MHz)

Imaging techniques in diabetic retinopathy

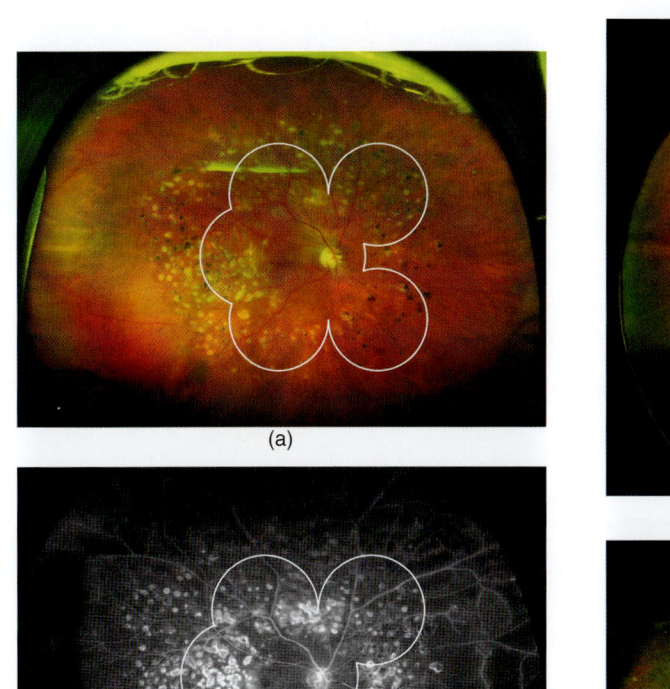

Fig. 5.15 (a) Optos UWF 200 degree image and (b) Optos UWF 200 degree fluorescein angiogram image. Schematic overlays depict the area captured in conventional seven-field photography.

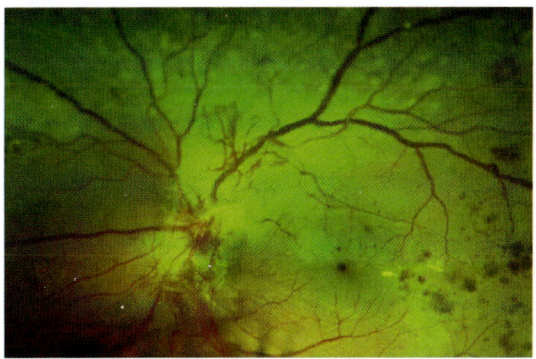

Fig. 5.16 Optos image showing NVD, NVE, macular HMas and exudate, venous beading and peripheral scatter laser scars.

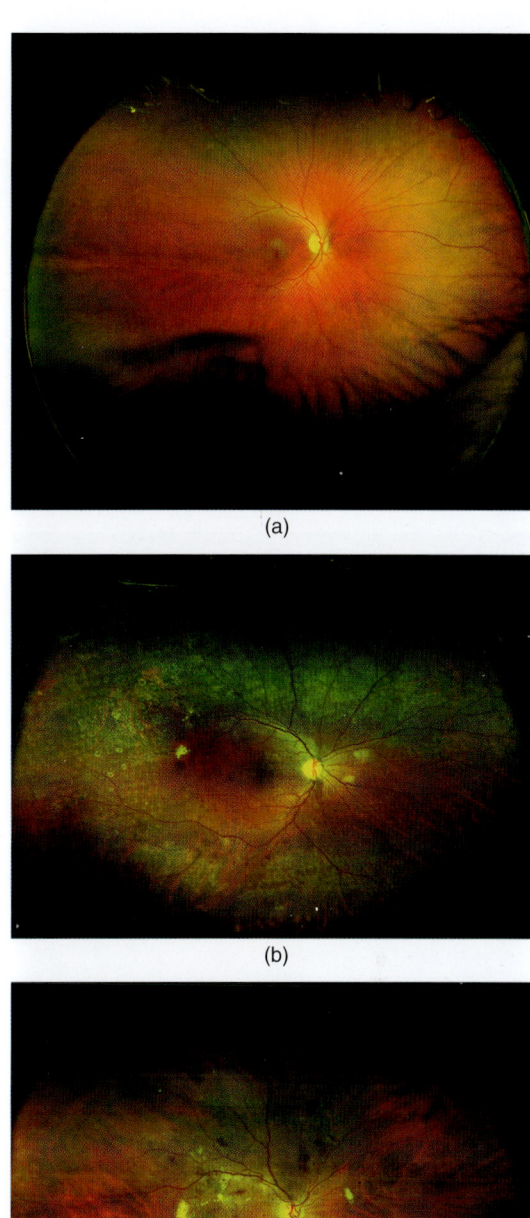

Fig. 5.17 (a) Optos UWF image showing eyelash artefact and peripheral distortion in a normal right eye. (b) Optos UWF image of a right eye that has had scatter laser treatment for proliferative DR. (c) Optos UWF image showing extensive exudates in the right macula.

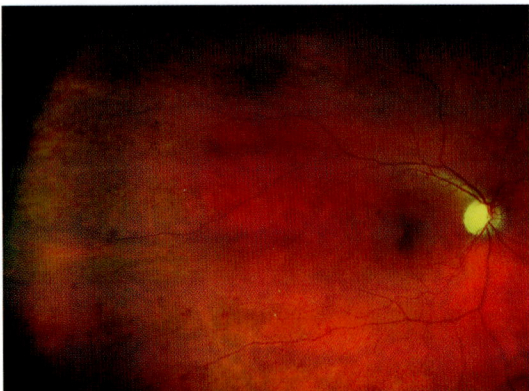

Fig. 5.18 Optos image of a right eye showing pathology in the temporal retina outside the conventional seven-field zone.

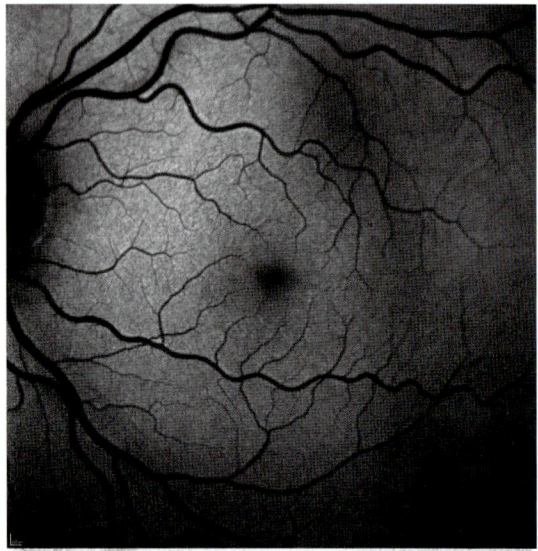

Fig. 5.20 Left macular fundus autofluorescence image exhibiting normal foveal hypoautofluorescence.

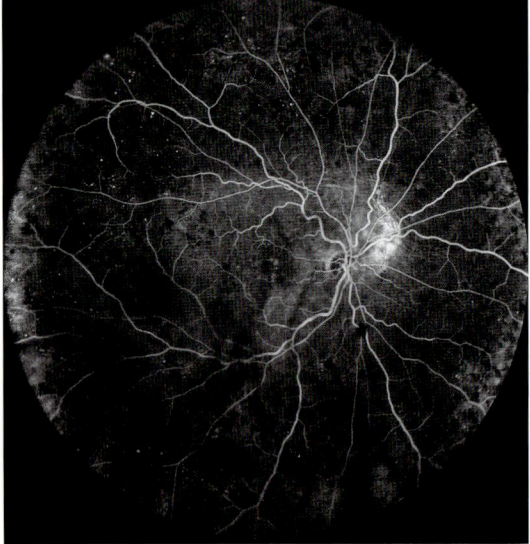

Fig. 5.19 Heidelberg UWF fluorescein angiogram image showing HMas and macular oedema.

in an oscillating probe to yield a two-dimensional (2D) acoustic section of the eye. Accordingly, B-scans provide cross-sectional images of the eye. Contact B-scan ultrasonography involves the use of a gel coupling agent, such as methyl cellulose, between the eyelid or ocular surface and the probe. Changes in gaze and probe position are used to achieve dynamic visualisation of ocular structures that can be helpful in identifying vitreous haemorrhage or evaluating vitreoretinal traction. This is particularly valuable in eyes with advanced diabetic retinopathy where fibrovascular membranes, tractional retinal detachments and vitreous haemorrhages often co-exist. As such, the technique constitutes an important tool in planning complex vitreoretinal surgery. Most B-scan ultrasound machines will provide an A-scan mode that superimposes an A-scan trace on the B-scan image to provide important reflectivity information than can be useful when distinguishing between lesion types (such as subretinal mass lesions). It is important to note that A-scans acquired via a B-scan probe are typically not standardised and should not be used for conventional biometry.

FLUORESCEIN ANGIOGRAPHY

Fundus fluorescein angiography or FFA has been an important diagnostic technique for diabetic retinopathy since its advent in 1959[14] (Figs 5.28, 5.29). The technique allows *in vivo*, real-time assessment of retinal and choroidal vascular anatomy and function. It involves the use of a specialised fundus camera or confocal scanning laser ophthalmoscope to capture high-resolution, rapid sequence photographs or digital videos (cSLO) to monitor the circulation of a fluorescent dye, sodium fluorescein, through the eye. The dye (typically 500 mg: 5 mL, 10% sodium fluorescein) is injected in a peripheral vein, usually in the antecubital fossa, forearm or hand, as a bolus injection over 5–6 s. The timer of the imaging system is started as soon as the fluorescein is injected and remains on for the duration of the angiogram, as accurate temporal information is important for the interpretation of images.

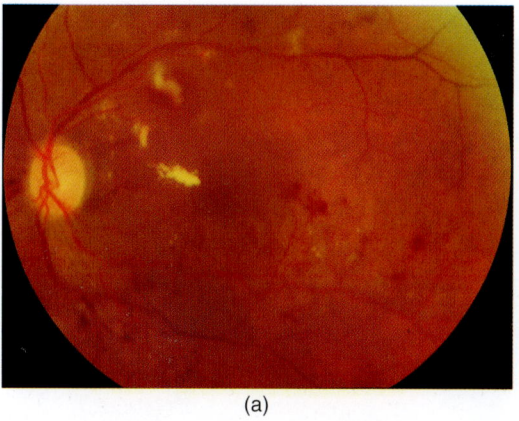
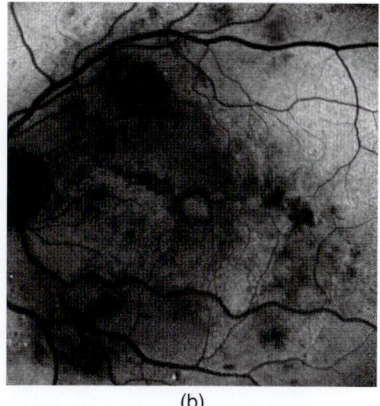

Fig. 5.21 (a) Colour fundus image of the left macular area in a patient with diabetic macular oedema. (b) Loss of foveal hypoautofluorescence is seen in this patient (same patient as in (a)) with diabetic macular oedema and poor vision. Haemorrhages are seen in the temporal macula and exudate in the nasal macula.

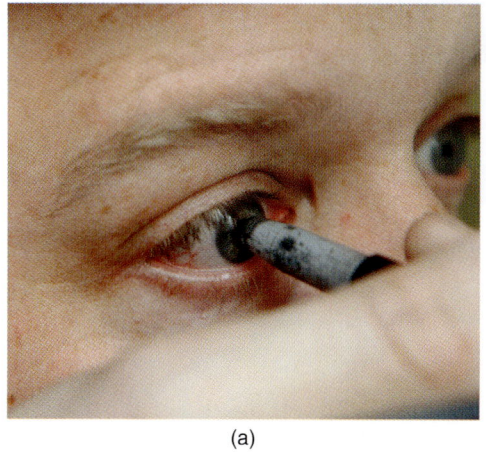
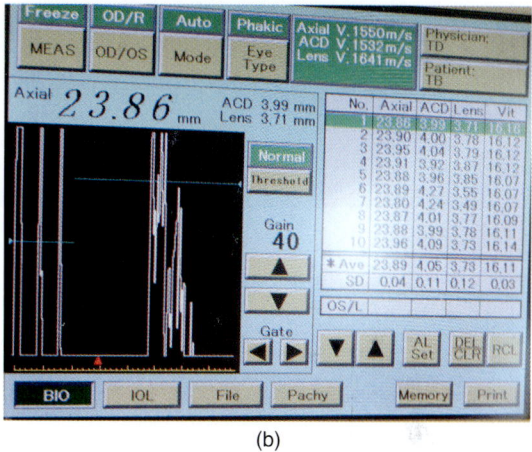

Fig. 5.22 An A-scan (a) being taken and (b) image.

The dye typically reaches the ocular circulation within 6–10 s of injection. Prolongation of arm-to-eye transit time may be procedural (e.g. due to slow fluorescein injection, injection into a distal vein, or extrinsic restriction of arm circulation due to arm positioning or tight clothing) or pathological (e.g. due to impaired ocular perfusion as a result of poor cardiac output, cerebrovascular disease, ophthalmic or retinal arterial obstruction).

Fluorescence (Fig. 5.30) is elicited with the use of narrow bandpass interference excitation filters or, in the case of cSLO, with narrow wavelength blue laser light that illuminate the fundus with light (typically 490 nm) corresponding to the excitation spectrum of fluorescein (465–490 nm). Emitted yellow-green fluorescence is detected with a barrier filter that only transmits light corresponding to the peak of the fluorescein emission spectrum (520–530 nm). In the case of cSLO angiography, a confocal aperture only allows image-forming light to reach the sensor. Angiography is a dynamic process and several cSLO imaging systems now offer video angiography, allowing the user to capture information that may be missed in static photography. Some cSLO systems allow simultaneous acquisition of fluorescein and indocyanine green angiographic images, providing enhanced visualisation of the choroidal and retinal circulations.

Following injection, a majority of fluorescein is bound to plasma proteins and does not fluoresce. Unbound fluorescein is unable to pass the intact blood-brain and blood-retinal barriers, but does diffuse across capillaries elsewhere, accounting for the temporary yellow skin

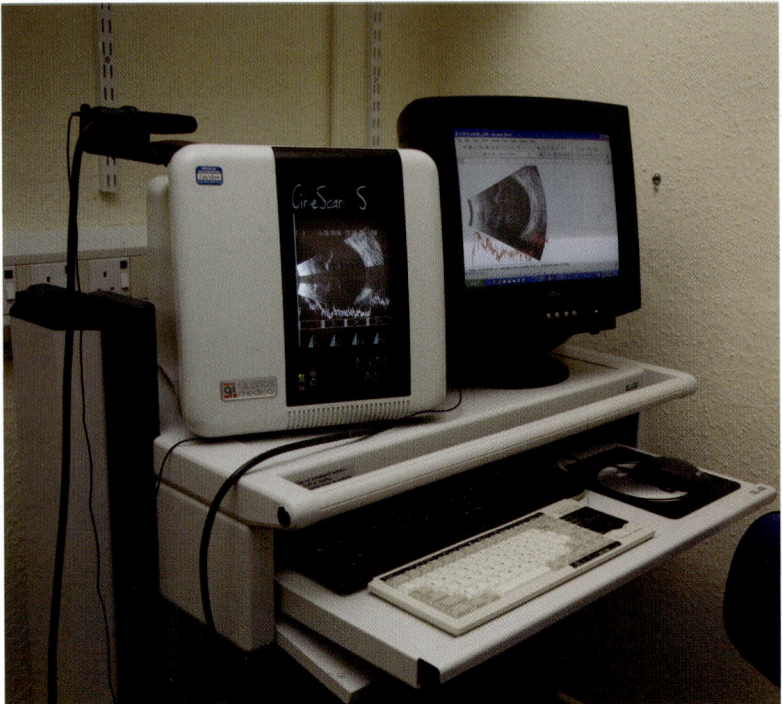

Fig. 5.23 An ophthalmic B-scan ultrasound machine.

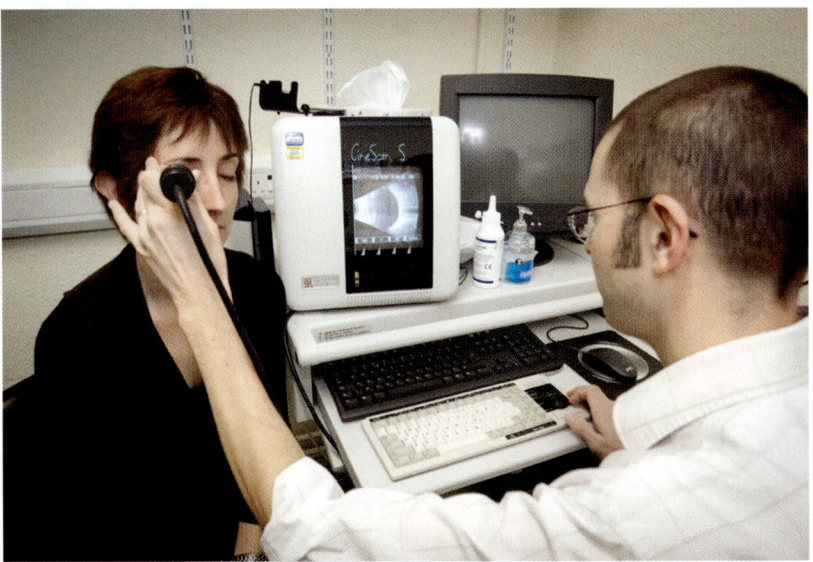

Fig. 5.24 B-scan being performed.

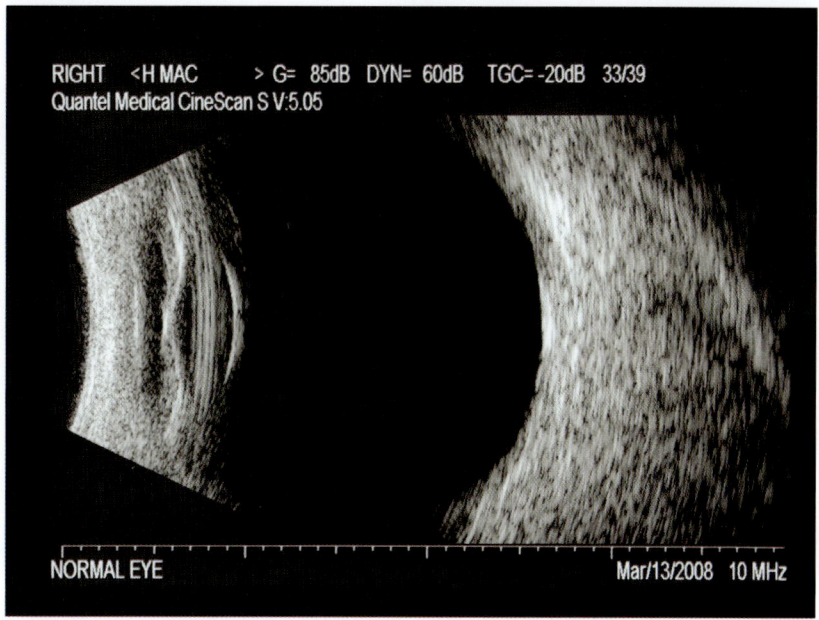

Fig. 5.25 A normal ultrasound B-scan image.

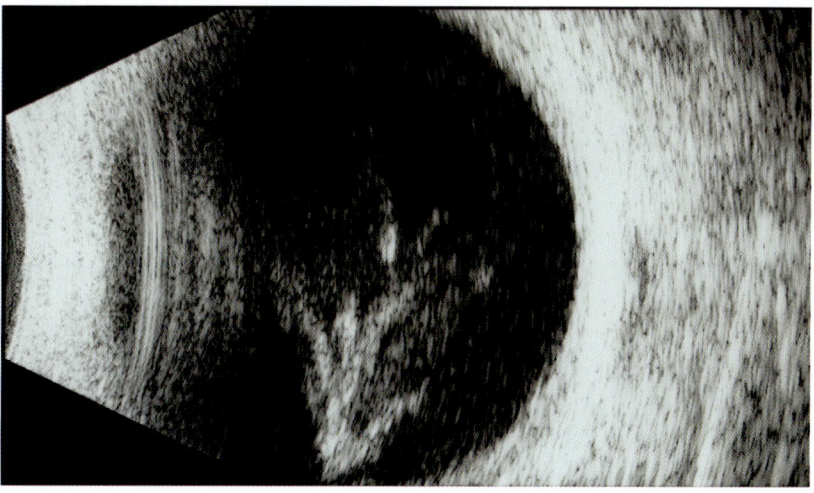

Fig. 5.26 Ultrasound B-scan showing intra-gel vitreous haemorrhage with attached retina.

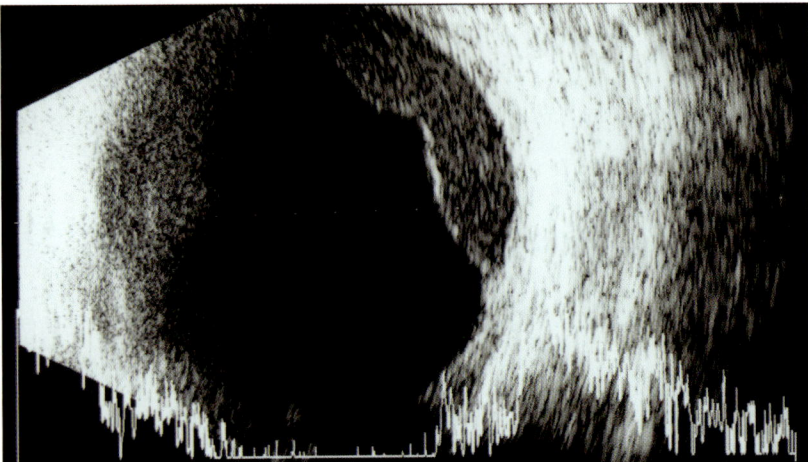

Fig. 5.27 Ultrasound B-scan showing retro-hyaloid vitreous haemorrhage with attached retina.

discolouration that occurs in people for several days after the procedure. Extravasation of fluorescein from the retinal vasculature is therefore a useful marker of blood-retinal barrier disruption that is used to identify diabetic macular oedema and retinal neovascularisation. Areas of capillary non-perfusion appear dark in fluorescein angiography and provide information about the severity of retinopathy and the risk of retinal neovascularisation. Macular ischaemia, defined as widening of the normal foveal avascular zone, disruption of the perifoveal capillary net and capillary non-perfusion in the central macula (within one disc diameter of the foveal centre), is an important sign that is associated with poor visual prognosis and poorer response to treatment[15]. The sequence of events in a normal fluorescein angiogram and commonly observed causes of hypo- and hyper-fluorescence are listed in Boxes 5.2 and 5.3.

Box 5.2: Sequence of events in a normal fluorescein angiogram

For colour and autoflourescence images pre-injection, see Figures 5.31 and 5.32.
- 0 s: fluorescein injection
- 6–10 s: choroidal flush (pre-arterial phase): the first appearance of fluorescein in the choroidal circulation; characteristic patchy and mottled appearance
- 8–12 s: arterial stage (Fig. 5.33)
- 12–15 s: maximum capillary transition stage
- 15–20 s: early venous stage (lamellar or early arterio-venous stage)
- 20–60 s: mid arterio-venous stage (Fig. 5.34)
- 1–10 min: late arterio-venous stage and venous stage (Figs 5.35–5.38)
- 3–10 min: late staining
- 30–60 min: little residual retinal appearance.

Box 5.3: Common causes of hypofluorescence and hyperfluorescence in fluorescein fundus angiography

Hypofluorescence
- Transmission defect
  - Commonly due to retinal or pre-retinal blood, pigment or hard exudates (Figs 5.39, 5.40).
- Filling defect
  - circulation abnormality such as occurs in an area of capillary non-perfusion (Fig. 5.41).

Filling defects can usually be distinguished from transmission defects by the ability to visualize underlying choroidal fluorescence—transmission defects block both retinal and choroidal fluorescence.

Hyperfluorescence
- Window defect
  - Loss of the blocking effect of the retinal pigment epithelium (RPE) in areas of RPE loss, results in the unmasking of choroidal fluorescence. Photocoagulation scars are common causes of window defects seen in patients with diabetic retinopathy (Fig. 5.42).
- Leakage of dye (Fig. 5.43)
  - retinal neovascularisation
  - macular oedema (Fig. 5.44)
  - choroidal neovascularisation
- Staining of retinal structures
  - blood vessel walls, as is seen in areas of retinal hypoxia or in retinal vasculitis (Fig. 5.45)
- Fluorescein pooling
  - retinal or RPE detachments
- Autofluorescence
  - optic disc drusen

Imaging techniques in diabetic retinopathy 67

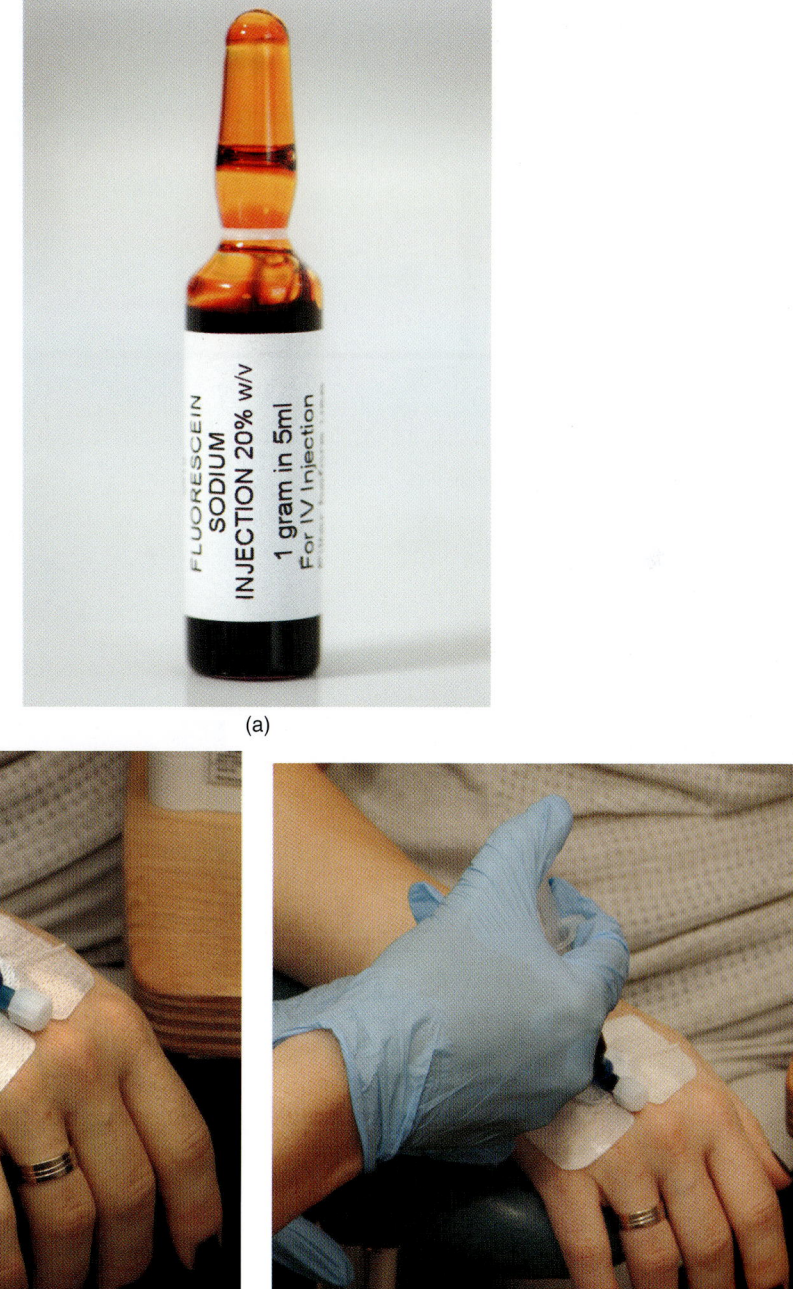

Fig. 5.28 (a) Fluorescein ampoule; (b) intravenous canula; and (c) fluorescein being injected intravenously.

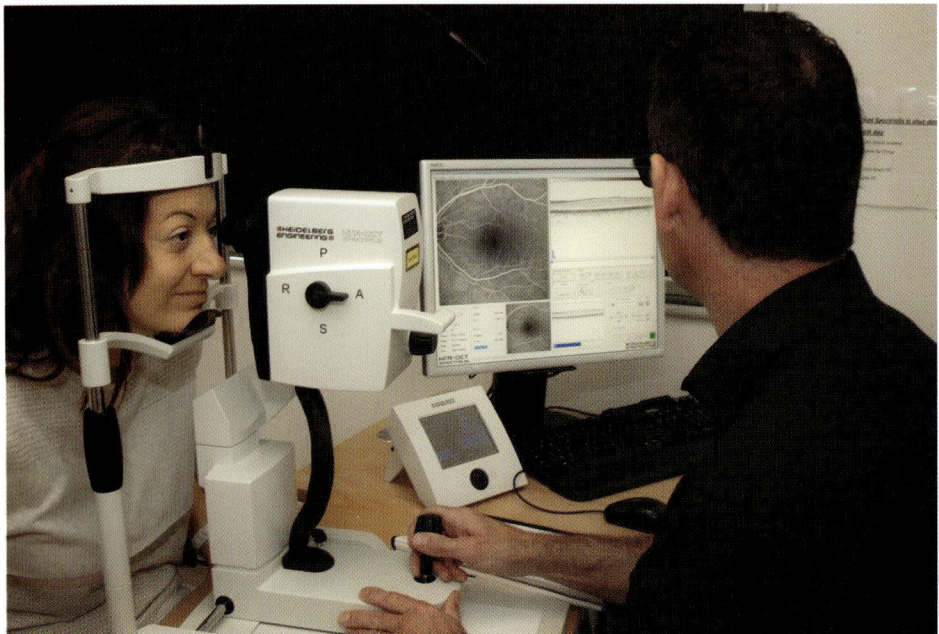

Fig. 5.29 A patient undergoing FFA.

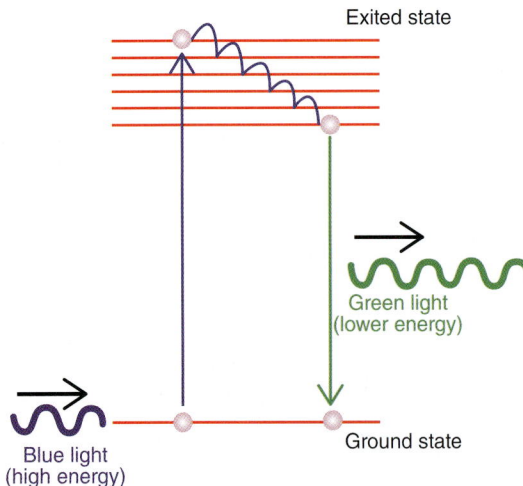

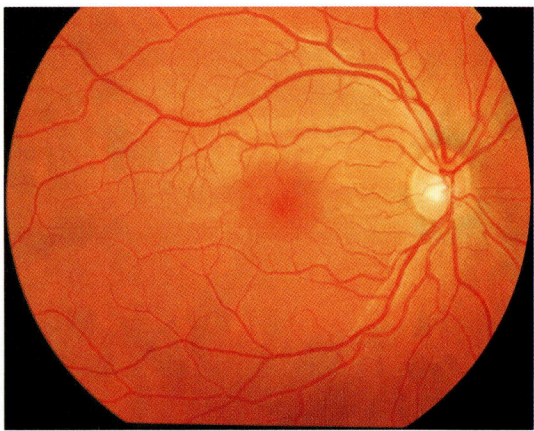

Fig. 5.31 A normal macular colour image.

Fig. 5.30 Fluorescence: a form of photoluminescence that occurs when certain molecules (fluorophores) absorb electromagnetic energy of a particular wavelength (excitation spectrum) and are temporarily excited into a higher energy state. When the fluorophore returns to its original energy state it releases electromagnetic energy, usually of a longer wavelength (emission spectrum). A characteristic feature of fluorescence is the requirement for continuous excitation; emission is extinguished rapidly upon the cessation of excitation.

While fluorescein angiography is generally safe and well tolerated, adverse effects can occur. Estimates of the occurrence of mild adverse effects range from 0.8–15%[16]. A recent large retrospective study reported adverse events in approximately 1% of cases[16]. Transient nausea and vomiting are the most common of these and rarely

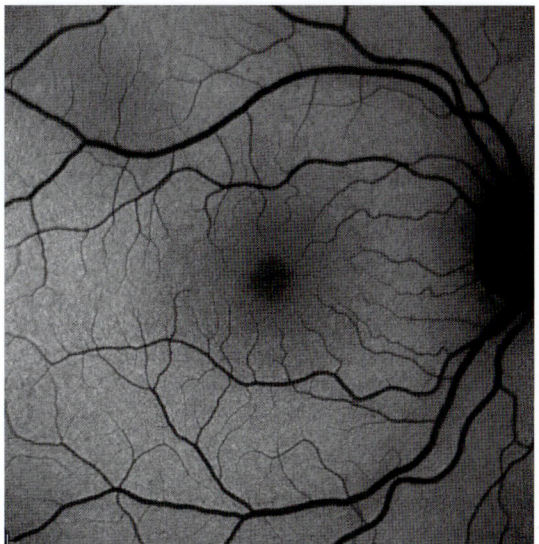

Fig. 5.32 A normal macular autofluorescence image.

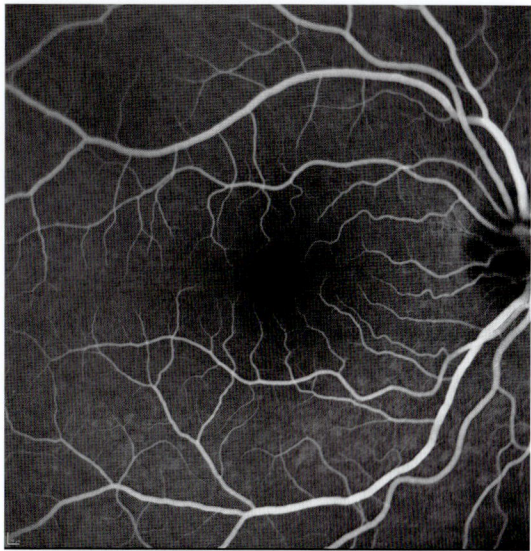

Fig. 5.34 Arteriovenous phase 58 s after injection.

require antiemetic treatment or significantly disrupt the successful conduct of the angiogram. Vasovagal syncope, rash (urticaria) and other mild allergic reactions are not uncommon. Cutaneous photosensitivity may occur and is likely to be under-recognised[17]. Bronchospasm and life-threatening anaphylactic reactions are rare. The risk of death from fluorescein angiography is thought to be between 1 in 49,557 and 1 in 220,000[18,19]. Accordingly, vascular access via an intravenous catheter is recommended during the course of the procedure to facilitate the management of these rare but significant adverse reactions. Administration is usually performed by a trained medical practitioner capable of dealing with any complications that may arise. Resuscitation equipment and emergency medicines should be close at hand. Careful consideration should be given before administering fluorescein to someone with a prior serious allergic reaction to the dye. Extravasation of fluorescein at the injection site may be painful and may lead to skin necrosis, subcutaneous granuloma formation and neuritis.

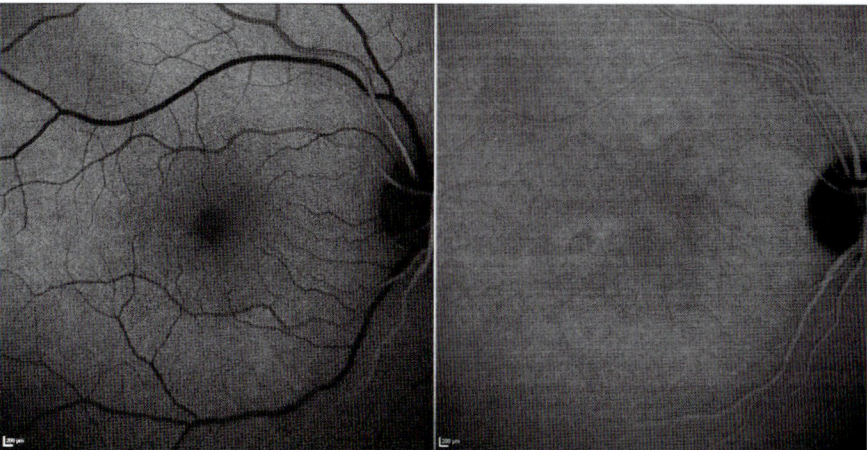

Fig. 5.33 Combined fluorescein and ICG angiograms demonstrating choroidal flush and early arterial filling, 11 s after injection.

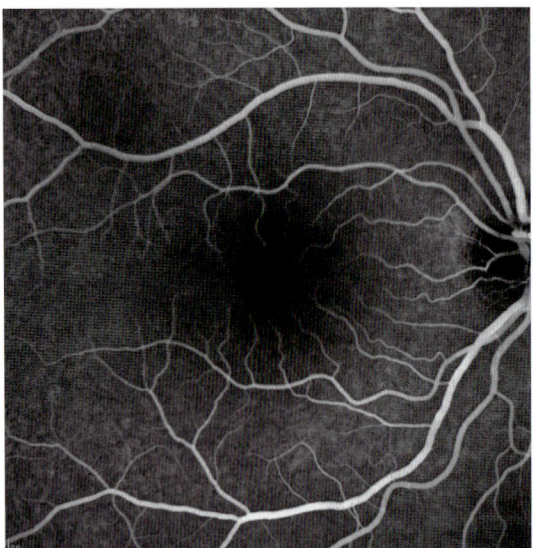

Fig. 5.35 Arteriovenous phase 2 min 11 s after injection.

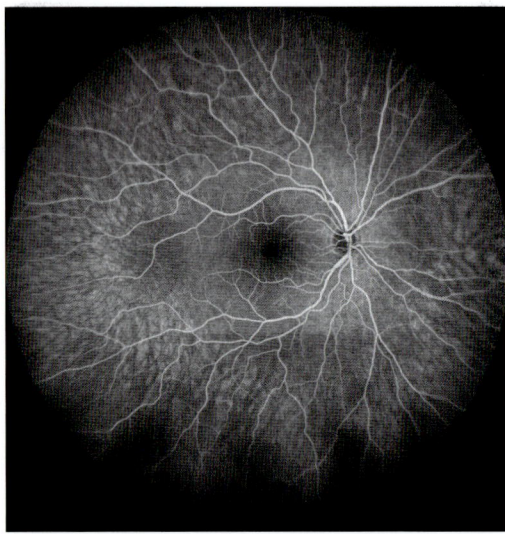

Fig. 5.37 UWF FFA image 5 min 42 s after injection, showing the late venous phase.

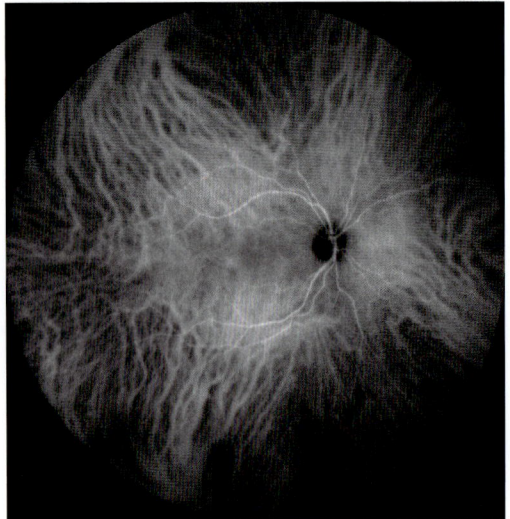

Fig. 5.36 UWF ICG angiogram image 3 min 22 s after injection, showing the normal choroidal vasculature.

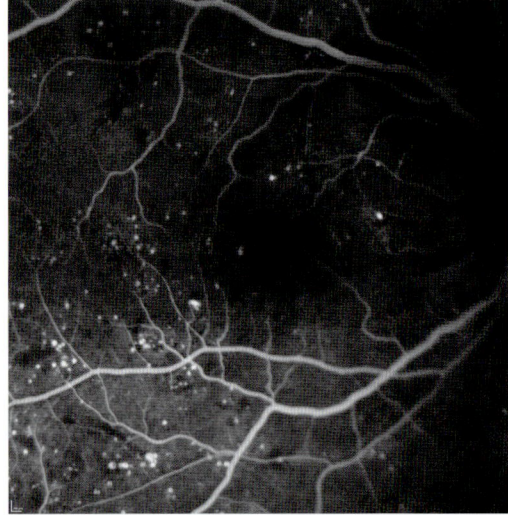

Fig. 5.38 HMas in arteriovenous phase of angiogram that leak at a later stage.

Fluorescein is excreted in urine, imparting an orange-yellow discolouration, and also in breast milk. Dose adjustment (250 mg) may be recommended by fluorescein manufacturers for subjects with renal impairment undergoing dialysis; however, there is limited evidence to support the need for this[20]. While no teratogenic effects of the dye have been identified, fluorescein angiography is generally avoided in pregnancy[21].

Given the persistence of fluorescein in the circulation for hours to several days following intravenous administration, it has the potential to interfere with blood tests that utilise fluorescence techniques. While fluorescein can minimally alter the accuracy of glucometer readings, the disparity between measured and actual glucose levels are unlikely to significantly alter insulin dosages in practice[22].

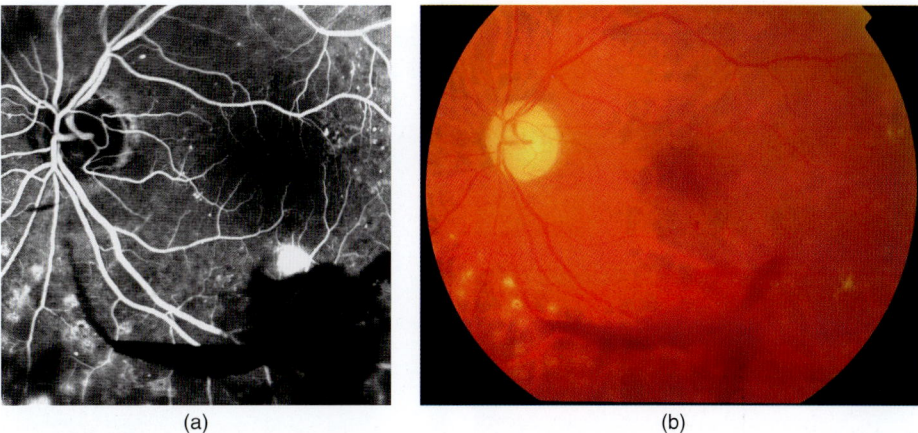

Fig. 5.39 (a) A preretinal haemorrhage masks underlying retinal fluorescence (FFA image). (b) A preretinal haemorrhage in the same patient (colour image).

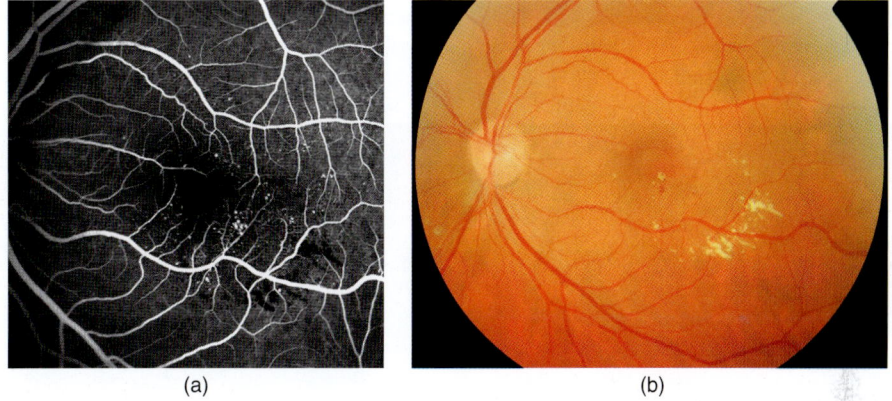

Fig. 5.40 (a) A crescentic area of hypofluorescence in the temporal macula due to masking of fluorescence by hard exudates. (b) A colour image of the same patient showing the crescentic area of exudate.

INDOCYANINE GREEN ANGIOGRAPHY

Indocyanine green (ICG) is a dye used in angiography to highlight the choroidal circulation (Fig. 5.36) as well as subretinal and sub-RPE vascular pathology. While ICG angiography is not commonly indicated in the investigation of diabetic retinopathy, it may be a helpful adjunct to fluorescein angiography in certain circumstances (e.g. to distinguish diabetic macular oedema from idiopathic polypoidal chorioretinal vasculopathy when macular oedema is accompanied by extensive haemorrhage and lipid exudation). ICG fluoresces when excited by near-infrared light (c. 800 nm). The long-wavelength emitted light can pass through the RPE and retina relatively unimpeded, in contrast to that of fluorescein which is largely blocked. ICG solutions used in angiography contain sodium iodide; accordingly, the dye is contraindicated in those with a history of iodine intolerance.

ULTRA-WIDEFIELD ANGIOGRAPHY

As for traditional retinal photography, conventional fluorescein angiography is constrained by the capacity to image a 30–50° field per exposure. While it is possible to perform the angiographic equivalent of seven-field photography and montage images to yield a wider field

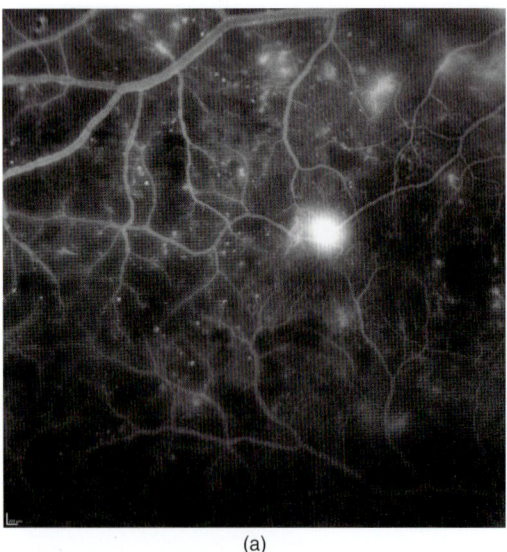
(a)

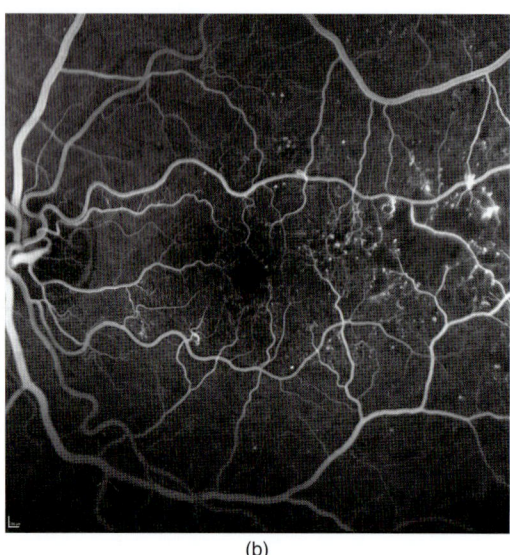
(b)

Fig. 5.41 (a) Extensive capillary non-perfusion (hypofluorescence) is seen peripheral to NVE in this angiogram image. (b) Capillary non-perfusion (hypofluorescence) temporal to left fovea in this FFA image. Note disruption of the perifoveal capillary net, a marker of macular ischaemia.

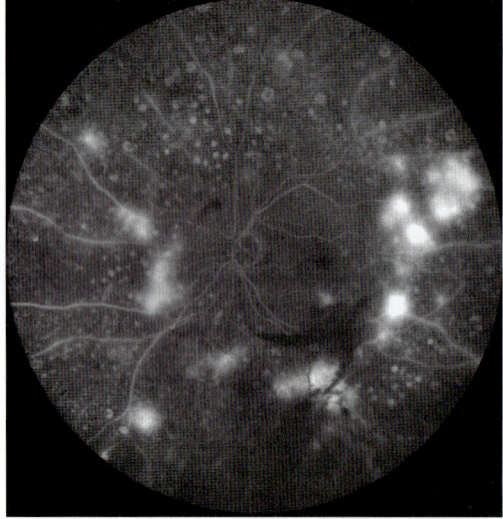

Fig. 5.42 UWF FFA image demonstrating window defects from photocoagulation scars. This patient has numerous NVE and a preretinal haemorrhage.

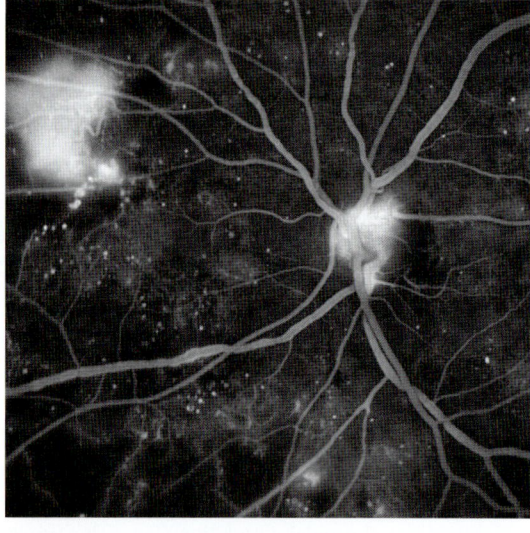

Fig. 5.43 Characteristic intense hyperfluorescence of NVD and NVE in the late arteriovenuos phase. Note areas of capillary non-perfusion adjacent to the NVE.

of view, the utility of this approach is diminished by the fact that the component images cannot be captured simultaneously. As angiography is a dynamic process, important information may be lost in the process of capturing images of each field. The development of confocal scanning laser ophthalmoscopy has enabled ultra-widefield fluorescein angiography with imaging fields of up to 200° (Figs 5.46–5.48). As is the case with ultra-widefield photography, the role of this new imaging technology in the management of diabetic retinopathy

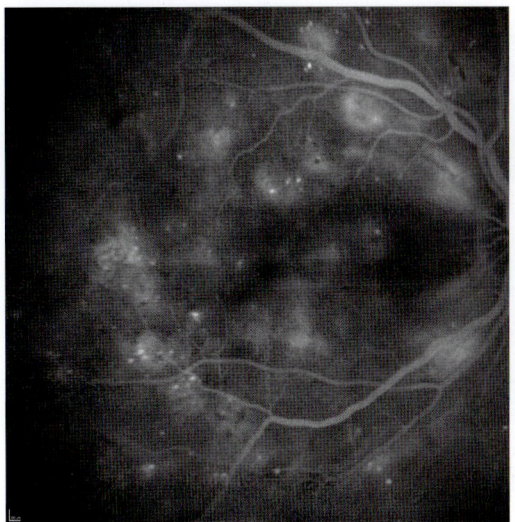

Fig. 5.44 DME with diffuse hyperfluorescence of the macula in later stages of angiogram (same patient as Fig. 5.38).

is still being defined. Ultra-widefield angiography may allow the identification of peripheral retinal pathology, including neovascularisation, which might otherwise be missed. Furthermore, it is well known that retinal ischaemia is associated with the risk of neovascularisation and therefore more complete identification of the extent of peripheral ischaemia afforded by ultra-widefield angiography may have advantages over conventional angiography for prognostication[23]. A recent study of 218 eyes of 118 patients with diabetes undergoing ultra-widefield angiography demonstrated the detection of 3.9 times more retinal non-perfusion and 1.9 times more retinal neovascularisation than was identified when an overlay approximating the area covered by conventional seven-field photography was superimposed on the image[24]. In 4% of eyes (17% of eyes with neovascularisation in the study) retinal neovascularisation was only apparent beyond the simulated seven-field zone.

OPTICAL COHERENCE TOMOGRAPHY

Optical coherence tomography (OCT) is a recently developed imaging modality that has transformed ophthalmic practice. OCT utilises optical interferometry to spatially resolve the different reflective layers of the retina at axial resolutions approximating histological detail, typically in the range of 3–8 μm for standard commercial systems. High axial resolution and the capacity for reproducible quantitative assessment of retinal thickness make OCT a powerful tool for diagnosing diabetic macular oedema and monitoring treatment responses. Thinning of the inner retina evident on OCT has been associated both with diabetic neuropathy and with retinal ischaemia[25–27]. Furthermore, diabetic macular ischaemia demonstrated on fluorescein angiography has been linked with the disruption of photoreceptors on OCT[28]. In cases of advanced proliferative retinopathy, OCT can provide valuable information about the vitreoretinal interface that can assist with surgical planning. Advances in image acquisition technology and data processing have provided clinicians with a growing array of tools including 3D projections, *en face* imaging (Box 5.4) and non-invasive, dye-free angiography.

OCT exploits low-coherence interferometry to generate retinal images. Broad bandwidth light sources

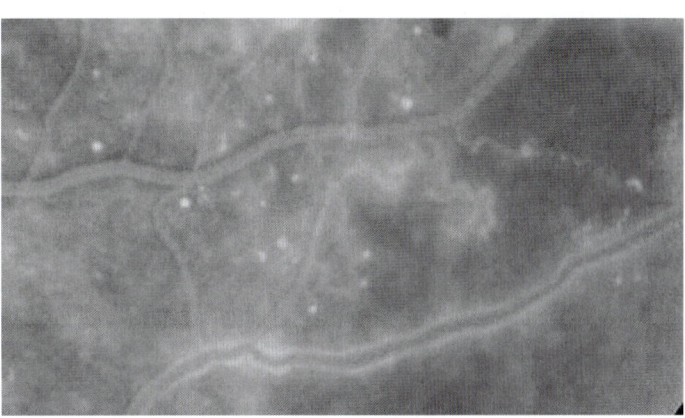

Fig. 5.45 Vessel wall hyperfluorescence/staining hyperfluorescence in an area with surrounding capillary non-perfusion (hypofluorescence).

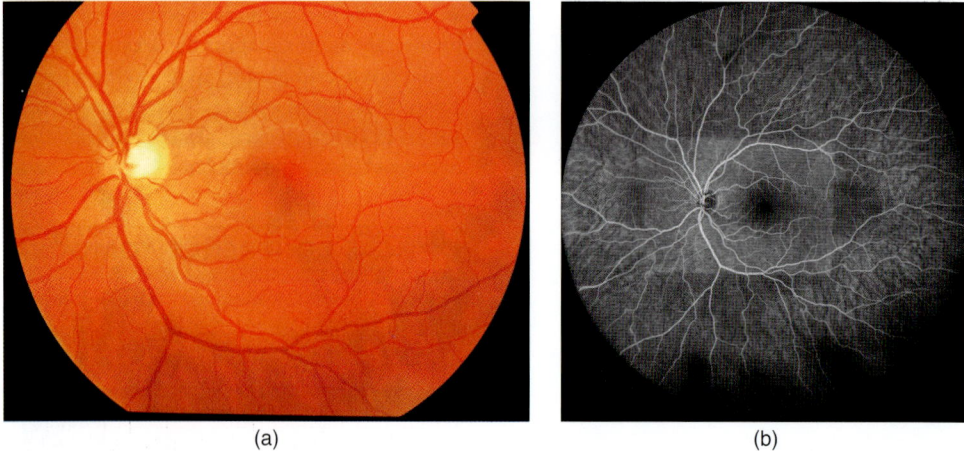

Fig. 5.46 Normal left eye (a) colour photograph and (b) UWF fluorescein image.

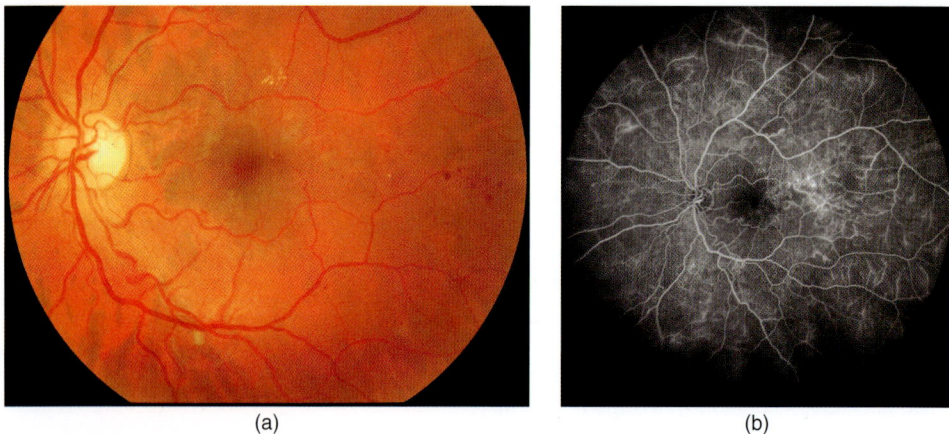

Fig. 5.47 (a) Central colour photograph and (b) UWF fluorescein image of the same patient, demonstrating capillary non-perfusion and vessel staining within the conventional seven-field zone.

(emitting light over a wide range of frequencies, generally in the near-infrared), typically superluminescent diodes or lasers with extremely short-pulse durations, are split into two arms; one of these is projected onto the retina and the other onto a reference mirror in the OCT device. Interference patterns, generated when reflected light from the retina and reference mirror combine, are measured and processed to generate a reflectivity profile of the retina. The resultant axial depth measure, or A-scan, provides spatial and structural information about the retina. A large number of adjacent A-scans are combined to generate a cross-sectional B-scan image.

Time-domain OCT, a technology used in most of the early commercial retinal OCT systems (Figs 5.49–5.51), employs a moving reference mirror to create interference patterns for light that is reflected from different depths of the retina. Reliance on this mechanical system limits the speed of data acquisition (approximately 400 A-scans per second) and consequently image quality.

Modern spectral-domain OCTs (Figs 5.52–5.58), otherwise known as Fourier-domain OCTs, do not rely on a moving reference mirror, but instead simultaneously measure a range of wavelengths of reflected light[29]. A common approach involves the use of a grating to split

Imaging techniques in diabetic retinopathy 75

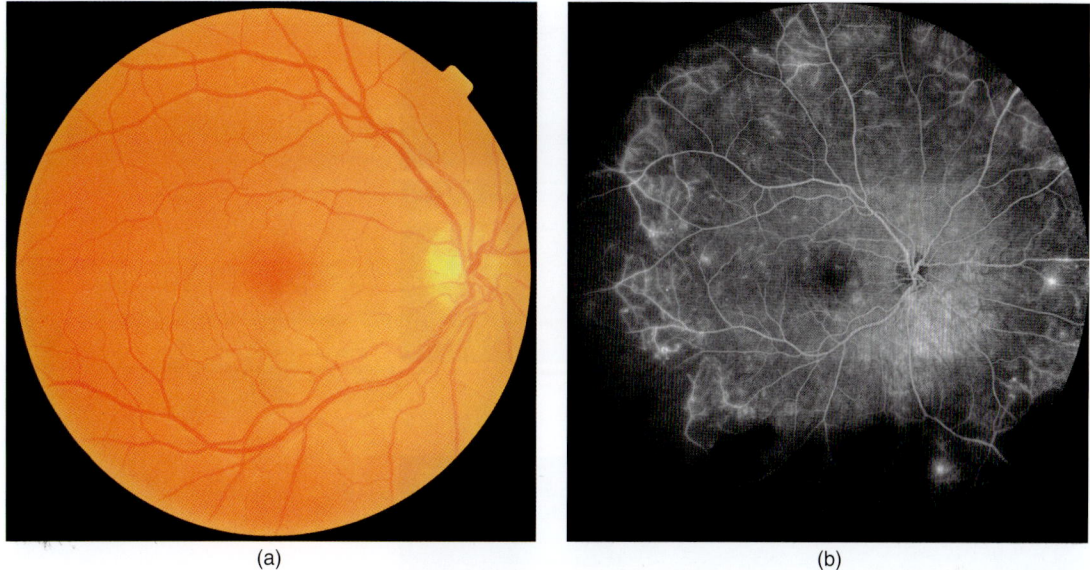

Fig. 5.48 (a) Central colour photograph and (b) UWF fluorescein image in the same patient, demonstrating pathology outside the zone of the 45 degree colour image in image (a).

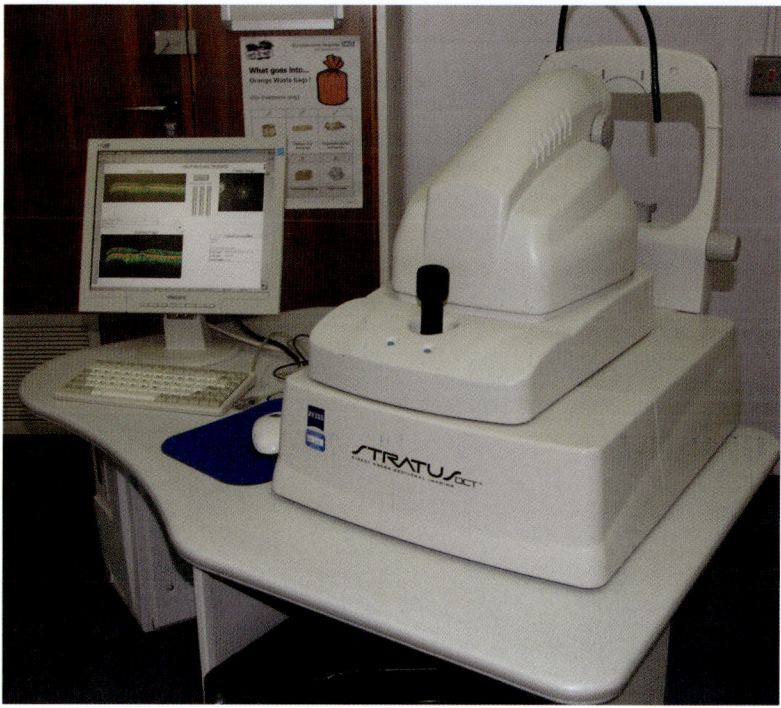

Fig. 5.49 Time-domain OCT machine.

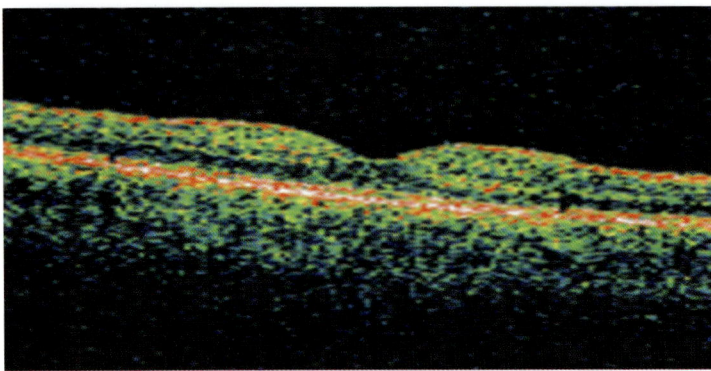

Fig. 5.50 TD-OCT image of a normal macula.

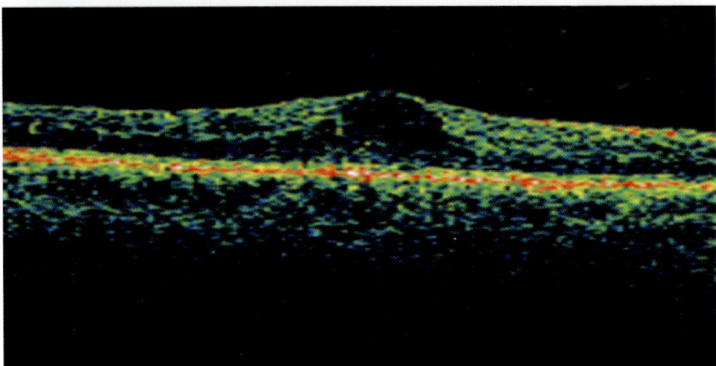

Fig. 5.51 TD-OCT image of diabetic macular oedema.

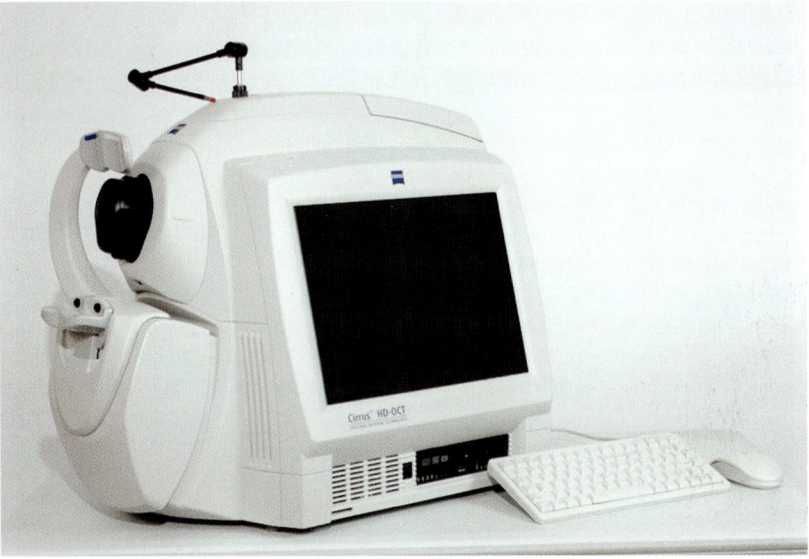

Fig. 5.52 Spectral-domain OCT machine.

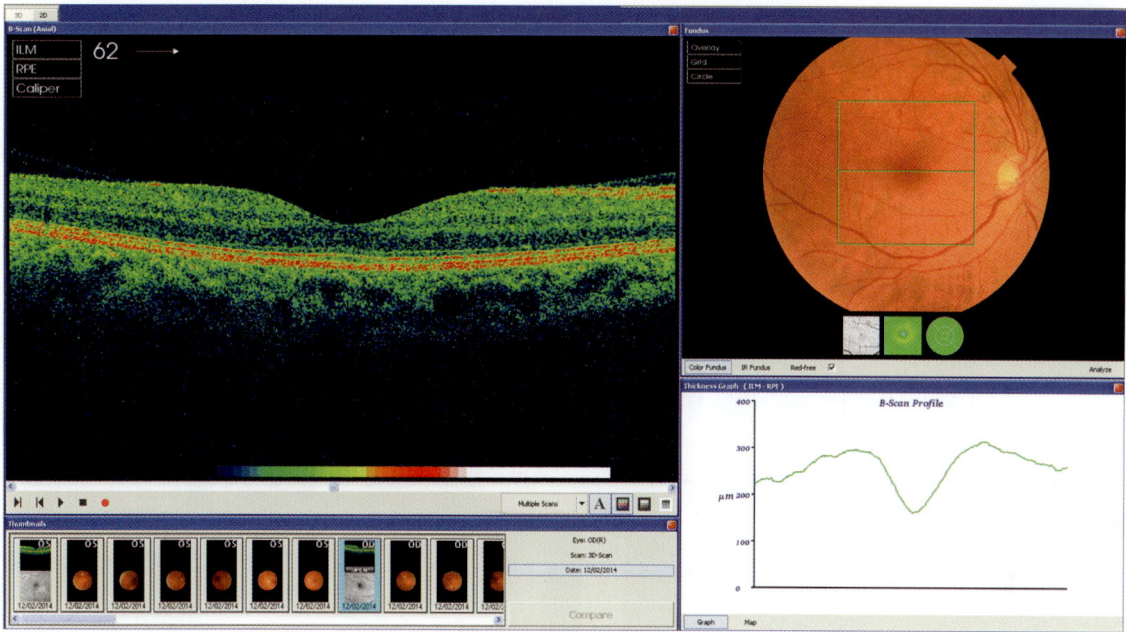

Fig. 5.53 SD-OCT image of a normal macula.

the interference pattern of reflected light into its component wavelengths, and these are simultaneously detected. The depth-resolved information (A-scan) is then retrieved using a mathematical transformation (Fourier transformation) of measured light frequencies. Each detected frequency corresponds to a particular depth in the retina. Accordingly, all points along each A-scan are captured simultaneously, greatly enhancing the rate of image acquisition (up to 40,000 A-scans per second) and allowing for higher A-scan density per B-scan and therefore superior transverse resolution[29]. The ability to rapidly acquire B-scans facilitates the generation of 3D datasets.

Swept-source OCT (Fig. 5.59a–d) is a recently developed variant of Fourier domain OCT which utilises a high-speed wavelength-scanning light source to acquire the interference pattern of reflected light as a function of time[30]. The technology employs longer wavelength light (1050 nm) than is used in spectral-domain OCT, allowing deeper tissue penetration for improved imaging of the choroid and anterior sclera. In addition, the lower signal-to-noise ratios and more rapid scan speeds (as many as 100,000 A-scans per second) allow for higher-resolution imaging and more accurate 3D reconstructions than can be achieved with conventional spectral-domain OCT. The technology allows for wider cross-sectional images (up to 12 mm) than can be captured with conventional OCT (typically 6–9 mm), meaning that the optic disc and macula can be imaged in a single scan. Taken together with its capacity for high-resolution vitreous imaging, swept-source OCT is well suited to imaging of the vitreoretinal interface in patients with proliferative retinopathy complicated by vitreoretinal traction.

Box 5.4: A matter of perspective

While most clinicians are accustomed to evaluating cross-sectional (*en coupe*) OCT projections, advances in image acquisition and processing mean that it is now possible to generate coronal (*en face*; C-scan; Fig. 5.60) OCT projections of the retina. *En face* images allow the clinician to assess each anatomical layer of the retina in turn, facilitating the localisation of retinal pathology in a highly intuitive fashion. Furthermore, *en face* OCT images are readily registered with retinal photos and angiograms, facilitating correlation between different imaging modalities.

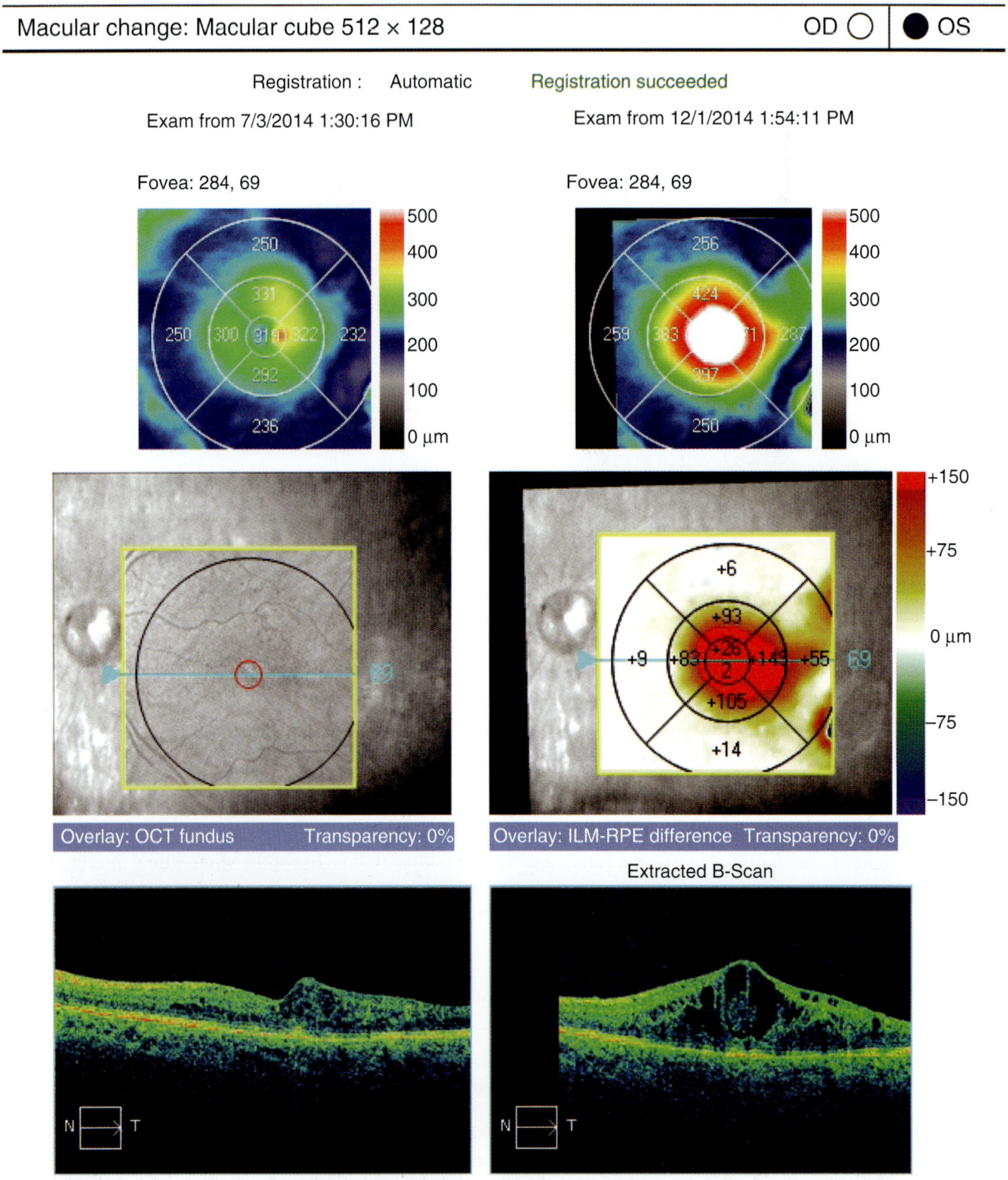

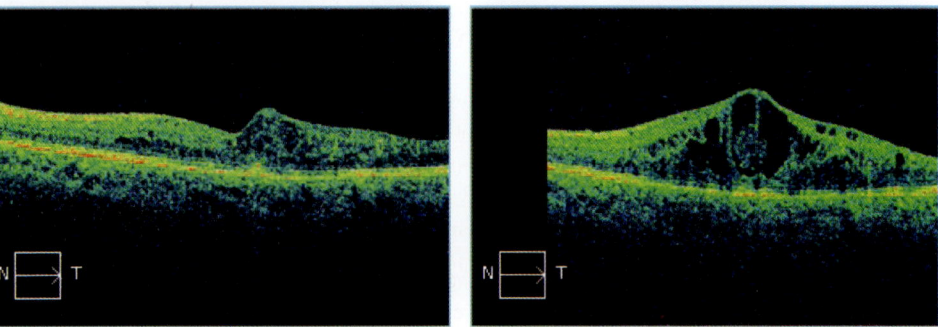

Fig. 5.54 SD-OCT image showing progression of DME.

Imaging techniques in diabetic retinopathy 79

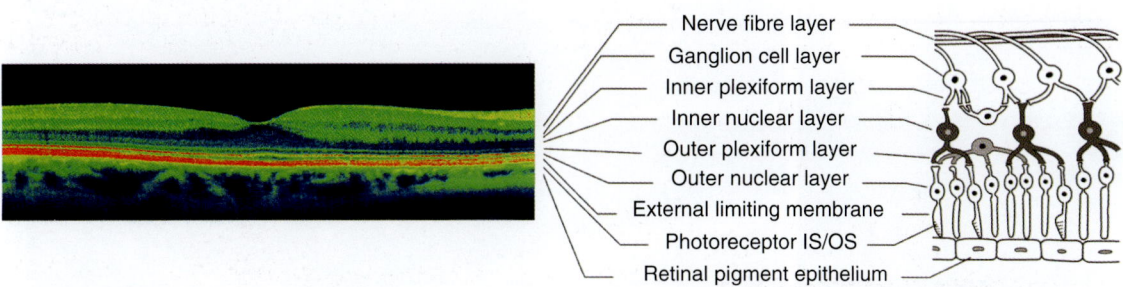

Fig. 5.55 (a, b) Correlation of histology layers of the retina to reflective layers on an OCT.

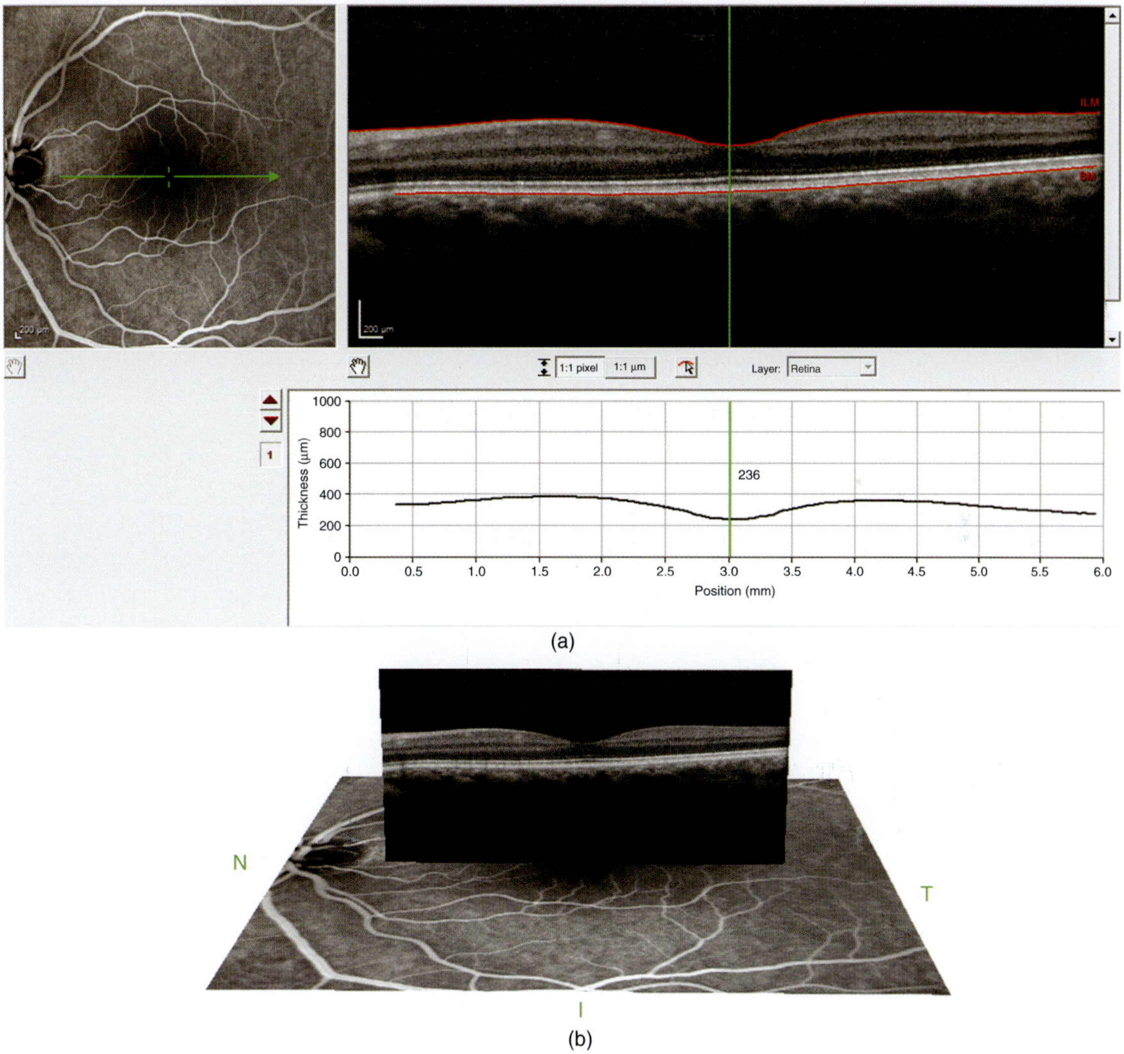

(a)

(b)

Fig. 5.56 (a) A 3D OCT image with (a) FFA (normal) and thickness measurements and (b) FFA (normal).

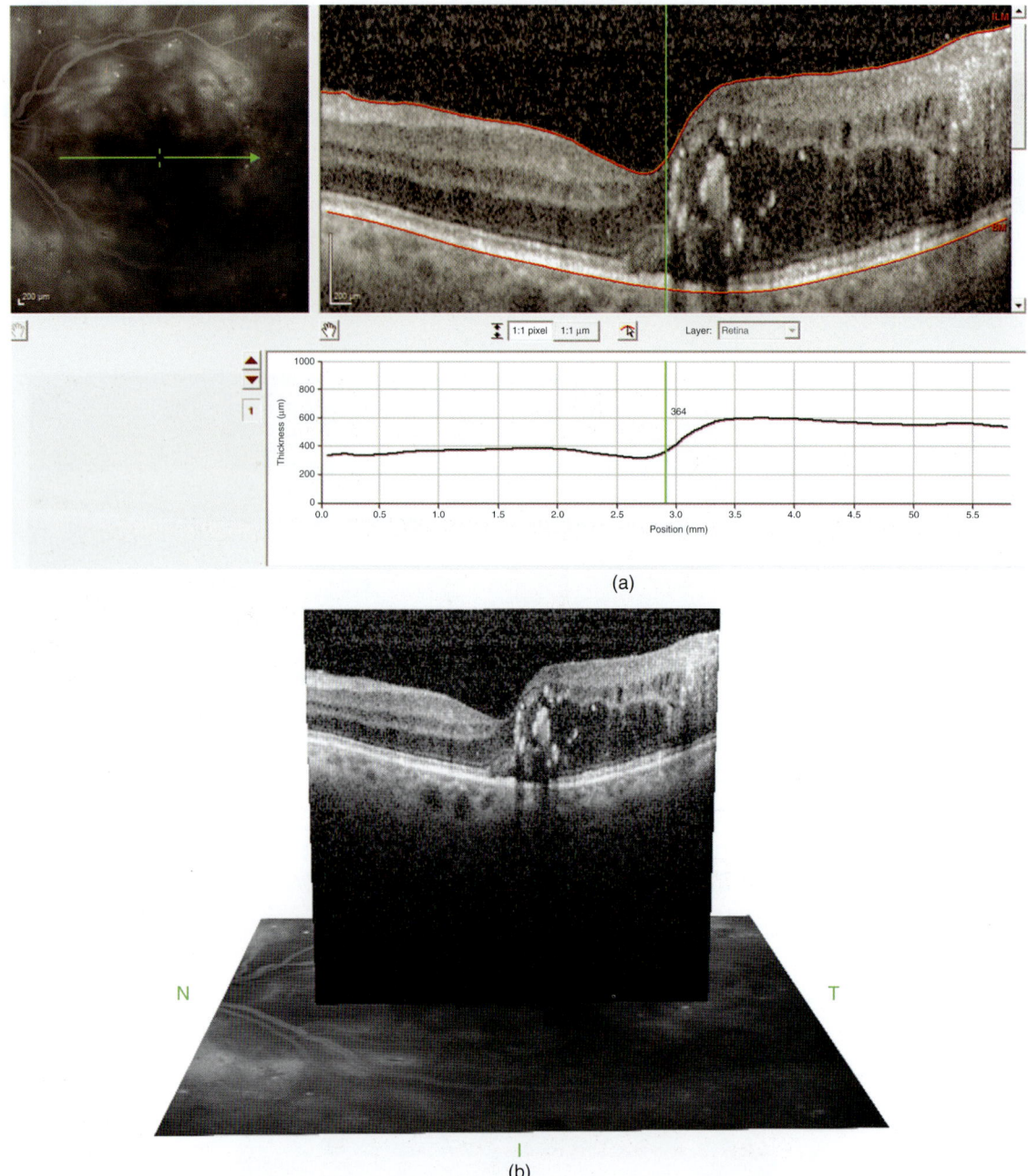

Fig. 5.57 3D OCT image with FFA showing DME.

Imaging techniques in diabetic retinopathy

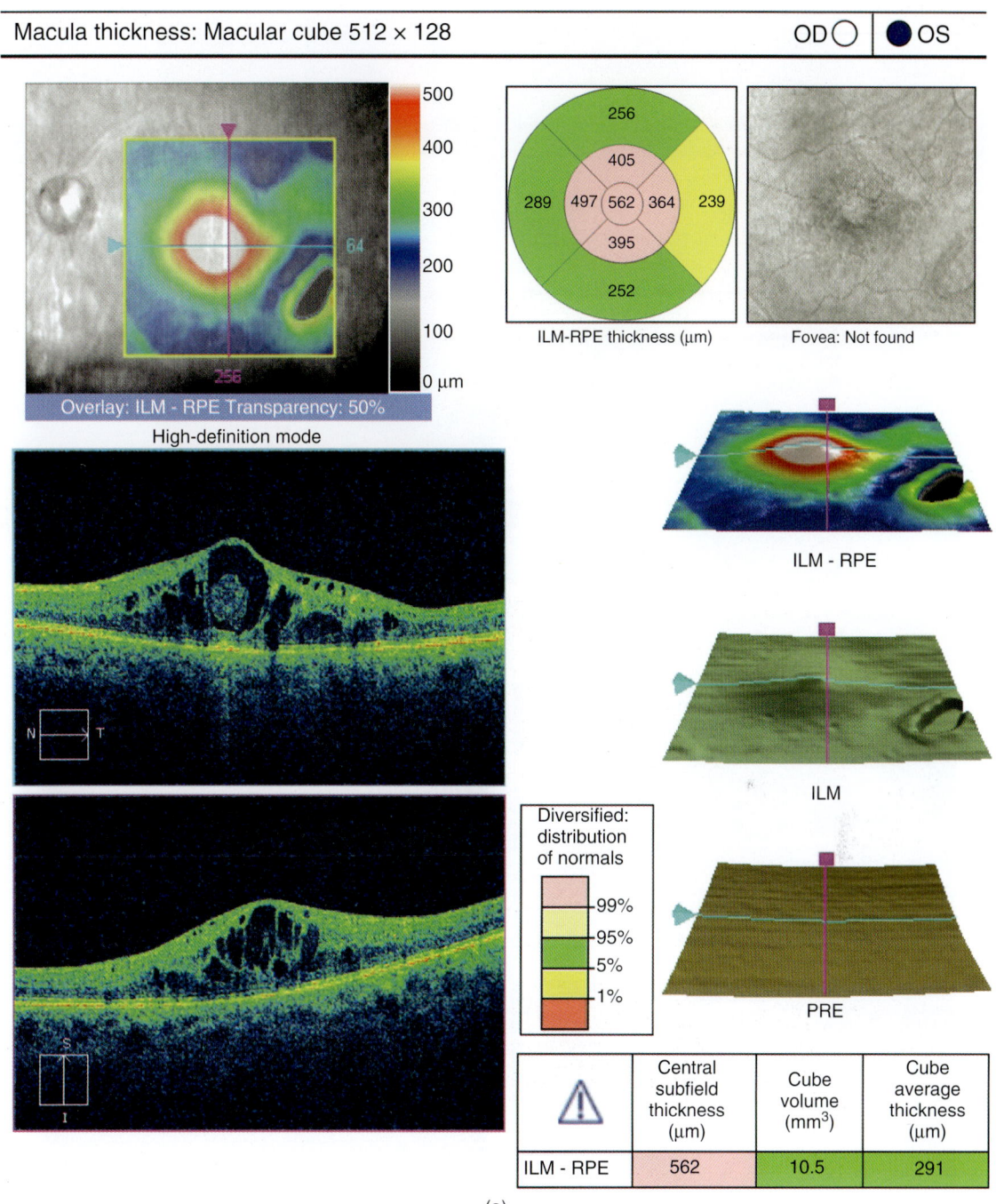

(a)

Fig. 5.58 For same patient as in Figure 5.53: (a) diabetic macular oedema and (b) 3D OCT reconstruction.

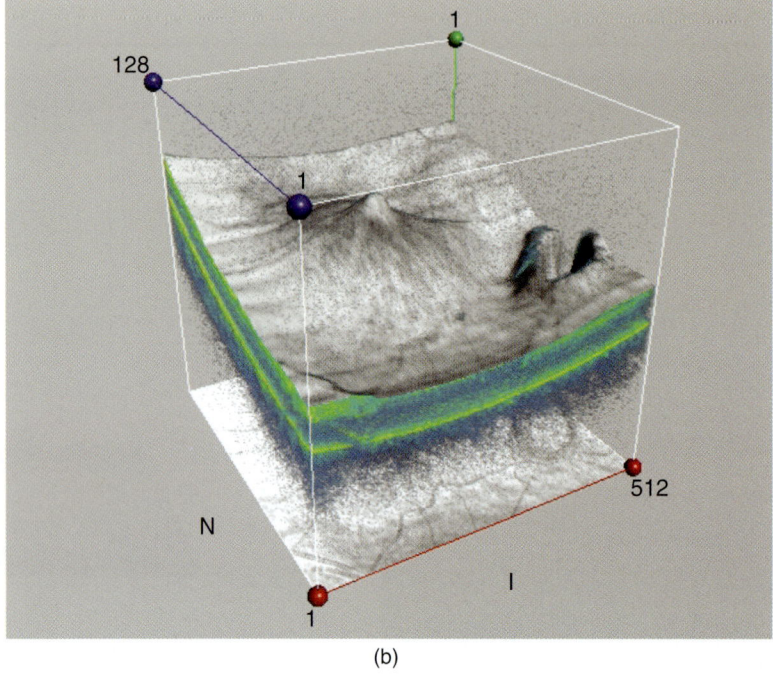

(b)

Fig. 5.58 (*Continued*)

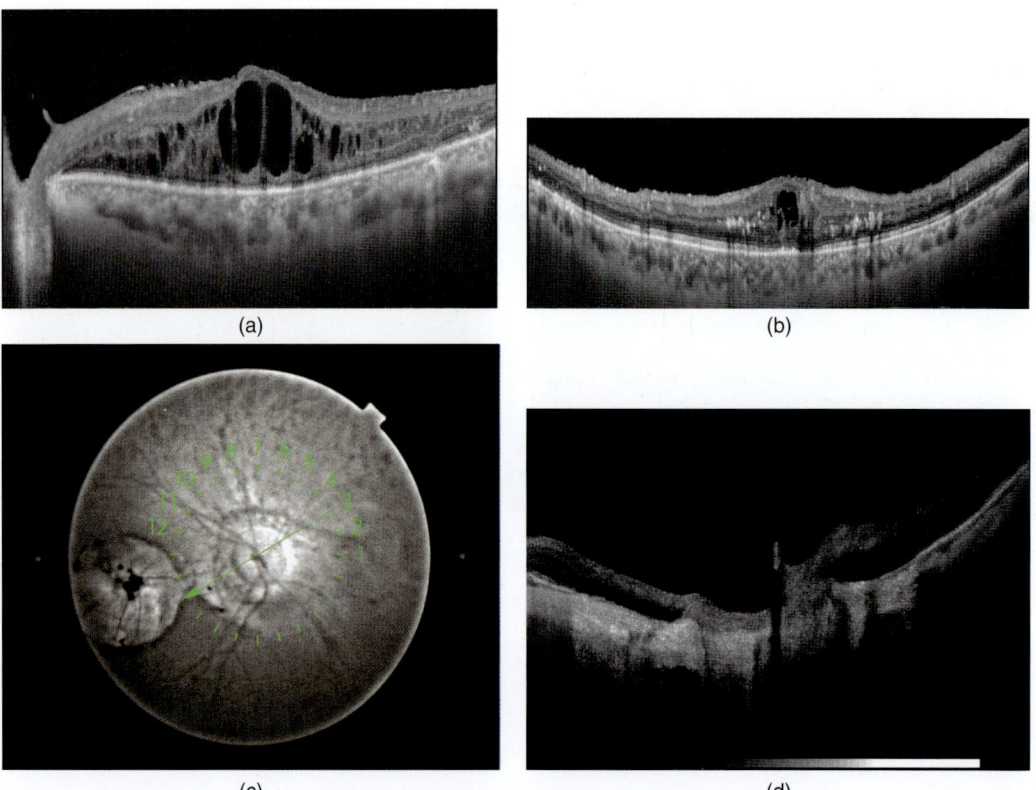

Fig. 5.59 SS-OCT images. (a, b) DME (courtesy of Professor Ogura, Japan). (c, d) Pathological myopia with peripapillary myopic retinoschisis (courtesy of Associate Professor Fred Chen, Australia).

Imaging techniques in diabetic retinopathy

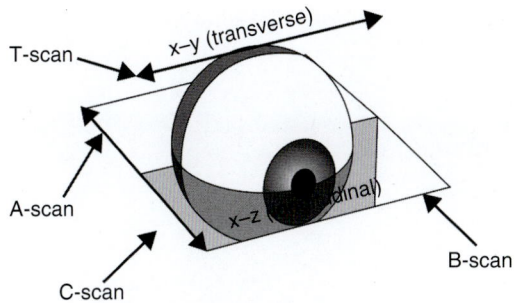

Fig. 5.60 Graphic comparing A-, B- and C-scans.

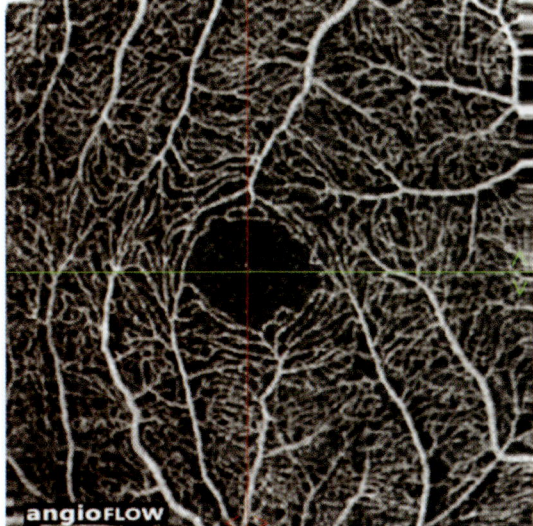

Fig. 5.61 Normal OCT angiography image showing the perifoveal vessels in exquisite detail (courtesy of Professor Ogura, Japan).

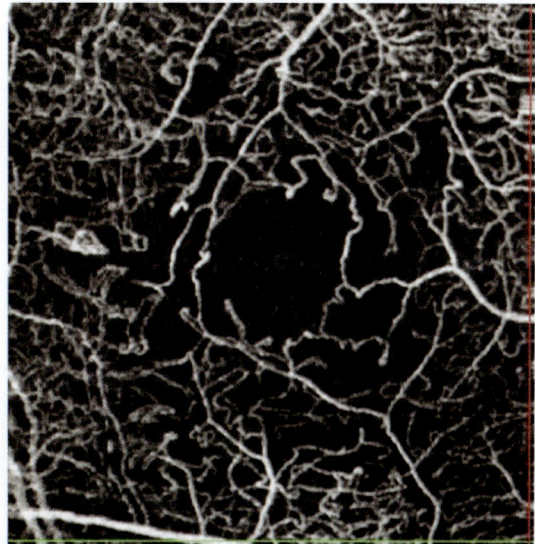

Fig. 5.62 OCT angiography image in mild NPDR. Note the loss of some perifoveal capillaries and early widening of the foveal avascular zone (courtesy of Professor Ogura, Japan).

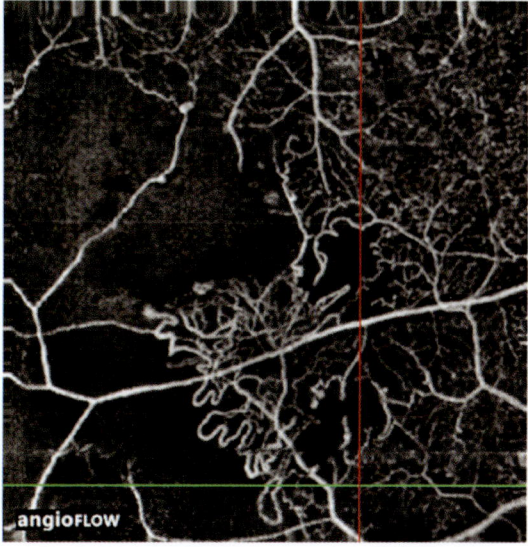

Fig. 5.63 OCT angiography image in proliferative DR. There is extensive capillary non-perfusion and coarsening of capillary networks (courtesy of Professor Ogura, Japan).

OCT ANGIOGRAPHY

Advances in OCT technology have seen the development of methods of non-invasive, dye-free angiography. These approaches extract information about axial motion associated with blood flow and use this to generate 3D reconstructions of the vasculature. A series of rapid A-scans is performed at each retinal location and motion

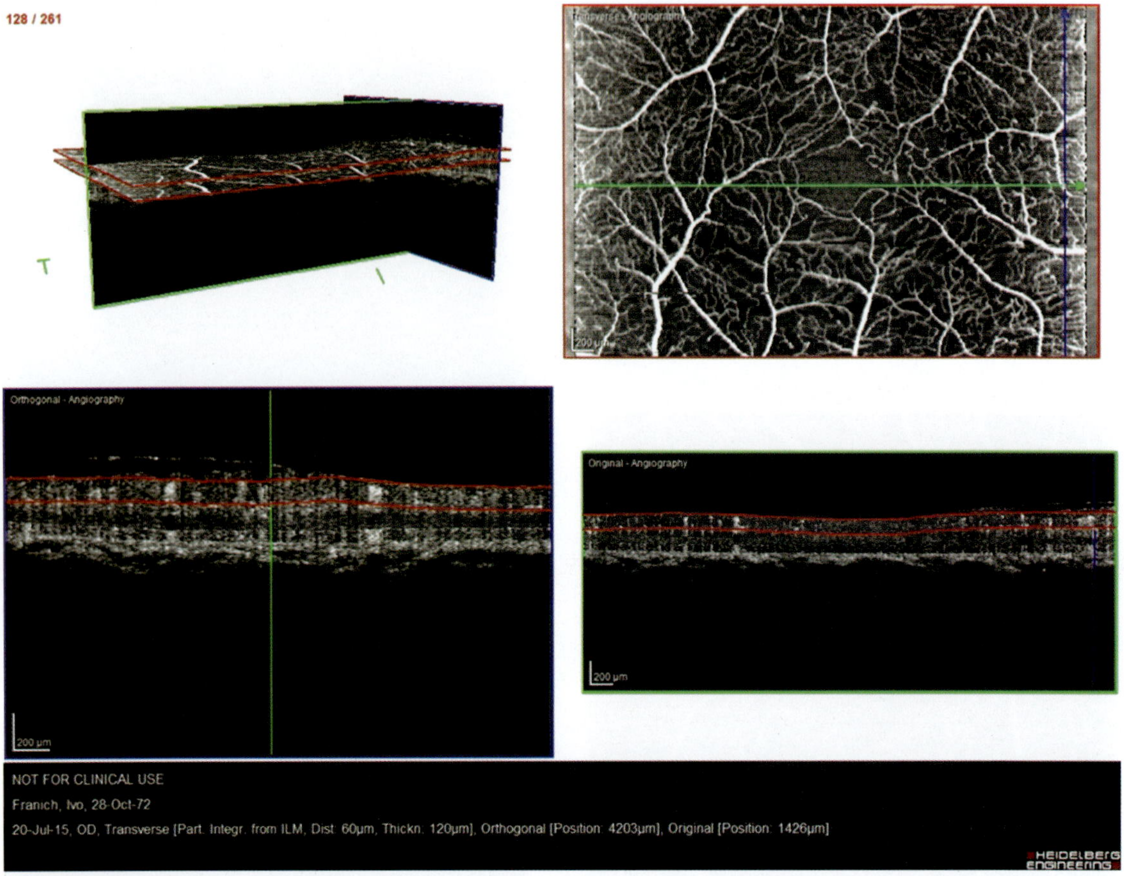

Fig. 5.64 OCT angiography of superficial retinal vessels (courtesy of Associate Professor Fred Chen, Australia).

is detected as phase change between adjacent A-scans for each depth position[30]. Given the speed of scan acquisition in Fourier-domain OCT, it is possible to extract motion data from adjacent B-scans using either phase change (spectral-domain OCT) or intensity change (swept-source OCT). Post-acquisition data processing algorithms are used to segment and visualise perfused vessels. High-speed image acquisition, gaze tracking and precise image registration are key to this technology. Spectral-domain and swept-source technologies are variously used in commercial systems; swept-source systems may offer improved visualisation of the choroidal circulation.

OCT angiography has a number of advantages over fluorescein angiography: it is non-invasive; does not require a contrast agent; and is quicker to perform. Furthermore, the technique facilitates 3D visualisation of the retinal and choroidal circulation and the ability to view the vasculature *en face* by anatomical planes for superior localisation of pathology. Quantitative measures of retinal and choroidal blood flow are attainable in research machines (Doppler OCT) and are likely to become available in

Imaging techniques in diabetic retinopathy 85

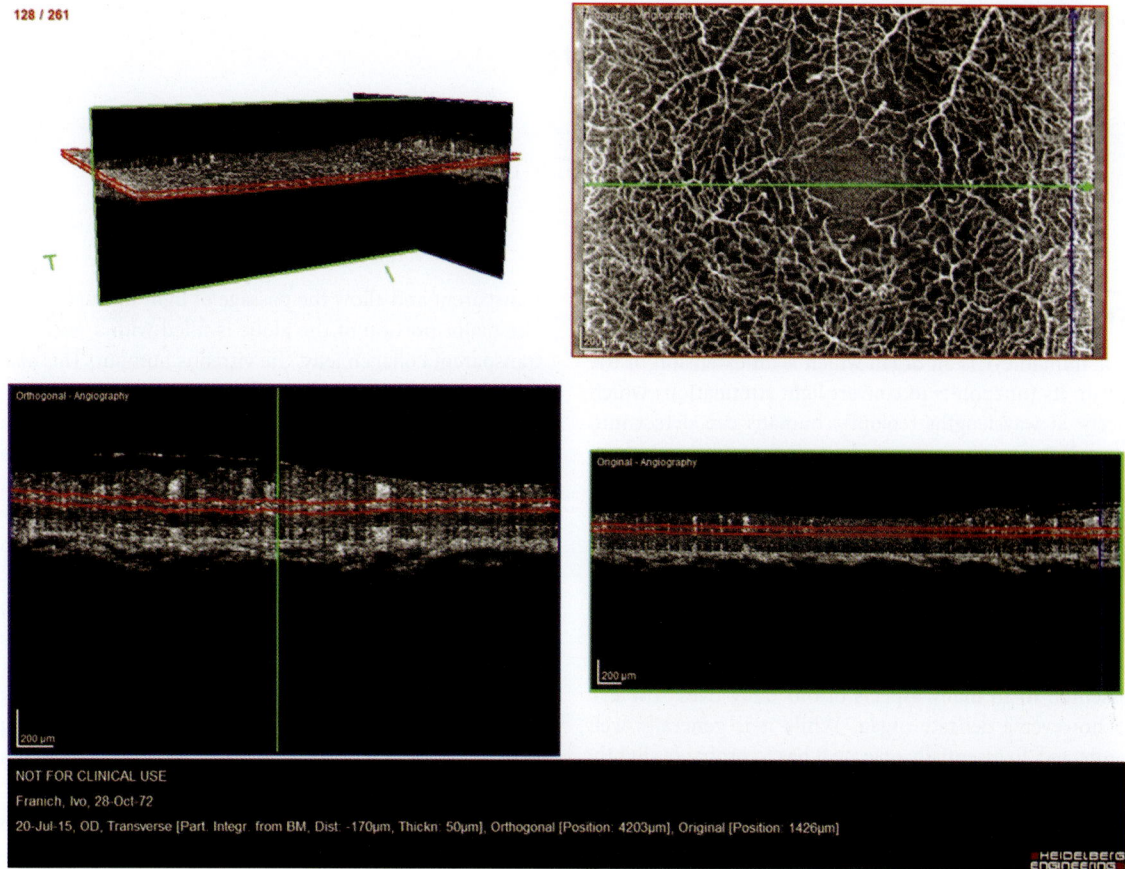

Fig. 5.65 OCT angiography of deeper retinal vessels (courtesy of Associate Professor Fred Chen, Australia).

commercial systems. While OCT angiography cannot be used to directly demonstrate vascular hyperpermeability, most systems include the capacity to present both angiographic and intensity projections so that important static features of the vasculature (Figs 5.61–5.65), such as leakage sites, can be observed in parallel with those derived from blood flow[30].

REFERENCE

Please visit www.wiley.com/go/scanlon/diabetic_retinopathy

6 The normal eye

Stephen J. Aldington

Gloucestershire Hospitals NHS Foundation Trust, UK; University of Warwick Medical School, UK

THE RELEVANT ANATOMY OF THE EYE

The human eye is an organ which is an extension of the brain. Its function is to convert light stimulations which occur at wavelengths (colours) humans can detect into electrical neurological impulses, and to transmit these impulses to specialised portions of the brain in order to generate an 'image'. Most people have two eyes, generally pointing forwards, so in health the two eyes work together to form a single full-colour detailed image comprising elements of shape, pattern, colour, tone and movement with which we are all, as adults, familiar. Our two eyes also give us the ability to 'see' depth and work out distances, essential in so many aspects of our daily lives. The eye is however a delicate organ. While it is generally well protected, to essentially operate it has to protrude slightly from the safety of the human body and so present its own beautiful manifestation, visible to the world at large. As such it also affords us, the viewer, an opportunity to look into the actual workings of the eye and indeed a representation of the workings of the body in health and disease.

The eye is an approximate globe, averaging 23 mm in horizontal and vertical diameters and 22–24 mm in axial length in emmetropes (normal-sighted persons). Long-sighted persons (hypermetropes) have slightly shorter eyeballs, while those with short-sightedness (myopes) are correspondingly slightly longer. As the primary function of the eye is to bring light rays into sharp focus onto the retina (the inside surface of the eye), short- or long-sighted people usually need the help of a pair of spectacles or other correction devices to achieve this. With the assistance of correction if required, most of us can see perfectly well and clearly.

The eyeball basically consists of three concentric major layers of tissue which, in their anterior aspect, are all transparent and allow the passage of light through them. The major portion of the globe is filled with a normally transparent collagen jelly, the vitreous humour. This also permits the passage of light from the anterior portions, allowing the light to fall onto the retina. The retina, the innermost surface of the posterior section of the eye, contains the specialised photoreceptor cells which, when light falls onto them, encode and transmit signals to the brain to convert the complex light stimuli into recognisable images (Fig. 6.1).

The outermost layer of most of the eye is the tough protective white sclera. At the front of the eye this outermost layer has developed to be completely transparent (in health) and forms the cornea. Inside the sclera, and hence not generally visible from the outside, is the uveal layer. Anteriorly this comprises the ciliary body and the iris (which is visible from outside) and posteriorly comprises the highly vascular choroid. Within the choroid is the innermost major layer, the retina, containing the photoreceptors. Lying between the choroid and the retina are the very thin Bruch's membrane and the pigment epithelium: both essential for normal retinal function. The choroid contains three vascular layers, the vessels in which become progressively smaller as the retina is approached. The retina also comprises several discrete layers which have relevance to many aspects of the development and presentation of diabetic eye disease, as shown in Figures 6.2 and 6.3.

The orientation of major structures within the anterior portion of the eye is shown in Figure 6.1b, which demonstrates the relationship between the anterior ocular structures and the production and flow of aqueous humour. The ciliary body and its processes, responsible for production of aqueous, lie within the posterior chamber with the inner surface in contact with the vitreous and outer surface in contact with the sclera and form a ring encircling the iris. The iris itself is internally separated from the cornea by the anterior chamber and from the lens of the eye immediately behind it by the much shallower posterior chamber. The iris edge rests onto the anterior surface

---

A Practical Manual of Diabetic Retinopathy Management, Second Edition. Edited by Peter Scanlon, Ahmed Sallam, and Peter van Wijngaarden.
© 2017 John Wiley & Sons Ltd. Published 2017 by John Wiley & Sons Ltd.
Companion Website: www.wiley.com/go/scanlon/diabetic_retinopathy

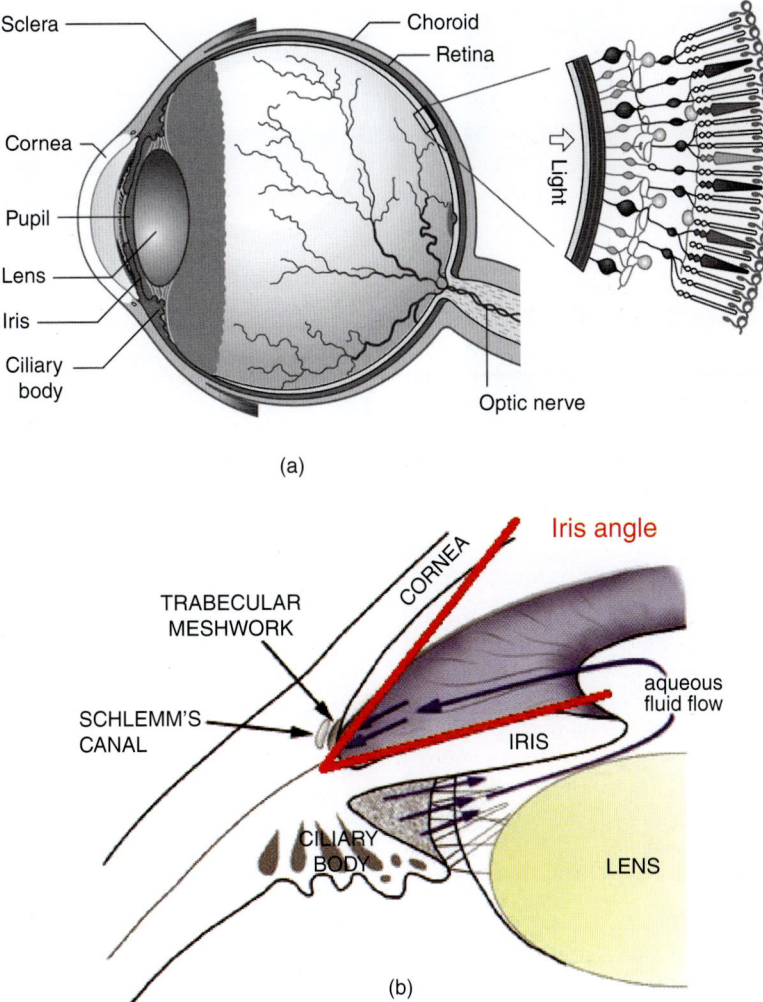

Fig. 6.1 Cross-section of (a) the eye and major structures and (b) anterior segment and aqueous flow.

of the lens capsule but allows aqueous humour to flow from the posterior chamber into the anterior chamber. Both chambers are therefore filled with aqueous humour, with the total quantity balanced through outflow from the anterior chamber of the eye through the trabecular meshwork and Sclemm's canal to connect to the aqueous and scleral veins. Anything which reduces the final outflow of aqueous from the anterior chamber, most particularly a narrow iris angle due to glaucoma, will cause a significant rise in the eye's intraocular pressure.

Through contraction of the circular and relaxation of the radial elements of the ciliary muscles, the eye causes the iris to expand and advance inwards towards the centre, diminishing the size of or constricting the apparent central pupil. This has the joint effect of limiting the amount of light falling on the retina and of increasing the depth of field of the optical viewing system (equivalent to 'stopping down' a camera lens). Conversely, through contraction of radial and relaxation of circular elements, the iris recedes outwards, enlarging or dilating the central pupil. This can be achieved either through normal reflex reaction in reduced light levels, through pharmacological intervention intentionally when desired or accidentally.

Moving posteriorly again but on the visual axis, the crystalline lens, lying within its elastic capsule, is situated

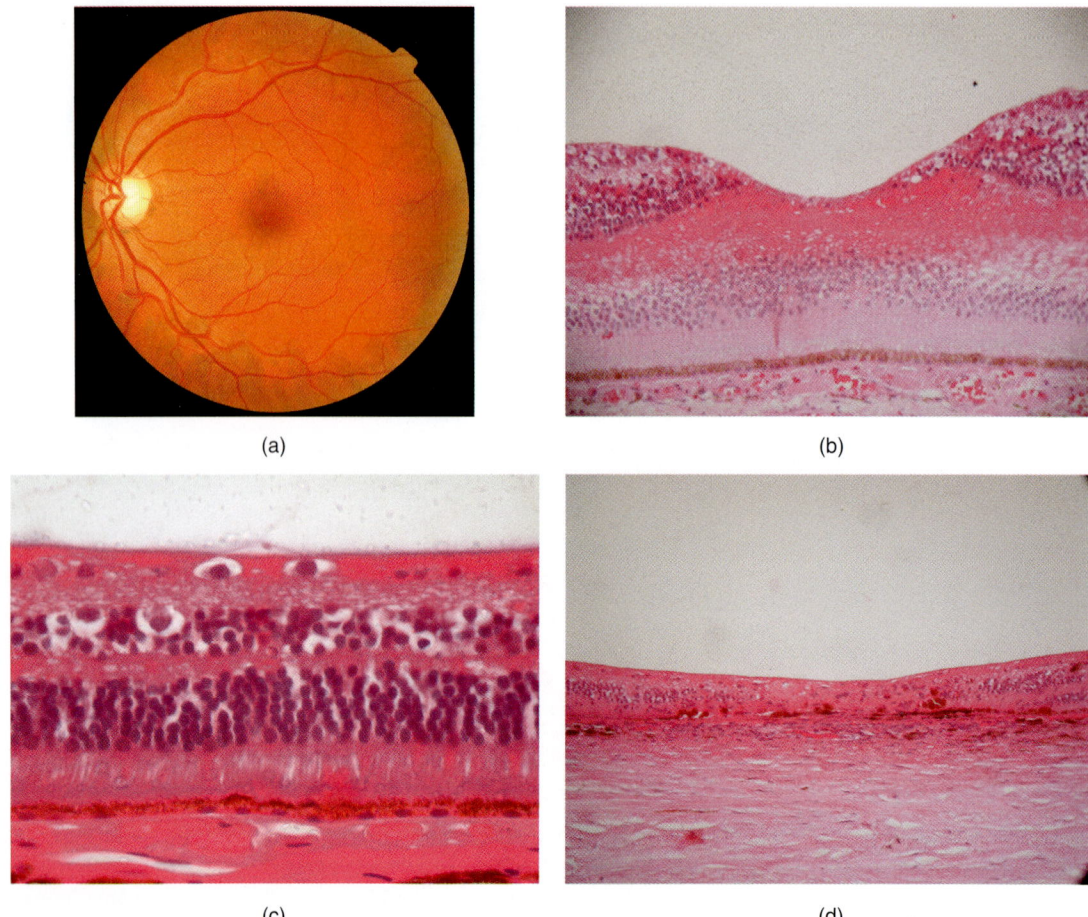

Fig. 6.2 (a) Basic retinal appearance on examination. (b) Normal human fovea: the inner and outer nuclear cell layers at the edge of the fovea and the concentration of cones centrally. (c) The receptive retina: the ganglion cell layer, the bipolar layer, the nuclei of the cones and rods, the pigment epithelium and the choroid. (d) The retina following laser treatment: the gliosis of the retina following laser treatment.

between the iris elements and the vitreous body and is suspended on a series of radial suspensory ligaments (the zonule) which, through contraction or relaxation, control the shape and thickness of the flexible lens they encircle. This affords the ability to finely focus light entering the eye onto the retina. Much of this fine focusing capability is lost with increasing age as the lens and capsule become more rigid.

Moving further backwards along the visual or optical axis through the vitreous, we encounter the retina. The retina is in intimate contact with and surrounds the vitreous outer surface layer, the posterior hyaloid (or internal limiting) membrane, and represents over 70% of the inside of the globe's surface. Normally largely transparent, the retina contains the light-sensitive photoreceptors along with an active blood supply, clearly visible by means of investigative techniques which illuminate and view the inside of the globe. The retina varies in thickness from approximately 0.1 mm (100 μm) in the periphery to over 0.6 mm (600 μm) at its thickest in the central regions of the posterior pole.

On viewing the retina through the central pupil formed by a dilated iris, the most apparent object is the yellow head of the optic nerve: the optic disc. This slightly off-centred feature with its associated pattern of radiating arteries and veins represents the point at which the major retinal blood supply enters and leaves the eye. It also provides the termination point for the eye's neurosensory

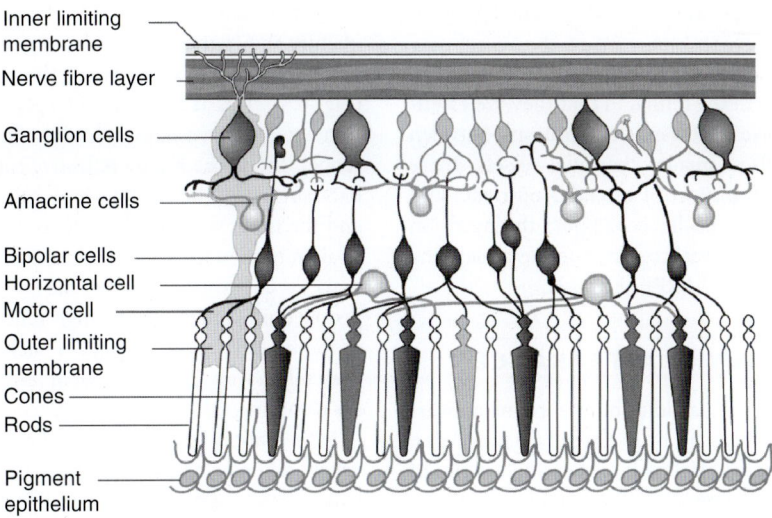

Fig. 6.3 Retinal structure cross-section diagram.

nerve fibres to coalesce and leave the eye for communication with the brain (Fig. 6.2a).

Lying approximately 3.5 mm temporal to the optic disc and close to the physical axis of the eye and, in health, exactly on its visual axis, is the fovea and the surrounding macular region. The macula, about 1.5–2.0 mm across, represents the area containing the macular pigments lutein and zeaxanthin. The <1 mm diameter foveal region is characterised by its high concentration of cone photoreceptors and much lower concentrations of rod receptors as compared to the retinal periphery (correspondingly where cones are less frequent). Cones provide the colour vision capabilities of the human eye and provide increasing acuity capability as the visual axis is approached. While loss of peripheral vision may go unnoticed for some time, any damage to the macula (particularly to the fovea) will usually result in loss of central vision, with immediately obvious results.

Within the central foveola, 200–250 µm in diameter and devoid of rods, the cones themselves within this region are narrower and tightly packed into a complex hexagonal pattern.

The majority of the retina, excepting the central foveal region, is provided with nourishment, oxygen and its waste-product removal system by means of the retinal vascular circulation. The central retinal artery, branching into the major and then minor arterioles, leads to a capillary network invisible to the naked eye, then through the minor and then more major venules and veins eventually to the central retinal vein. This leaves the eye approximately down the centre of the optic nerve and hence completes the major retinal circulation.

In the foveal region, however, where high acuity and accurate colour perception are generated, there are no extraneous objects such as blood vessels within the retinal layers. The foveola is responsible for the highest acuity capabilities associated with reading, detailed working and driving, etc. The central foveal region is thinner (normally approximately 150–250 µm thick) and importantly and uniquely is devoid of retinal blood supply. The supply is provided through diffusion from the choriocapillaris of the innermost choroidal layer and through intimate contact between the fovea and the retinal pigment epithelium. By this means, light being 'focused' at the fovea will not be adversely affected by retinal blood vessels before its presentation to the densely packed foveal cone photoreceptors.

The blood vessels in the retina, like those in the brain and much of the central nervous system, exhibit tight junctions between adjacent cells. This is important as it prevents leakage of blood components, fluids, chemicals or drugs (endogenous or exogenous) through the retinal blood vessel wall and hence maintains the aptly termed blood-retinal barrier formed by both the tight-junctions in retinal cell walls and those in the unilayer retinal pigment epithelium (RPE) immediately outside the retina. The RPE is itself supported by the adjacent layer of Bruch's membrane, damage to which is frequently manifest as (among other things) drusen and ultimately as age-related macular degeneration (AMD) with its associated progressive visual loss.

The cells of the choroidal circulation are however quite different from those in the retina, in that they are essentially designed to have small gaps (fenestrations) between the cells in the walls of smaller choroidal vessels. These fenestrations allow transport of essential nutrients and other small molecules and hence support the nutrition and oxygenation of the foveal region from the underlying choriocapillaris through the RPE (Fig. 6.3).

THE PHOTOGRAPHIC APPEARANCE

On examination the normal adult human retina appears as an orange-red (Caucasian) or green-red (Indian Asian and African Caribbean) mottled layer bearing a series of branching retinal blood vessels which originate from the near-circular yellow-white head of the optic nerve or optic disc as it enters/leaves the eye and spread across the entire visible retinal surface (Fig. 6.4).

Retinal examination in juveniles and young adults frequently shows there to be a very distinct and bright reflection across and surrounding the entire macular region (Fig. 6.5). This is a feature of light from the examination equipment (usually a fundus camera or ophthalmoscope) hitting the highly reflective interface between the back surface of the vitreous body (the posterior hyaloid) and the inner surface of the retina, which then bounces straight back to the viewer/recording medium. This often makes accurate assessment of the macular region in these people quite difficult as the high reflectivity masks much of the underlying pathology. In such cases multiple images, taken with slightly different angles onto the macula, are recommended.

Examination or imaging of the right eye shows the yellow-white or occasionally pinkish-coloured optic disc lying to the right of (i.e. nasal to) the darker-coloured macular region, itself demarcated by the superior and inferior retinal vessel 'arcades' curving respectively above and below the macula. The centre of the macula is slightly

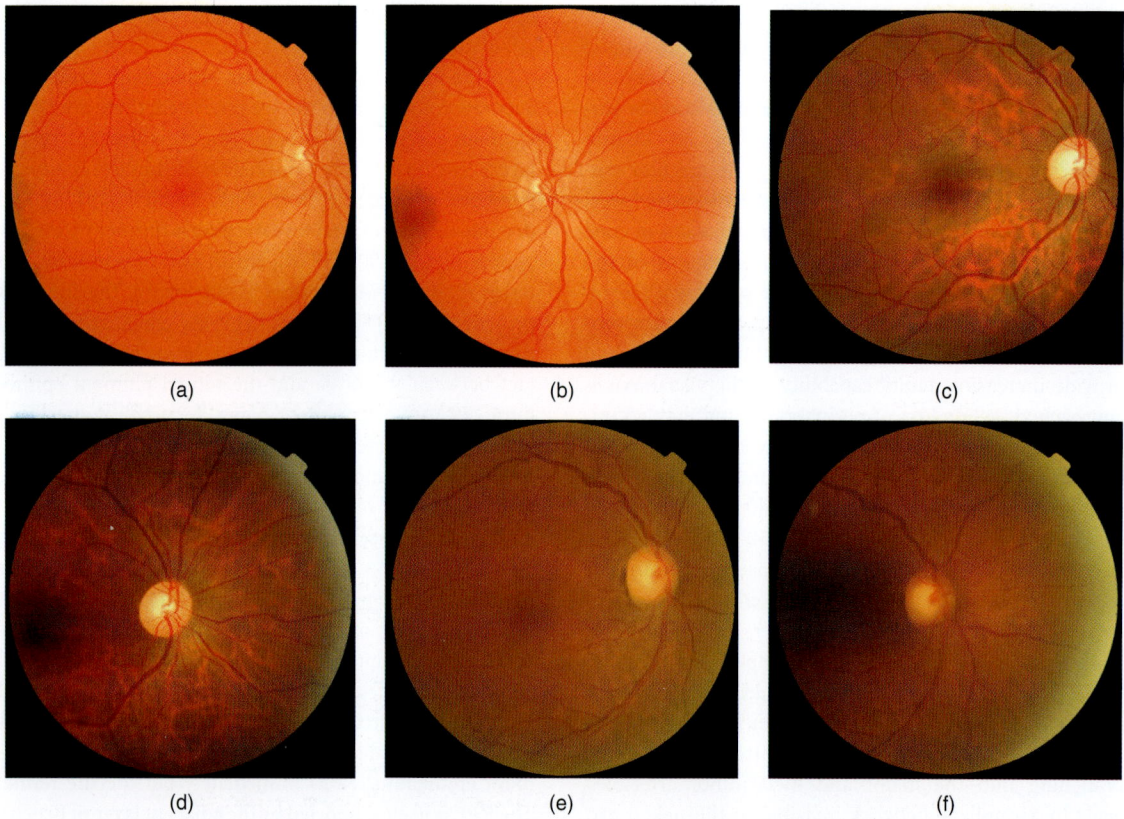

Fig. 6.4 Normal Caucasian retinal appearance: (a) macular view and (b) nasal view. Normal Asian Indian retinal appearance: (c) macular view and (d) nasal view. Normal Caribbean retinal appearance: (e) macular view and (f) nasal view.

The normal eye

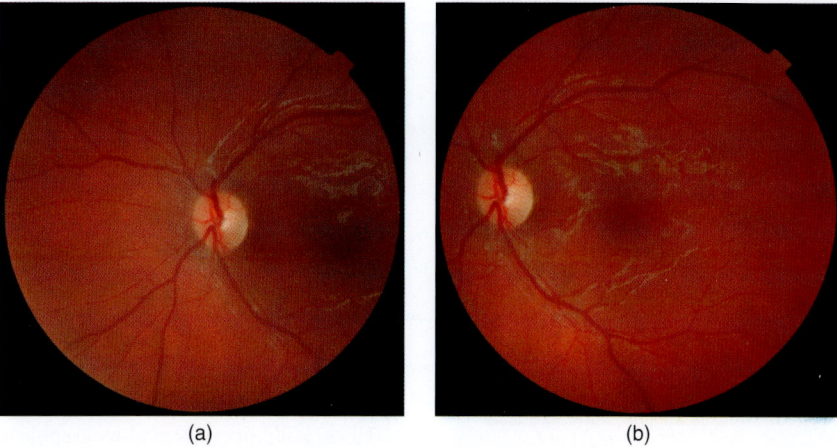

Fig. 6.5 Image of young person's retina: (a) nasal view, showing posterior hyaloid reflections and (b) macular view, showing posterior hyaloid reflections. There are also some mild changes of diabetic retinopathy in each image.

darker still in colour, often appearing dark grey, and represents the foveal region where pigmentation is densest.

The superior and inferior temporal vessel arcades meet lateral to the macular region at a point on the horizontal meridian of the globe, termed the lateral or temporal retinal watershed. While the retinal blood vessels supplying the central and temporal aspects of the eye are formed as curving arcades, vessels supplying the nasal portions of the eye leave the optic disc and traverse the retina in straighter, less deviating patterns. The overall pattern of the visible retinal vessels is the same as that for the usually invisible retinal nerve fibres; temporally the nerve fibres follow the curved arcades to meet laterally beyond the macular region while nasally they radiate straight out towards the retinal periphery (Figs 6.6 and 6.7).

The central retinal artery and retinal vein usually enter and leave the eye at a point which lies slightly towards the nasal aspect of the optic disc, that is, slightly further away from the fovea than the centre of the disc. At or around the surface of the optic disc, the central retinal artery bifurcates into two branches and then, before reaching the outer margin of the optic disc, each again branches to form the four major retinal artery branches serving the superior temporal, superior nasal, inferior nasal and inferior temporal quadrants of the retina. These are usually geographically followed by the retinal veins which, as they return from the retinal periphery to the optic disc, sequentially join to form the four retinal quadrant venous branches before finally forming the central retinal vein leaving the eye through the optic disc.

Retinal veins and arteries generally alternate around the circumference of the optic disc, veins generally having larger diameters than the corresponding retinal artery at that point, and are slightly darker in colour. While both

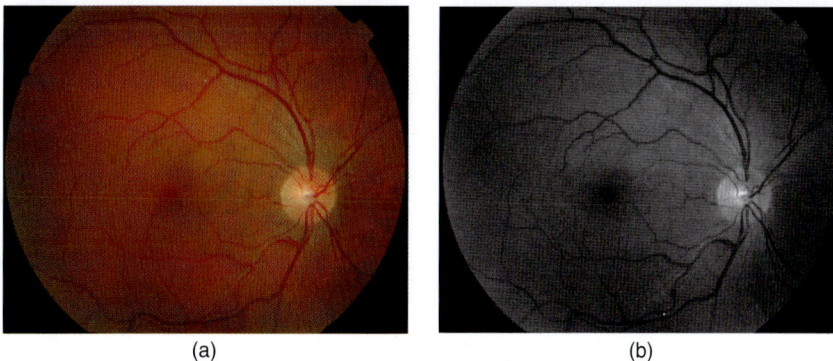

Fig. 6.6 Image of nerve fibre layer patterns: (a) colour photograph and (b) red-free photograph.

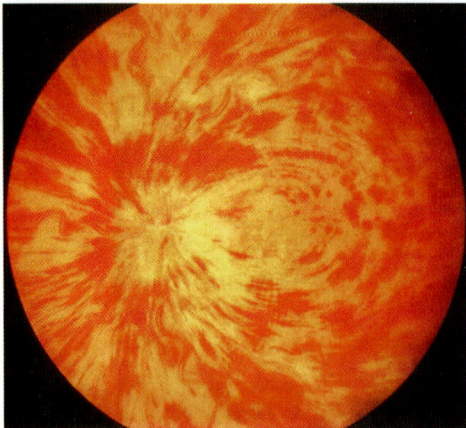

Fig. 6.7 Image of nerve fibre layer patterns from a patient who has had a left central retinal vein thrombosis with haemorrhages under the nerve fibre layer.

veins and arteries can display a central light 'reflex' along their length, constant or interrupted, which is literally a reflection of the illuminating light source from the topmost surface of the circular vessel, this is more usually apparent from arteries. It is important to note that this normal light reflex from vessels is quite common and must not be confused with threading or white-lining of vessels, which is a feature of vessel occlusion in advanced disease states.

Normal, non-diseased retinal blood vessels can be seen to evenly and gradually reduce in diameter as they are followed away from the optic nerve head and out towards the retinal periphery. This is a traditional form of vascular bed with decreasing diameters of arterioles down to the level of the invisible capillary bed, followed by increasing diameters of venules and then veins. Assessment of changes in vessel calibre, locally or generally, can be a crucial indicator of advanced or progressing retinal vascular disease and damage.

The areas of retina lying between retinal vessels are, in absence of disease, generally relatively featureless and are reasonably homogenous in colour and pattern. It is uncommon to see individual vessels within these areas, as capillaries in the normal eye are too fine to be seen on colour images or by direct examination of the retina.

It is however quite normal and common to see variously sized predominantly greenish- or darker-coloured striations within the areas between major vessels. These are vessels of the underlying major choroidal circulation, visible as indistinct 'shapes' through the pigment epithelium and retina. The lighter skinned the patient, and hence the lighter the retinal pigment epithelium, the more apparent can be the choroidal vessels when viewing the retina. Albino and even blond patients can have extremely apparent choroidal vessels. It tends not to be possible to see the choroidal vessels of dark-skinned and heavily pigmented individuals. Very highly myopic patients usually have thin retinae and RPE and, in these cases, it is sometimes possible to actually see the white sclera.

Historically, permanent photographic recording of retinal appearance was carried out by means of colour transparency ('diapositive') films. During the late 1990s and into the twenty-first century, colour film recording has been almost if not entirely replaced by digital image recording. Among the many advantages of digital imaging (discussions on which are largely beyond the remit of this publication), a most significant aspect relates to the ability to simply select and view individual colour 'channels' of the image. This allows examination of the 'normal' retinal appearance across differential 'slices' of the colour spectrum generated by the retinal camera illumination flash source and recorded by the digital imaging sensor. As such, the red-free or green images which potentially provide much useful additional information are routinely available without requiring additional patient imaging. A fuller discussion on this, including normal fluorescein and normal OCT appearance, is covered in Chapter 5 on Imaging Techniques in Diabetic Retinopathy.

PRACTICE POINTS

The uniqueness of appearance and layout of each individual's retinal vasculature is both a blessing and a curse. While it certainly affords opportunities for high-level biometric security systems based on retinal vascular pattern analysis, it also indicates the immensely wide range of parameters which must be taken into account when defining an eye as being normal. As such, more correctly, the term 'normal eye' (or patient) should be considered to be that which is not displaying or manifesting the particular characteristic or disease under study or investigation.

7 Diabetic macular oedema

Ahmed Sallam[1] & Abdallah A. Ellabban[2]

[1]University of Arkansas for Medical Sciences, USA
[2]Suez Canal University, Egypt

DIABETIC MACULOPATHY

Diabetic maculopathy may be classified into: focal (subdivided into focal exudates and focal/multifocal oedema); diffuse; and ischaemic types.

In focal maculopathy (Fig. 7.1) focal leakage tends to occur from microaneurysms, often with extravascular lipoprotein in a circinate pattern around the focal leakage[1].

In the diffuse variety (Fig. 7.2) there is a generalised breakdown of the blood-retina barrier and profuse early leakage from the entire capillary bed of the posterior pole[2], often accompanied by cystoid macular changes[1]. As well as considering macular treatment, it is important to consider correction of systemic abnormalities such as hypertension and severe fluid retention.

In ischaemic maculopathy (Fig. 7.3), enlargement of the foveal avascular zone (FAZ) due to capillary closure is found but may not have any visual consequences. However, extensive capillary and arteriolar closure is more serious and is more commonly associated with visual loss. The ischaemic areas appear hypofluorescent with capillary drop-out in fluorescein angiography and may show late leakage. Severe ischaemic maculopathy (Fig. 7.4) is often suspected when the level of vision loss does not correlate with the extent of DMO. Foveal ischaemia may also be associated with visual field defects, reduction in contrast sensitivity and poor functional response to intravitreal pharmacotherapy despite anatomical improvements[3-7]. Macular ischaemia usually correlates with the severity and duration of hyperglycaemia and is more common in patients with systemic circulatory disturbances, particularly hypertension[8-10]. Fluorescein angiography is the standard method for evaluation of macular ischaemia; however, OCT may depict some changes as photoreceptor outer segment shortening, inner segment ellipsoid band disruption and thinning of the retinal nerve fibre layer[11,12].

OPTICAL COHERENCE TOMOGRAPHY

The development of optical coherence tomography (OCT) has been described in detail in Chapter 5 on imaging techniques. Nowadays, optical coherence tomography is an indispensable tool for the assessment and monitoring of patients with diabetic macular oedema in clinical practice, providing unprecedented information on retinal thickness and detailed anatomy of the retinal layers.

In early stages, DMO appears as a reduction of the reflectivity of the retinal layers and increased retinal thickness on OCT. Later, intraretinal fluid accumulates into more well-defined spaces mainly located in the outer plexiform, inner nuclear layer, foveal and parafoveal region. The arrangement of the cystoid spaces is mainly governed by the orientation of Muller cell fibres. The fluid may sometimes leak into the subretinal space, leading to localised subretinal serous detachment.

Fluid accumulation in DMO may take one of several morphologic patterns on OCT although, in many cases, a combination of more than one pattern exists[13,14]: (1) diffuse (sponge-like) retinal thickening, characterised by diffuse retinal swelling with low internal reflectivity (Fig. 7.5); (2) cystoid macular oedema with multiple cystoid spaces (Fig. 7.6), mainly in the fovea and parafoveal regions, separated by highly reflective septa; (3) subfoveal serous detachment (Fig. 7.7), with accumulation of a cuff of subretinal fluid under the detached neurosensory retina; or (4) foveal traction by antero-posterior vitreomacular traction (Fig. 7.8), taught posterior hyaloid or epiretinal membrane (Fig. 7.9).

The morphological pattern of oedema on OCT may influence the visual outcome after treatment of DMO[15-17]. It is also important to identify eyes with significant tractional component, as these could require surgical intervention. Examples are shown in Figures 7.8 and 7.9.

A Practical Manual of Diabetic Retinopathy Management, Second Edition.
Edited by Peter Scanlon, Ahmed Sallam, and Peter van Wijngaarden.
© 2017 John Wiley & Sons Ltd. Published 2017 by John Wiley & Sons Ltd.
Companion Website: www.wiley.com/go/scanlon/diabetic_retinopathy

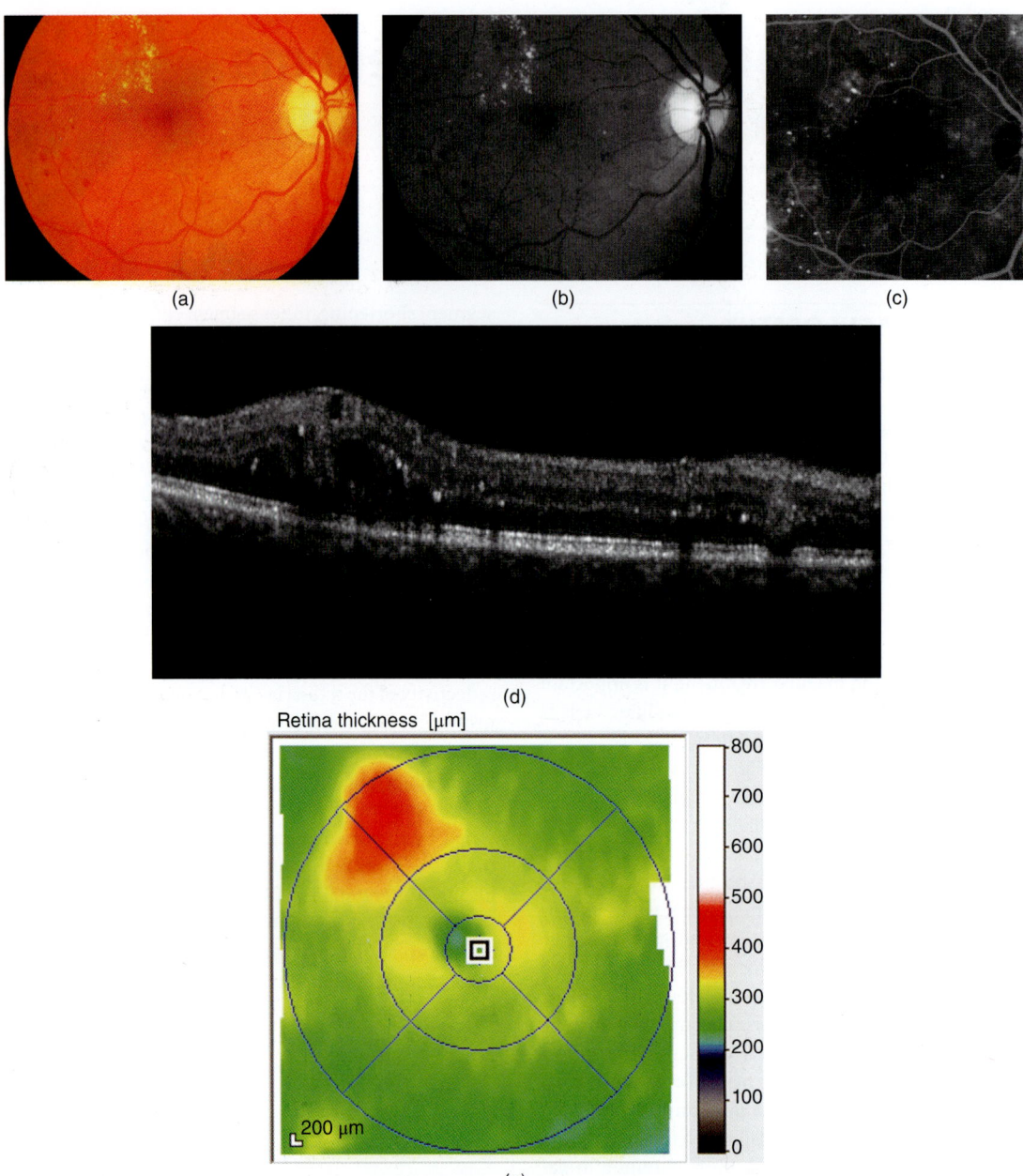

Fig. 7.1 Focal maculopathy. (a) Colour fundus and (b) red-free showing focal leakage and hard exudates superiotemporal to the fovea. (c) Fluorescein angiography, late phase, depicting some leaking microaneurysms superiotemporal to the fovea. (d) OCT scan through the area of leakage showing focal retinal thickening. (e) Macular thickness map shows only localised retinal thickening.

Diabetic macular oedema

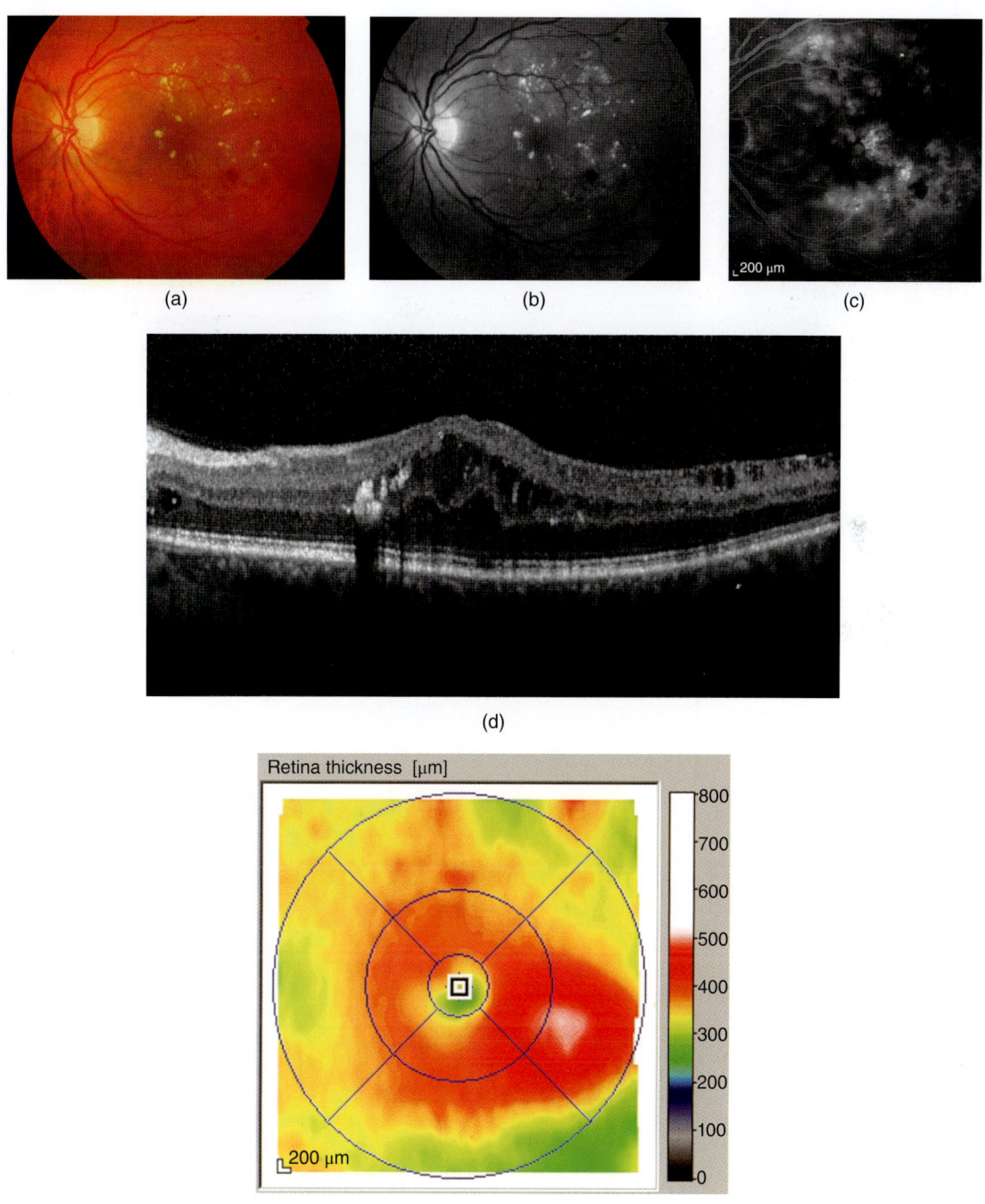

Fig. 7.2 Diffuse maculopathy. (a) Colour fundus and (b) red-free showing diffuse maculopathy. (c) Fluorescein angiography depicting multiple areas of leakage. (d) OCT scan through the fovea showing focal diffuse retinal thickening. (e) Macular thickness map shows diffuse oedema.

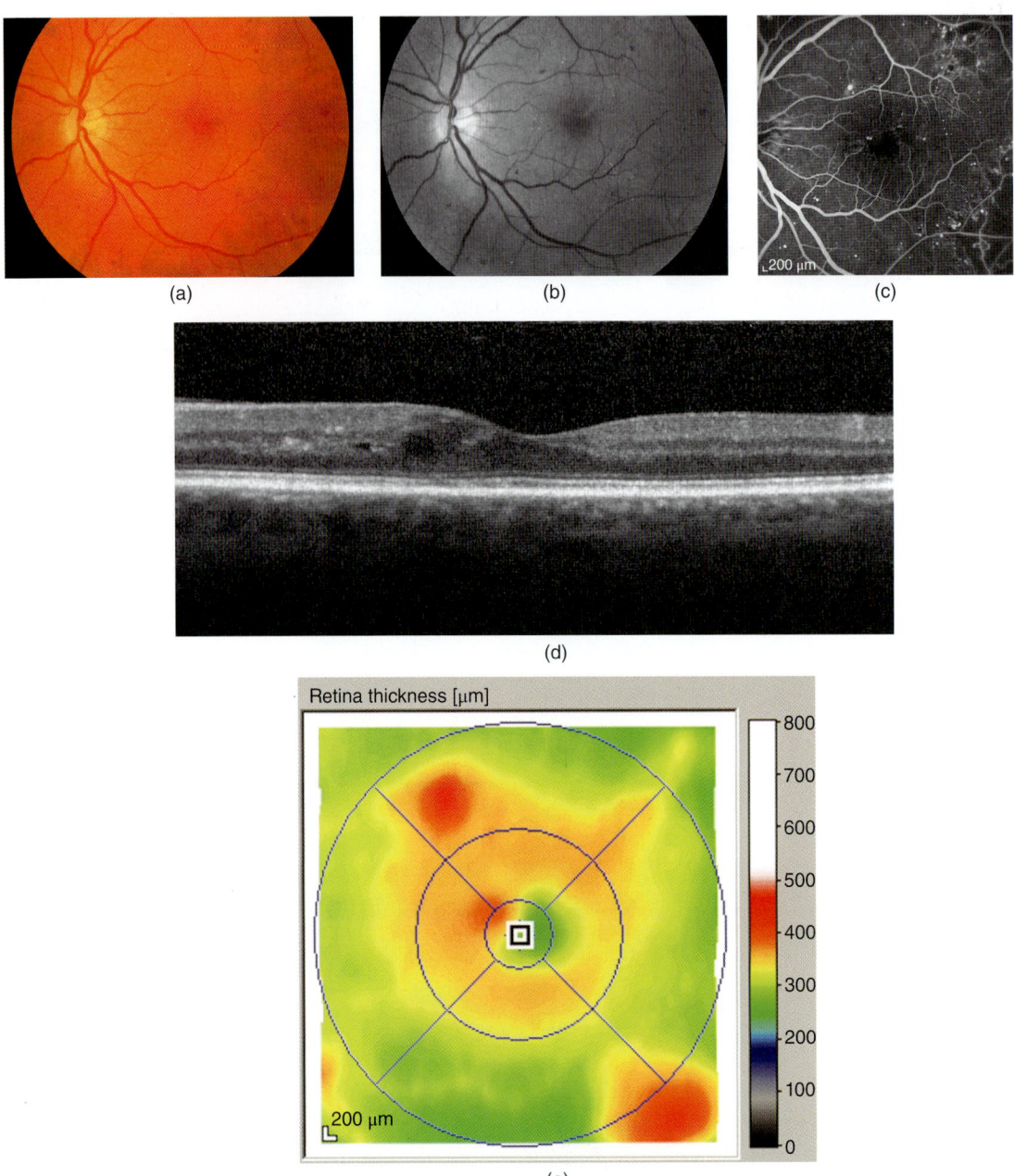

Fig. 7.3 Ischaemic DMO. (a) Colour fundus and (b) red-free showing minimal mid-diabetic changes at the macula. (c) Fluorescein angiography, early phase, depicting ischaemic changes with widening of the foveal avascular zone, pruning of perifoveal vessels and capillary drop-out at the fovea. There are multiple areas of capillary drop-out temporal to the fovea. (d) OCT scan through the fovea showing only mild oedema. (e) Macular thickness map shows only minimal retinal thickening.

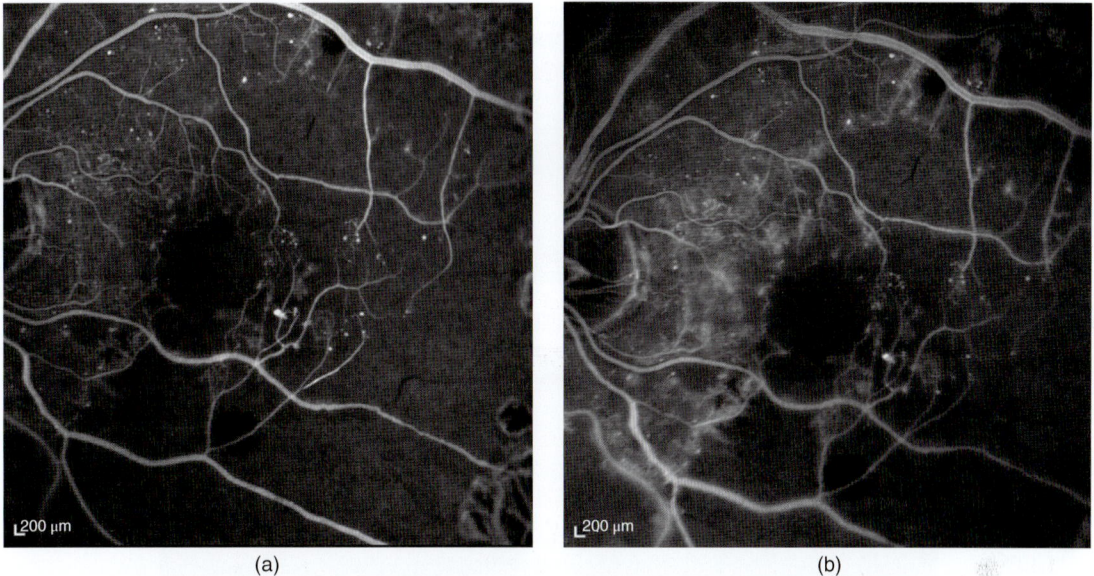

Fig. 7.4 Severe ischaemic maculopathy. Fluorescein angiography left eye (a) 54 s and (b) 4 min 20 s showing marked capillary drop-outs at the macula and irregular foveal avascular zone in a patient with markedly uncontrolled diabetes and hypertension.

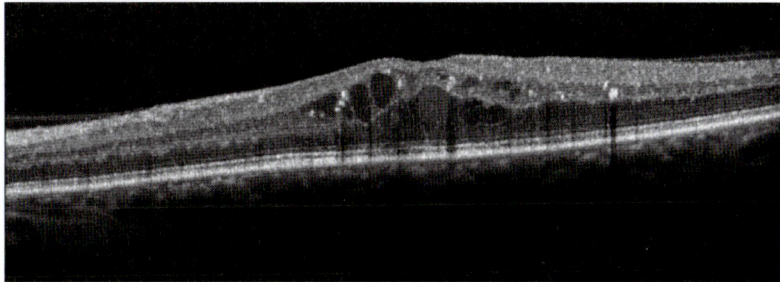

Fig. 7.5 Diffuse (sponge-like) retinal thickening.

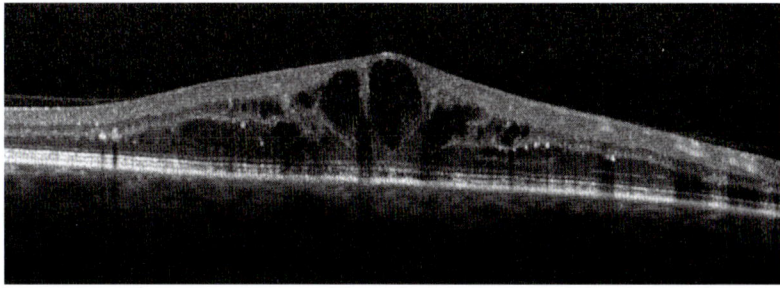

Fig. 7.6 Cystoid macular oedema.

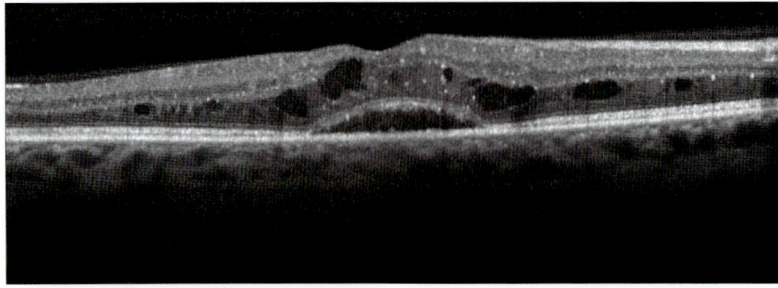

Fig. 7.7 Subfoveal serous detachment (in addition to cystic inner and outer retinal spaces).

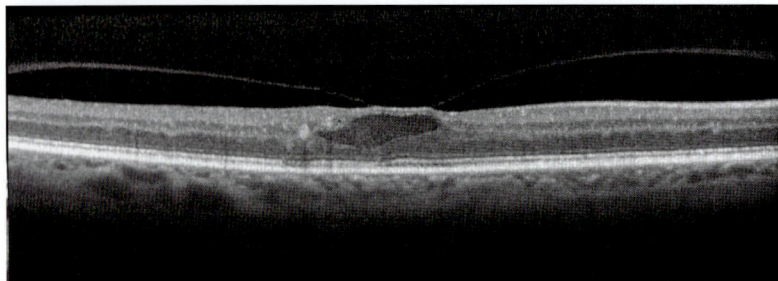

Fig. 7.8 Foveal traction due to antero-posterior vitreomacular traction.

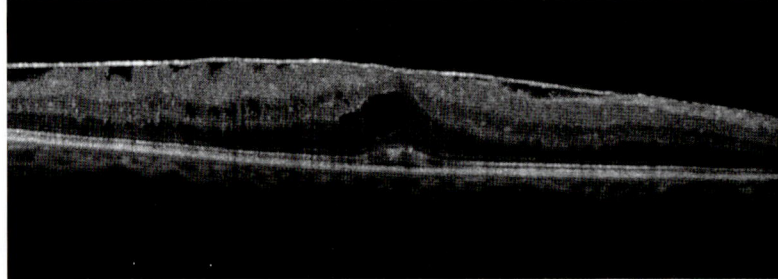

Fig. 7.9 Foveal traction due to epiretinal membrane.

TREATMENT OF ASSOCIATED RISK FACTORS

Systemic hypertension

The importance of good control of blood pressure, blood glucose and blood lipid on the progression of diabetic retinopathy is explained in Chapter 2.

> **Case History 7.1: Hypertension in diabetic maculopathy**
>
> A 39-year-old man (BMI 21) presented on an emergency admission under the physicians with symptoms of tiredness, weight loss and blurring of vision. On admission his blood glucose was 20.7, HbA1c 13.7 and B/P 220/109. He gave a 1-year history of symptoms including neuropathic symptoms in his feet, which made it more likely that he had type 2 diabetes. He had a strong family history of diabetes in his father, maternal grandmother and two maternal uncles. He was commenced on insulin during this admission. He was seen in the eye department when his visual acuity was found to be right 6/36 (20/180) and left 6/18 (20/60). Red-free photographs (Fig. 7.10a and b) and a fluorescein angiogram (Fig. 7.10c–i) show haemorrhages and extensive signs of ischaemia in both macular areas, but also ischaemic signs in the peripheral retinal areas, particularly the left nasal retina where signs of severe intraretinal microvascular abnormality (IRMA) are shown.

Diabetic macular oedema

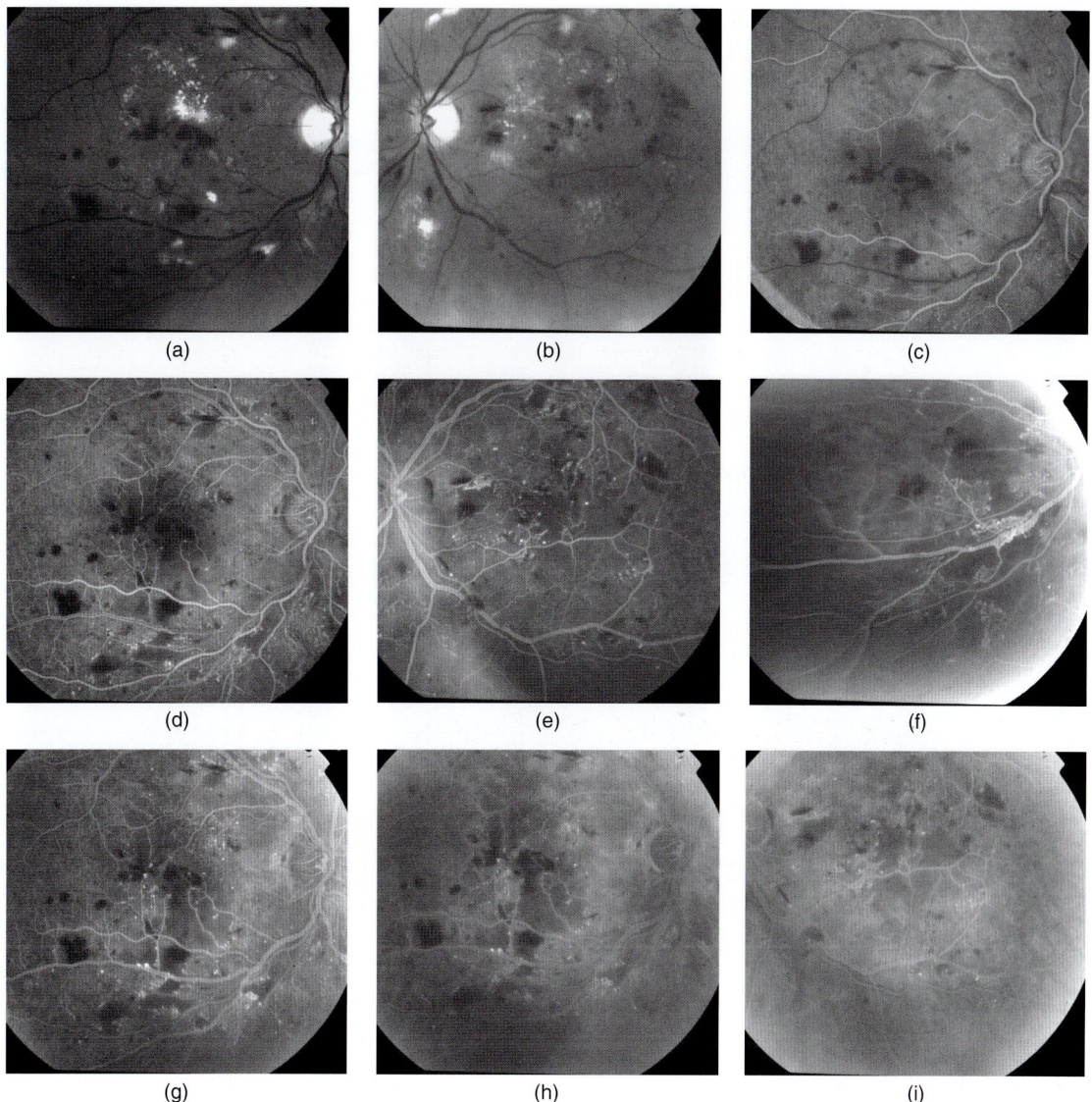

Fig. 7.10 (a) Right and (b) left macula red-free. Flourescein right macula (c) 15 s; (d) 19 s; and (e) 40 s. (f) Fluorescein left nasal 1 min 9 s. Fluorescein right macula (g) 1 min 16 s and (h) 4 min 4 s. (i) Fluorescein left macula 4 min 13 s. Year 4: (j) colour right macula; (k) colour left macula; (l) venous phase fluorescein right macula; and (m) colour venous phase fluorescein left macula.

The hypertension was treated with Ramipril 10 mg daily, and Lacidipine 4 mg, Furosemide 20 mg and Dixasocin MR 4 mg were subsequently added. His other medication was Actrapid 10 + 10 + 12, Insulatard 18, Simvastatin 40 mg and Aspirin 75 mg.

Six months after presentation, his BP had improved to 122/75 and HbA1c to 6.8, but his VA had remained the same in his right eye at 6/36 (20/120) and deteriorated in his left to 6/60 (20/200). A decision was made to treat both eyes with panretinal photocoagulation. The left eye was treated first with 2518 burns of 350 micron size, power 250–290 mW, duration 0.1 s, Transequator lens (magnification factor 1.44), argon laser. The right eye was then treated with 2331 burns of 350 micron size, power 210–260 mW, duration 0.1 s, Transequator lens (magnification factor 1.44), argon laser.

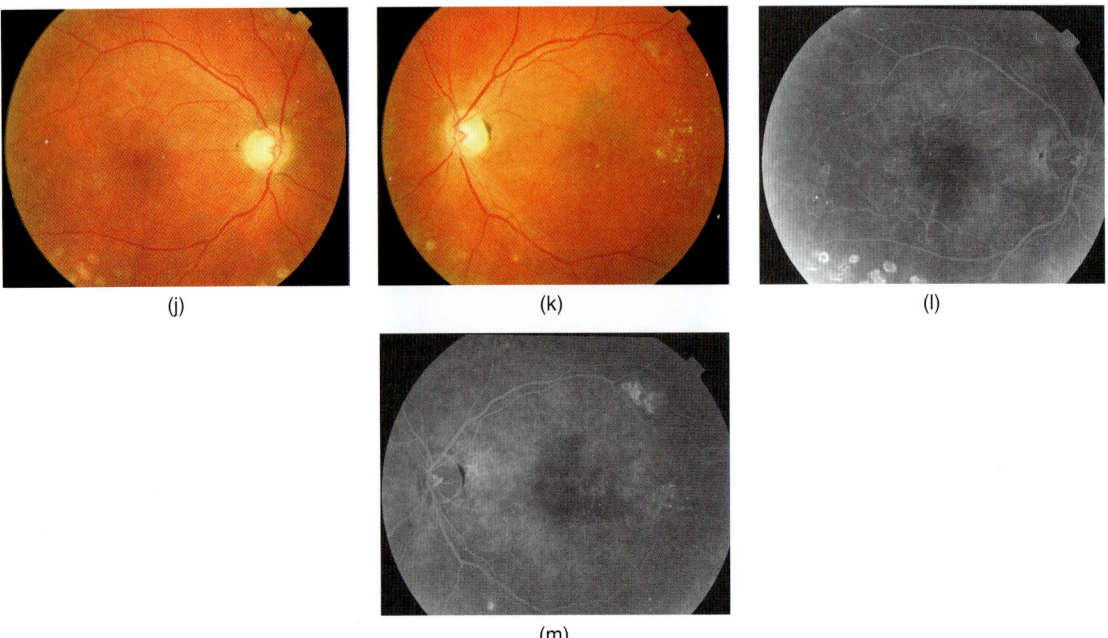

(j)   (k)   (l)

(m)

Fig. 7.10 *Continued*

One year after presentation, a small area of leakage in the left macular area was treated with 16 burns, 100 micron size, 230 mW, 0.1 s, Area centralis lens, argon laser. 18 months after presentation the VA had improved to right 6/18 (20/60) and left 6/36 (20/120). Two years after presentation, the VA had improved to right 6/12 (20/40) and left 6/24 (20/80). Three years after presentation, the VA had improved to right 6/9 (20/30) and left 6/18 (20/60). Four years after presentation, the VA had improved to right 6/9 (20/30) and left 6/12 (20/40). The photographs in Figure 7.10j–m were taken at the year 4 visit.

We believe that the primary reason for the improvement in appearance of the macular areas and the improvement in VA was control of the BP. BP readings over this 4-year period were: 122/75, 165/72, 132/80 and 154/87. His HbA1c results were 6.7, 7.4, 6.6 and 6.8.

Current attempts to manage patients with diabetic maculopathy are aimed at preserving vision and reducing progression of the disease by appropriate management of glucose, blood pressure, weight and lipids, and laser treatment at the appropriate stage in the disease process. Ongoing studies on the use of ACE inhibitors, angiotensin receptor blockers, fenofibrate and PKC inhibitors are discussed in Chapter 17 on future advances.

LASER FOR DIABETIC MACULAR OEDEMA

While previously considered as first-line treatment of diabetic macular oedema, macular laser treatment has been currently surpassed by anti-VEGF therapy.

Spalter[18] first described the photocoagulation of circinate maculopathy in diabetic retinopathy in 1971 and subsequent reports appeared by Whitelocke et al.[19] in 1979 and a British Multicentre Study Group[20] in 1983. However, it was in 1985 that the Early Treatment Diabetic Retinopathy Study[21] (ETDRS) demonstrated that focal (direct/grid) laser photocoagulation reduces moderate vision loss caused by diabetic macular oedema (DME) by 50% or more and described 'clinically significant macular oedema', which defined the parameters for treatment.

The ETDRS[21] reported the results of 754 eyes that were randomly assigned to focal argon laser and 1490 eyes to deferral, which showed that focal photocoagulation of 'clinically significant' diabetic macular oedema (CSMO) substantially reduced the risk of visual loss. Clinically significant macular oedema was defined in a further report from the ETDRS[22] study group as follows:

1. thickening of the retina at or within 500 microns of the centre of the macula;

2. hard exudates at or within 500 microns of the centre of the fovea, if associated with thickening of the adjacent retina (not residual hard exudates remaining after disappearance of retinal thickening); and
3. a zone or zones of retinal thickening 1 disc area or larger, any part of which is within one disc diameter (1DD) of the centre of the macula.

Focal and grid treatment were used singly or in combination as was considered appropriate for each treated eye, and were not compared with one another. Focal treatment was recommended for focal lesions located between 500 and 3000 microns from the centre of the macula and believed to be causing retinal thickening or hard exudates.

The majority of focally treated lesions were microaneurysms, treated with 50–100 micron burns of moderate intensity, preferably to produce a whitening or darkening of the larger microaneurysms ($\geq$40 microns) or mild to moderate whitening of the adjacent retinal for smaller microaneurysms (<40 microns), at 0.05–0.1 s duration.

Grid treatment was recommended for areas of thickened retina that showed diffuse fluorescein leakage or capillary drop-out. Burns of 50–200 micron spot size were placed one burn width apart in areas of intense leakage and more widely spaced in areas of less intense leakage. Grid treatment was not recommended within 500 microns of the centre of the macula or within 500 microns of the disc margin, but could be placed in the papillomacular bundle. Grid treatment could extend in all directions up to two disc diameters from the centre of the macula.

Follow-up treatment was recommended for 6 weeks later, to determine whether obvious treatable lesions had been missed during the initial treatment, and at subsequent 4-month intervals if macular oedema persisted.

ETDRS results

Among eyes with clinically significant macular oedema not involving the centre of the macula, approximately 8% of the control group eyes had visual loss at the 1 year visit and 16% at the 2 year visit. Treatment reduced these percentages to 1% and 6%, respectively. When the centre of the macula was involved visual loss was more frequent, reaching 33% in the control group after 3 years. Treatment reduced this frequency by approximately 60% to 13%.

After 5 years of this 9-year study, the accumulating data showed that focal photocoagulation was effective in reducing moderate visual loss. The protocol was therefore changed to allow focal photocoagulation for clinically significant macular oedema whenever it occurred. Moderate visual loss was defined as the loss of 15 or more letters between baseline and follow-up visit, equivalent to doubling of the visual angle.

The 'early worsening' phenomenon

In 1998 the Diabetes Control and Complications Trial[23] (DCCT) described the effect of early worsening of diabetic retinopathy at the 6- and/or 12-month visit in 13.1% of 711 patients assigned to intensive treatment. Early worsening led to clinically significant macular oedema in three patients in the DCCT. The most important risk factors for early worsening were higher haemoglobin A1c level at screening and reduction of this level during the first 6 months after randomisation.

> **Case History 7.2: The early worsening phenomenon soon after commencing insulin treatment**
>
> This man with type 2 diabetes (BMI 39) was diagnosed at the age of 41 years. He was initially treated with diet and his blood glucose levels were between 6 and 10 in the first 2 years, but in the subsequent 5 years these were recorded at levels of 10–12 mmol/L and he was therefore started on Glibenclamide 2.5 mg o.d. at the age of 48 years. Over the next 13 years the Glibenclamide was gradually increased to 15 mg and at the age of 51 years Metformin 500 mg b.d. was added. Six months later, his blood glucose was varying over 10–14 mmol/L during the day, the HbA1c was 10.5, a foot ulcer had formed on his right foot and a decision was made to commence insulin, stop the Glibenclamide and continue the Metformin. At that time, he had had some laser treatment for circinate areas of maculopathy but the VA was 6/9 before commencement of insulin. Within a few days of starting insulin VA dropped to rightt 6/18 and left 6/24 and slit-lamp biomicroscopy confirmed that both macular areas had developed a cystoid type of macular oedema. The HbA1c improved over the next 3 months to a reading of 7.5 and has subsequently remained at a level below 8.5. Red-free photos taken at the time are shown in Figure 7.11a and b.
>
> The vision gradually returned to a level of 6/9 (20/30) in each eye over the next 7 months as the cystoid macular oedema subsequently resolved spontaneously. Eighteen months later, NVD were developing at both discs as shown in Figure 7.11c and d.
>
> Despite panretinal photocoagulation to both eyes, vitrectomies were required for both eyes at the age of 66 years. Following the vitrectomies, the visual acuities have stabilised at right 6/9 (20/30) and left 6/60 (20/200). The left vision is reduced due to an ischaemic maculopathy. Colour photos are shown in Figure 7.11e and f.

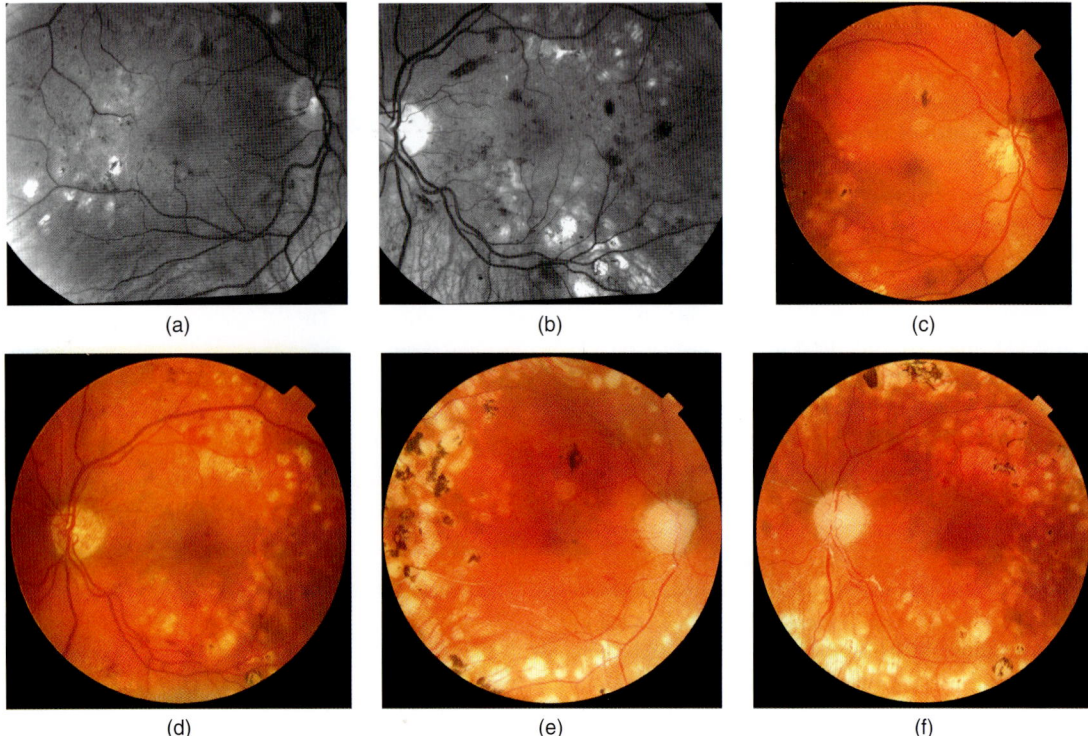

Fig. 7.11 Red-free image at 3 months of (a) right macula and disc and (b) left macula and disc. Colour image at 18 months of (c) the right macula and disc and (d) left macula and disc, showing the development of new vessels at the disc (NVD). Colour image of the (e) right and (f) left macula post-vitrectomy.

The key point in this case history is that control of glycaemia has been shown to be linked to microvascular complications. If a person has had poor control for years and is placed on insulin to control the glycaemia there is a risk of early worsening of VA, particularly due to an effect on the macular area. However, the long-term benefits outweigh any short-term disadvantages of improving control. Good communication between the diabetologist and ophthalmologist is essential for this group of patients.

Case History 7.3: Focal maculopathy left eye

This 25-year-old man with type 1 diabetes (BMI 25) from the age of 3 years was referred from the retinal screening service. His HbA1c levels had improved from 10.8 to 7.8 over the previous 5 years and his BP was normal at levels averaging 133/67. He was found to have clinically significant macular oedema in his left eye as shown in the colour and red-free photographs (Fig. 7.12a). A colour and red-free photograph taken within a few minutes of the laser treatment (Fig. 7.12b) shows the pale spots produced by the laser from blanching of the retina. A colour and red-free photograph taken 4 months after the laser treatment (Fig. 7.12c) shows clearing of the exudates and the clinically significant macular oedema.

Case History 7.4: Diffuse maculopathy

This 39-year-old man with type 2 diabetes (BMI 25) for 10 years controlled on insulin presented with a maculopathy in his right eye and VA of 6/9 (20/30) (Fig. 7.13a). Treatment was given to the right macular area of right 44 burns 100 micron size, 180 mW, 0.1 s using an Area Centralis lens and argon laser. This resulted in some initial clearing in the right macular area but there was a subsequent increase in leakage; Figure 7.13b was taken 7 months later and a drop in his right VA to 6/18 (20/60) was observed.

Treatment was given to the right macular area of right 45 burns 100 micron size, 170 mW, 0.1 s using an Area Centralis lens and argon laser, and subsequently treatment

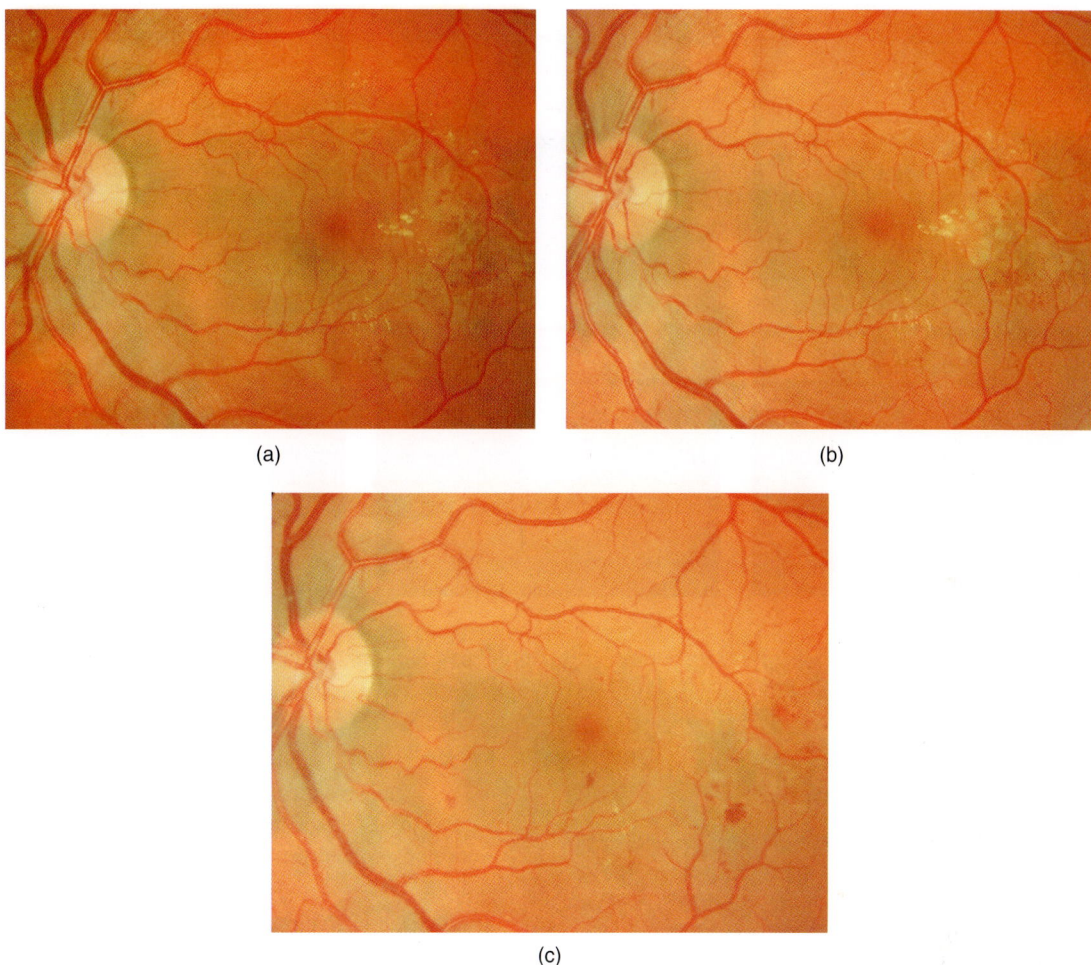

Fig. 7.12 Left macula colour (a) pre-laser, (b) immediately post-laser and (c) 4 months post-laser.

was given to the right macular area of right 27 burns 100 micron size, 220 mW, 0.1 s using an Area Centralis lens and argon laser. This resulted in an improvement in VA to 6/12 (20/40) and clearing of much of the exudates and thickening as shown in Figure 7.13c–e, and this improvement was maintained 8 years after the initial presentation (Fig. 7.13f).

During the last 9 years of laser treatment, his HbA1c has fluctuated between 8.5 and 9.5 with his most recent result being 8.9. His BP has been difficult to control, running at 152/88 at the beginning of the period and the most recent recording is 167/71. His Cholesterol is 3.6 and Ch:HDL ratio 4.5.

Mechanisms of action of conventional laser for macular oedema

The effectiveness of focal laser treatment may be partly due to the closure of leaky microaneurysms, but the specific mechanisms by which focal photocoagulation reduces macular oedema is not known. Studies have shown histopathological changes[24] and biochemical changes[25,26], which have been suggested as mechanisms for improvement in macular oedema. Some investigators have suggested alternative mechanisms for clearance of the oedema, such as the application of Starling's law and improved oxygenation[27].

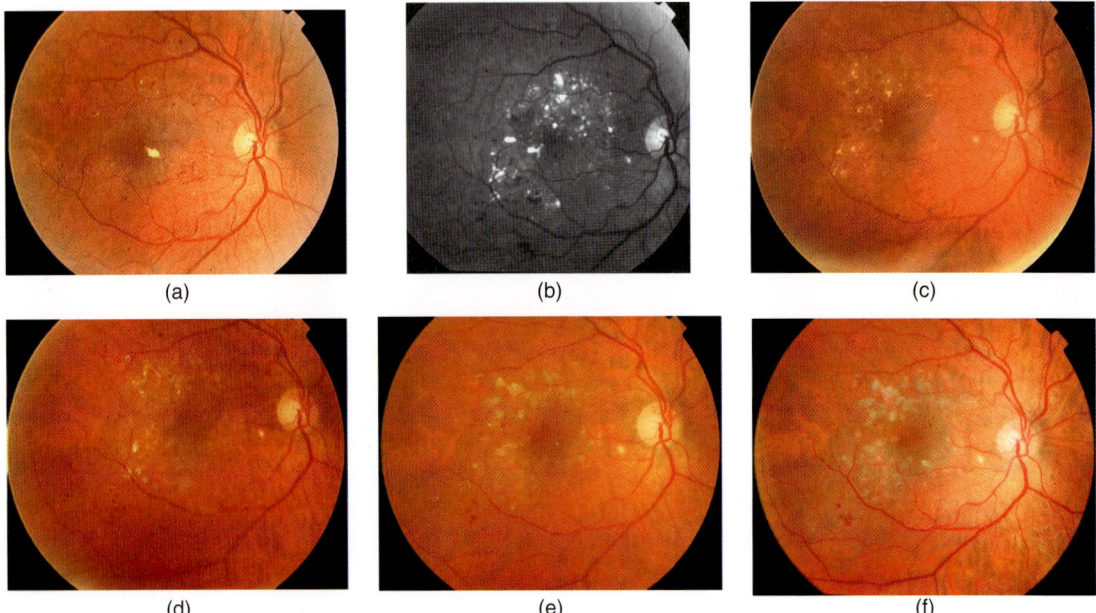

Fig. 7.13 Right macular area: (a) colour photo at presentation; (b) red-free image 7 months after presentation; and colour photo (c) 10 months, (d) 19 months, (e) 27 months and (f) 8 years after presentation.

Limitations and adverse effects of macular laser treatment

The advantages of macular laser have been made clear by the ETDRS, in which laser photocoagulation was shown to halve the risk of moderate visual loss over 3 years. However, only a small percentage of patients (less than 5%) achieved better visual acuity[21]. Macular photocoagulation is also not suitable for foveal involving macular oedema and in eyes with significant foveal ischaemia and foveal avascular zone disruption.

Adverse effects of laser have been principally covered in Chapter 10 on panretinal photocoagulation in the treatment of proliferative diabetic retinopathy. However, potential side-effects specific to macular laser are as follows.

1. *Laser close to the central fovea, resulting in a drop in VA immediately after laser treatment or a visible scotoma or laser scars increasing in size over time to involve a more central area of fovea than the original lasered area.* Laser burns may be associated with para-central scotomas and may become larger than the original spot size[28] and encroach on fixation. In an attempt to reduce adverse effects, many retinal specialists now treat patients using burns that are lighter and less intense than what was originally specified in the ETDRS. In 2005, Bandello et al.[29] reported the results of a prospective randomised pilot clinical trial in which 29 eyes of 24 diabetic patients with mild to moderate non-proliferative diabetic retinopathy (NPDR) and CSMO were randomised to either 'classic' or 'barely visible' green laser. Comparison of reduction of oedema and visual improvement showed no statistical difference between the groups at 12 months. This study suggested that 'light' photocoagulation for CSMO is likely to be effective as 'classic' laser treatment.

2. *Choroidal neovascular membrane developing in an area that has received laser treatment.* This complication is extremely rare and in fact people with diabetic maculopathy do seem to get less choroidal neovascular membranes than one might expect.

Macular laser for DMO is likely to continue to be part of the management of DMO in a selected subset of patients with non-centre-involving macular oedema. This would be of particular importance in the developing world, due to the lower cost of laser treatment and the less intensive management requirements compared to newer intravitreal therapeutics. Focal/grid laser could also be used in conjunction with anti-VEGF therapy, as will be described in the section 'Anti-vascular endothelial growth factor treatment'.

The pattern argon laser

Optimedia Corporation introduced the PASCAL (pattern scan laser) photocoagulator in June 2006, which is a frequency-doubled Nd: YAG diode-pumped solid-state laser producing a wavelength of 532 nm. The operator can select different arcs, circular grid patterns or sectors of grids for treatment, or use a rectangular array. With the patterned scanning laser photocoagulation, the laser pulse time can be reduced from 100 ms to just 10–30 ms and automated multiple spots are produced with each depression of the foot pedal. However, higher power is required where burns of shorter duration are applied.

The main advantage of the PASCAL laser when used for macular treatment over conventional long-pulse laser is that the short-pulse durations may result in less destruction to the outer retina because of reduced axial and lateral thermal spread[30]. Results of studies using standard or lower fluency 'barely visible' short-pulse laser demonstrated comparable clinical effectiveness in reduction of macular oedema compared to conventional ETDRS laser[30,31].

The authors would advise caution in using the grid patterns with four concentric rings in one treatment session, as this could potentially drop vision in a macula that has extensive capillary or arteriolar closure and had previously maintained a reasonable visual acuity or produce annoying scotomata, as patients found in the study by Olk[32].

Subthreshold micro-pulse laser photocoagulation

The term 'subthreshold' refers to photocoagulation that does not produce visible intraretinal damage or scarring either during or after treatment. In fact, burns are undetectable not only by clinical examination, but also on fluorescein angiography and fundus autofluorescence[33].

The subthreshold laser imparts more tissue-sparing treatment in order to decrease the collateral retinal tissue damage observed with standard fluency conventional and even short-pulse macular laser. In this technique, micropulse diode laser (810 nm) treatment is delivered as a train of short pulses, allowing the tissue temperature to cool between pulses. The subthreshold laser treatment is thought to be selectively absorbed by the retinal pigment epithelium with no or minimal effect on the outer retinal layers. Each laser pulse has an on and off duration and the ratio between them is defined as the 'duty cycle'. The duty cycle can be controlled and the lower the duty cycle, the lower the thermal effect in tissues. The laser parameters can be titrated to achieve the desired subthreshold level.

Similar to conventional laser, the mechanism of subthreshold micropulse laser (SMPL) is not completely understood. It is speculated that SMPL produces its effect by photostimulation of the retina pigment epithelium pump, hence improving intraretinal fluid resorption[34-36]. There is some evidence to suggest that SMPL may have comparable clinical effectiveness to modified ETDRS macular laser, with better preservation of retinal functions[34-40].

Vujosevic et al.[35] conducted a prospective randomised clinical trial including 62 eyes randomised to SMPL versus modified ETDRS grid. They reported improved retinal sensitivity in the central 4° and 12° in the SMPL group as compared to worsening in the modified ETDRS laser group. There was no significant difference between both groups in terms of BCVA or central retinal thickness ($P=0.48$ and $P=0.29$, respectively).

Sivaprasad et al.[39] reported the 3-year outcome of 25 eyes treated by SMPL. They reported that BCVA stabilised or improved in 84% by the end of first year and 92% maintained their vision by the third year. Ohkoshi and Yamaguchi[40] treated 43 eyes with CSMO and CRT <600 μm with SMPL and BCVA was improved or at least maintained within 0.2 LogMAR for 12 months in 94.7% of their patients.

The effect of SMPL may be related to the severity of macular oedema. Mansouri et al.[41] found that SDMP is more effective in treating mild to moderate DMO (CRT <400 μm) and less effective if CRT >400 μm.

Micropulse laser can be delivered directly over areas of oedema, including the central fovea. The effect of the laser is slow and may require several months to obtain the desired result, but appears to be longer lasting. While the technique has its proponents, the technique does have the disadvantage that there is no ophthalmoscopically visible endpoint to confirm the effect of treatment.

Navigating laser treatment

Navigating laser treatment (Navilas) is a new technology for delivering retinal laser with integrated imaging and navigation systems. Similar to PASCAL, this technology is capable of delivering both conventional, long-pulse and short-pulse laser for macular treatment in different patterns. The built-in camera system provides a 50° view of the posterior pole capturing true-colour, infrared and fluorescein angiography images. The system can also import external images such as OCT maps or ICG images to add relevant diagnostic information. Treatment can be pre-planned by graphically designating future treatment areas on the selected images. Laser treatment is then delivered onto the patient's retina by overlaying prepositioned points on the live fundus image. The eye-tracking system stabilises the position of the aiming beam and the laser onto the retina to take into account eye movements during treatment. The Navilas system also documents laser spots and patterns delivered to the retina, which can help ensure complete treatment and avoid over-treating. This is of significant benefit when using subthreshold laser where laser spots are invisible during and even long term after treatment. Treatment accuracy in DMO using Navilas was found to be superior to conventional laser, with a microaneurysm hit rate of more than 90% as compared to 72% with conventional laser[42].

ANTI-VASCULAR ENDOTHELIAL GROWTH FACTOR TREATMENT

Intravitreal pharmacotherapy based on VEGF inhibition is currently the mainstay of treatment for DMO. In eyes of patients with diabetes, chronic hyperglycaemia results in oxidative damage to the vascular endothelial cell. The ensuing ischaemia leads to overexpression of a number of growth factors, including VEGF as well as insulin-like growth factor-1, angiopoeitin-1 and -2, stromal-derived factor-1, fibroblast growth factor-2 and tumor necrosis factor[26]. Synergistically, these growth factors mediate angiogenesis, protease production, endothelial cell proliferation, migration and neovascularization. VEGF also increases vascular permeability by relaxing endothelial cell junctions. While blockade of all involved growth factors be necessary to completely suppress the detrimental effects of ischaemia and vascular leakage, isolated blockade of VEGF was shown to have significant beneficial effects on DMO[27,28].

Currently, there are four anti-VEGF intravitreal treatments being used in clinical practice: pegaptanib, ranibizumab, bevacizumab and aflibercept.

Pegaptanib sodium

Pegaptanib sodium (Macugen®, Eyetech Pharmaceuticals, Melville, NY) is an anti-VEGF aptamer that blocks the effects of VEGF165, one isoform of the VEGF family of molecules. Pegaptanib is one of the earliest anti-VEGF inhibitors trialled in clinical studies for both AMD and DMO. However, because of limited clinical effectiveness compared to other anti-VEGF agents, this drug is much less used nowadays in clinical practice[43,44].

Ranibizumab

Ranibizumab (Lucentis™, Genentech, San Francisco, CA) is an antibody fragment that also binds to and blocks the effects of VEGF. Unlike pegaptanib, ranibizumab binds and inhibits all isoforms of VEGF. Ranibizumab use in DMO is approved by the FDA (0.3 mg dose) and in Europe (0.5 mg dose). In the UK, The National Institute for Health and Care Excellence (NICE) has also recommended ranibizumab as an option for treating visual impairment due to DMO only if associated with a central retinal thickness of at least 400 μm. Ranibizumab has consistently been shown to be effective in treating DMO by a series of phase 2 and phase 3 randomised clinical trials:

The study on 'Safety and efficacy of ranibizumab in diabetic macular edema' (RESOLVE) is a phase-2, placebo-controlled, randomised, multicentre study[45]. In this study, 151 patients were randomised to ranibizumab monotherapy at a dose of 0.3 mg or 0.5 mg or sham treatment. Rescue laser photocoagulation treatment was offered with persistent disease activity after 3 months. Patients received an initial treatment of 3 consecutive monthly injections and were followed monthly with an as-necessary regimen (prn) from month 3 to month 12. At month 12, a mean increase in BCVA of 11.8 letters was achieved in the 0.3 mg group and 8.8 letters in the 0.5 mg group, as compared to a reduction in BCVA of 1.4 letters in the sham group.

In the RESTORE study, a phase-3, randomised, multicentre study, 345 patients were randomised to either 0.5 mg ranibizumab, 0.5 mg ranibizumab plus active laser, or active laser. Ranibizumab treatment was administered as required after three initial loading injections and laser was applied at day 1 and repeated as needed[46]. At months 12, mean change in BCVA was +6.1 letters in the ranibizumab monotherapy group, +5.9 letters in the group receiving combination therapy with ranibizumab and laser and +0.8 letters in the laser alone group. In year 2 and 3 extension studies, laser patients were crossed over to ranibizumab resulting in gradual improvement of vision to +5.4 letters in this cohort at year 2 (compared to +7.9 for ranibizumab monotherapy; +6.7 for ranibizumab and laser) and +6 letters at year 3 (compared to +8 for ranibizumab monotherapy; +6.7 for ranibizumab and laser)[47,48].

RIDE and RISE studies are two identically designed, parallel, double-blind, 3-year clinical trials which were placebo-treatment–controlled for 24 months[49]. A total of 759 patients were randomised into three groups to receive rigorous monthly treatment with 0.3 mg ranibizumab (n=250), 0.5 mg ranibizumab (n=252) or placebo injection (control group, n=257) with rescue laser being available from month 3. More patients who received ranibizumab were able to read at 15 ETDRS letters (RIDE, 34% in the 0.3 mg group and 46% in 0.5 mg group v. 12% in the control group; RISE, 45% in the 0.3 mg group and 40% in 0.5 mg group v. 18% in the control group). Furthermore, the ranibizumab group had average vision gain exceeding 10 letters at 24 months (RIDE, 10.9 letters in the 0.3 mg group and 12 in 0.5 mg group, v. 2.3 letters in the control group; RISE, 12.5 letters in the 0.3 mg group and 11.9 in 0.5 mg group, v. 2.6 letters in the control group). The data published from the extension study showed that vision improvements observed with ranibizumab treatments at 24 months were maintained with continued treatment through 36 months. However, although the sham cohort was crossed over to ranibizumab, improvements in vision seen at the 36-month time point (4.7 letters in RIDE and 4.3 in RISE) were considerably smaller than those achieved in originally treated ranibizumab groups[50].

Bevacizumab

Bevacizumab (Avastin®, Genentech, San Francisco, CA) is the full antibody from which ranibizumab is derived. Bevacizumab is FDA approved for systemic treatment of metastatic colon cancer, but not for any ophthalmic indications. Its use in conditions such as age-related macular degeneration, diabetic retinopathy and DMO is currently off-label. The use of bevacizumab for the treatment of DMO has been investigated by several studies. The intravitreal bevacizumab or laser therapy in the management of diabetic macular oedema (BOLT) study was a prospective, single-centre, randomised, 2-year study of 80 patients with centre-involving DMO who had received at least one prior macular laser treatment[51]. The study aimed to compare the efficacy of repeated intravitreal bevacizumab against 4 monthly modified macular laser treatments. Results of this study were not different from those obtained with ranibizumab indicating that, compared to laser where most patients did not gain vision, anti-VEGF inhibition by bevacizumab was associated with significant visual gain. The mean change in ETDRS visual acuity at 12 months in the laser group was −0.5 letters, while the bevacizumab group gained a mean of 8 letters during the same period. Similar results were observed at the 24-month time point of the study[52].

Aflibercept

Another anti-VEGF agent that has been currently approved for intravitreal use in DMO is aflibercept (Eylea; Bayer HealthCare, Whippany, NJ). Aflibercept is an engineered fusion protein that consists of key binding domain of VEGF receptors 1 (VEGFR1) and a key binding domain of VEGFR2 fused to Fc portion of the human immunoglobulin-G1. Two dual-domain arms are used for each aflibercept molecule to confer tight binding affinity for both VEGF-A isomers. Aflibercept also binds placental growth factor (PIGF), which is known to potentiate the angiogenic action of VEGF[53].

Aflibercept has a vitreous half-life of 3.63 days, which is longer than that of ranibizumab (2.51 days) but shorter than bevacizumab (6.99 days). Because of its high binding affinity to VEGF receptors, the drug was found to have a long duration of clinical activity than other anti-VEGF therapies available, and can be injected every 8 weeks[53].

Recent data from two controlled, randomised, phase-3 trials (VISTA and VIVID) showed that intravitreal aflibercept use in a dose of 2 mg/0.05 mL was associated with significant superiority in functional and anatomical endpoints over macular laser, with similar efficacy when used monthly (2q4) or bimonthly (2q8). Mean BCVA gains from baseline to week 52 in the aflibercept 2q4 and 2q8 groups v. the laser group were, respectively, 12.5 and 10.7 v. 0.2 letters in VISTA, and 10.5 and 10.7 v. 1.2 letters in VIVID. The 52-week visual and anatomical superiority of aflibercept over laser control was sustained through week 100, with similar efficacy in the 2q4 and 2q8 groups[54,55].

VEGF inhibition represents an important component of current DMO therapy resulting in significant anatomical and visual improvements. Eyes with DMO usually exhibit early visual improvement as anti-VEGF treatment is commenced and continue to improve with repeat treatments, but may require up to 1 year to reach their best visual potential[49]. Once this is achieved, the visual outcome is usually maintained albeit the need for further intravitreal treatment in many patients. Rigorous monthly treatment regimen used in certain studies as RIDE and RISE appears to be associated with superior outcomes when compared to more flexible treatment protocols. However, this regimen is difficult to follow in real-world clinical practice, particularly as DMO patients usual require long-term treatment with a significant proportion (around 40%) requiring treatment in both eyes. Regarding treatment frequency, results of DMO studies using flexible treatment regimens indicate a trend towards reduction of the number of injections with time. In the first year, it is expected that 7–9 anti-VEGF injections would be required, 2–4 in the second year, 1–3 in the third and approximately 1 injection per year in years 4 and 5[56,57].

In general, intravitreal therapy with anti-VEGF therapy has an acceptable ocular side-effects profile. Repeat therapy with intavitreal anti-VEG has, however, been suspected of causing sustained elevation of intraocular pressure and/or an increased risk of glaucoma. A report from the Diabetic Retinopathy Clinical Research network (DRCR.net) found that, in eyes receiving repeat anti-VEGF treatment for DMO, the cumulative probability of sustained IOP elevation requiring treatment by 3 years was 9.5% (compared to 3.4% in the control group; hazard ratio, 2.9; $P=0.01$)[58]. The risk of endophthalmitis with repeat injections also remain a concern, although the risk in patients with diabetes (0.04–0.06/injection) appears to be as low as in those without diabetes[50]. While there have been some variations in published rates of cardiovascular events between studies, results of a meta-analysis of six randomised controlled studies of intravitreal ranibizumab therapy in DMO found no difference in rates between eyes receiving ranibizumab and the control group (relative risk = 0.94, 95% CI 0.25–3.5, $P=0.92$)[59].

There is current evidence to inform the choice of anti-VEGF in DMO: the Diabetic Retinopathy Clinical Research network published the results of Protocol T study comparing the efficacy and safety of anti-VEGF drugs for centre-involving DMO[60]. The multicentre study included 660 patients randomised to receive 2 mg aflibercept ($n=224$), 1.25 mg bevacizumab ($n=218$) or 0.3 mg ranibizumab ($n=218$). All patients were followed up every 4 weeks, with a repeat injection administered if BCVA or OCT improved or worsened.

At 1 year, the mean improvement in letter score vision was 13.3 with aflibercept, 9.7 with bevacizumab and 11.2 with ranibizumab. All three drugs had almost similar ocular and systemic safety profile. However, a subgroup analysis of eyes that had vision of less than 69 letters (approximately ≤6/15) showed that aflibercept was more effective at improving vision: mean improvement was 18.9 with aflibercept, 11.8 with bevacizumab and 14.2 with ranibizumab. At year 2, this difference in visual acuity between aflibercept and ranibizumab that was noted at 1 year in eyes with poor initial vision had decreased and was no longer statistically significant[61].

> ### Case History 7.5: Favourable response after intravitreal anti-VEGF treatment
>
> This 45-year-old woman with type 1 diabetes controlled by insulin had moderate non-proliferative diabetic retinopathy in the right eye. The colour fundus photograph (Fig. 7.14) of the right eye (top, left) and red-free photograph (top, middle) highlight centre-involving DMO. The infrared image depicts the diabetic changes (top, right), with the green line indicating the position of the OCT scan. The foveal OCT scan (middle, left) and macular thickness map (middle, right) at baseline show centre-involving DMO with central subfield thickness (CST) of 420 μm and VA of 6/12. Following three consecutive intravitreal injections of ranibizumab, her macular oedema has markedly improved (bottom, left) with the CST decreasing to 272 μm and vision improving to 6/7.5. Her vision and OCT remained stable over 1 year of follow up.

> ### Case History 7.6: Persistent DMO despite multiple intravitreal anti-VEGF treatment
>
> This 53-year-old man with type 2 diabetes controlled by tablets for 14 years had moderate non-proliferative diabetic retinopathy. The colour fundus photograph (Fig. 7.15) of the left eye (top, left) and infrared fundus image (top, middle) show diffuse maculopathy. The late-phase fluorescein angiography shows diffuse macular leakage (top, right). The OCT scan and macular thickness maps (topographic and numerical) at baseline show centre-involving DMO with retinal thickening, particularly in central and temporal subfields (VA = 6/9, central subfield thickness (CST) = 411 μm, temporal subfield thickness = 514 μm) (second row). The macular oedema did not respond well to six consecutive monthly intravitreal ranibizumab (VA = 6/12, CST = 366 μm, temporal subfield thickness = 487 μm) (third row). After three further ranibizumab injections, his vision slightly improved but the macular oedema remained unchanged (VA = 6/9, CST = 374 μm, temporal subfield thickness = 463 μm) (fourth row). In DMO patients that are partially unresponsive to intravitreal anti-VEGF therapy, switching to another anti-VEGF or using intravitreal steroid implant would be the most appropriate strategy. However, this patient was not able to access these alternative treatments due to funding constraints.

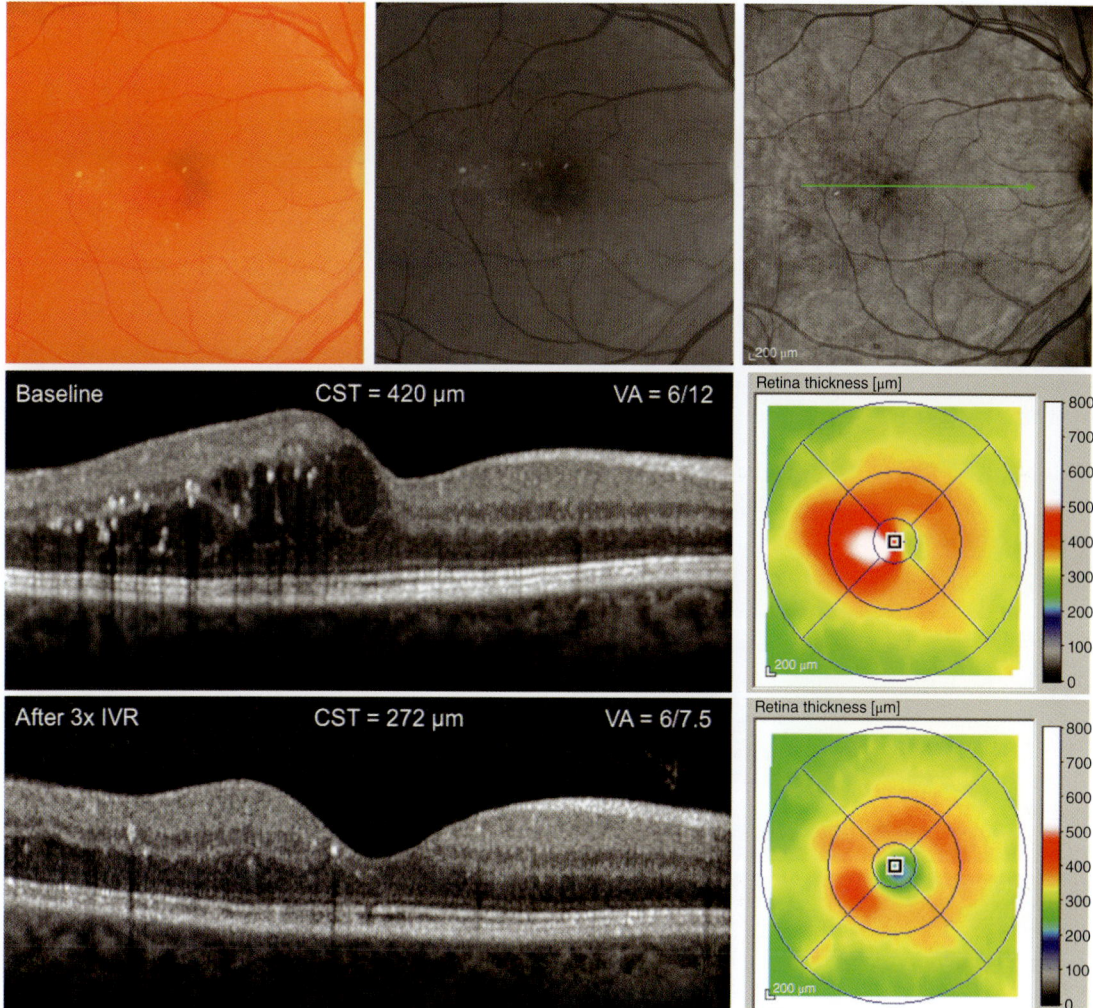

Fig. 7.14 Colour fundus photograph of the right eye (top, left) and red-free photograph (top, middle) showing centre-involving DMO. Infrared image depicting the diabetic changes (top, right) with the green line indicating the position of the OCT scan. Foveal OCT scan (middle, left) and macular thickness map (middle, right) at baseline and following three consecutive intravitreal injections of ranibizumab (bottom, left). CST, central retinal thickness; IVR, intravitreal ranibizumab; VA, visual acuity.

Predictors of visual outcomes after anti-VEGF therapy

Several factors could influence the visual outcome after anti-VEGF treatment. As expected, poor baseline vision (≤6/36) predicts poor visual outcome (≤6/30) after treatment with ranibizumab[62]. Regarding the effect of retinal fluid, resolution of macular oedema is more likely to occur if retinal oedema is mild than when it is severe. While the presence of macular cystoid spaces in untreated eyes is associated with reduction in final visual acuity and is worse with large spaces, their presence does not seem to affect the visual outcome after anti-VEGF treatment. Similar to retinal cysts, the presence of subretinal fluid is associated with loss of vision in untreated eyes, but seems to respond well to anti-VEGF treatment; its presence may be a predictor for achieving good vision with treatment[63]. The presence of macular exudates in eye with DMO does not appear to correlate negatively with baseline BCVA or influence the visual response to anti-VEGF. Therapy

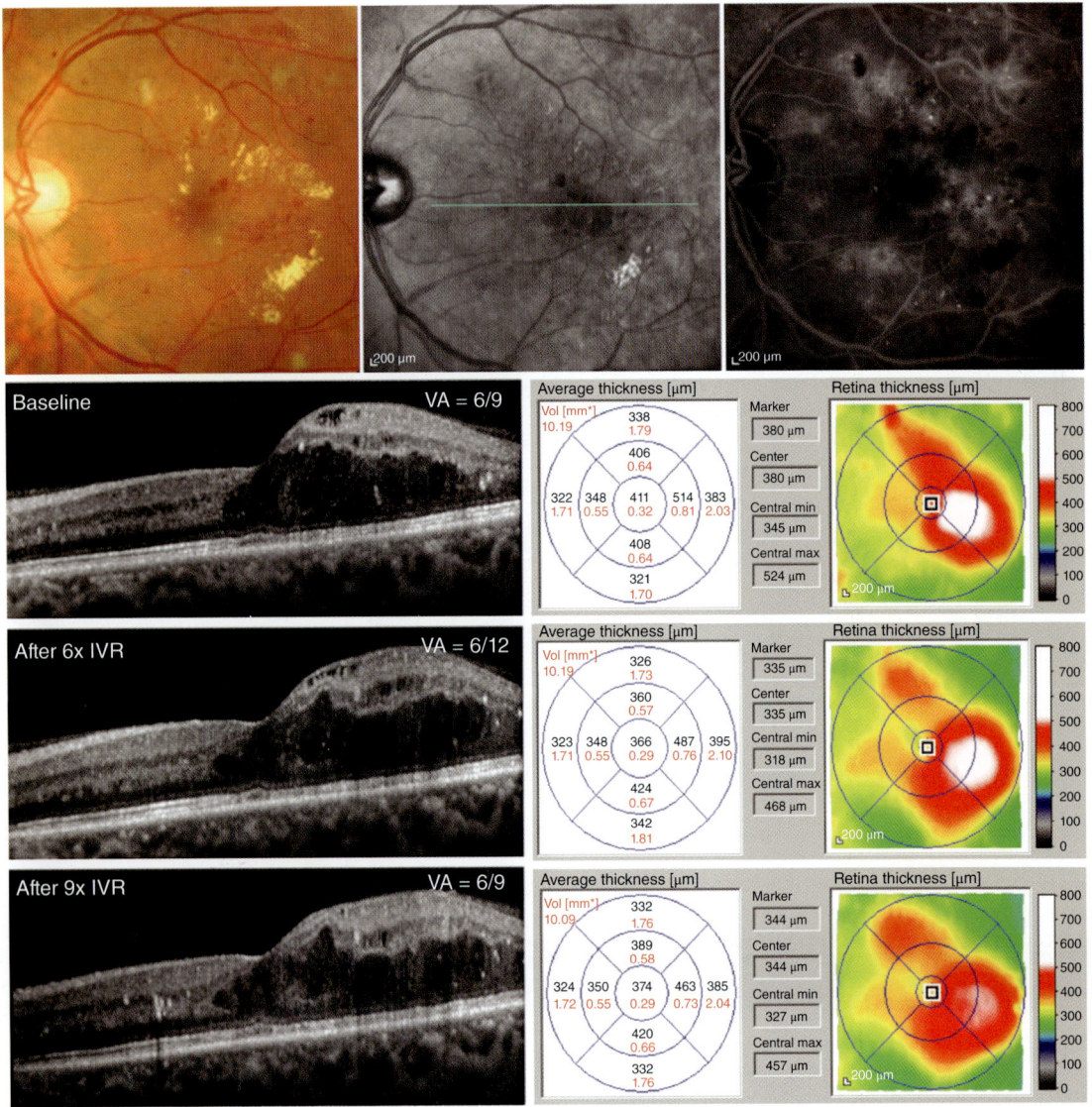

Fig. 7.15 Colour fundus photograph of the left eye (top, left) and infrared fundus image (top, middle) showing diffuse maculopathy. Late-phase fluorescein angiography showing diffuse macular leakage (top, right). In addition, OCT scan and macular thickness maps are shown at baseline and following 6 months and 9 months of intravitreal treatment with intravitreal ranibizumab. CST, central retinal thickness; IVR, intravitreal ranibizumab; VA. visual acuity.

with anti-VEGF enhances the absorption of exudates, but this takes a significantly longer time compared to retinal fluid absorption[64]. In 1997, Fong et al.[65] described the characteristics of and risk factors for subretinal fibrosis in patients with diabetic macular oedema, and found the strongest risk factor for the development of fibrosis to be very severe hard exudates. Intraretinal fibrosis in exudative diabetic macular oedema after ranibizumab treatment has also been reported[66].

Mismatch between retinal thickness and vision is sometimes seen during treatment with anti-VEGF therapy[63] and has also been observed after laser treatment and intravitreal steroid therapy. In chronic DMO, reduction of macular thickness without improvement in vision can signify structural photoreceptor damage. Conversely, vision can improve despite the presence of significant macular thickening in early cases where macular oedema has not been prolonged[62].

An assessment of outer retinal layers on OCT could also provide useful information regarding post-treatment vision. Alasil et al.[67] demonstrated significant correlation between visual acuity and tomographic data on photoreceptor outer segment thickness and volume.

Whether macular ischaemia negatively influences the visual outcome remains unclear. Some studies suggested that the presence of macular ischaemia may be associated with a trend towards worse visual outcome after anti-VEGF treatment[46], whereas others reported the absence of any independent association with vision[62]. Furthermore, while concerns remain regarding the use of anti-VEGF in eyes with pre-existing macular ischaemia, DMO studies that included eyes with significant macular ischaemia did not find any definitive causal relationship between use of anti-VEGF therapy and progression of ischaemia[51,68].

Regarding the influence of systemic factors on visual outcome after DMO treatment, increasing age and the presence of cardiovascular disease were found to be associated with poorer visual outcome after treatment. Patients with renal impairment and DMO also appear to have a higher likelihood of having <6/12 vision if untreated, but could achieve a good outcome with anti-VEGF treatment[63].

INTRAVITREAL CORTICOSTEROIDS

There is a growing body of evidence to indicate that leukocyte-induced inflammation plays a significant role in the development of macular oedema in patients with diabetes[69]. Given the role of steroids in modulating inflammation, there is a good rational for their use in DMO, particularly when the oedema is chronic. It is possible that the mode of action of steroids in DMO may be also dependent on their ability to inhibit the expression of VEGF and other growth factors that result from hypoxia and promote vascular leakage and ischaemia[70,71].

Intravitreal triamcinolone acetonide

Intravitreal triamcinolone acetonide is an off-label treatment that is not approved for ocular use. Triamcinolone acetonide was one of the first steroid preparations to be used for intravitreal injection and, while more frequently used in the past for treatment of DMO, the advent of VEGF-blocking therapy and recent corticosteroids implants has dramatically reduced its use. Short-term improvement of the vision in eyes with chronic diabetic macular oedema unresponsive to conventional laser treatment and reduction of macular thickness after treatment with intravitreal triamcinolone have been reported in studies by Ciardella et al.[72], Jonas et al.[6,73], Lam et al.[74], Massin et al.[75], Micelli Ferrari et al.[76], Ozkiris et al.[77], Sutter et al.[78], Chieh et al.[79], Er and Yilmaz[80], Islam et al.[81], Khairallah et al.[82], Negi et al.[83], Ozdemir et al.[84], Patelli et al.[85], Zacks and Johnson[86] and Avci et al.[87].

Two further randomised controlled trials by the DRCR.net have investigated the use of intravitreal triamcinolone in the treatment of DMO. In the first of these two studies, the use of focal/grid laser was compared to treatment with 1 mg or 4 mg of intravitreal triamcinolone, with retreatment possible every four months in each arm of the study. At 4 months, the triamcinolone arms showed superiority in terms of visual acuity, at one year laser and intravitreal triamcinolone treatments appeared equivalent, and at the 2-year time point laser was found to be superior to both intravitreal steroid arms and these results were held after 3 years[88].

In the second of these trials, focal/grid laser alone was compared to 4 mg of intravitreal triamcinolone plus laser. The study also included two additional arms utilising intravitreal ranibizumab. Similar to the previous study, the triamcinolone plus laser arm showed superiority compared to laser alone in terms of visual acuity at 24 weeks follow-up. However, at 1 and 2 years, all treatments appeared fairly equivalent in terms of visual acuity outcome, but with increased rates of cataract and elevated intraocular pressure in the triamcinolone plus laser group[89]. Results from these studies reflect the pharmacokinetics of intravitreal triamcinolone with the drug effect being short lived (3 months); it does not provide sustained treatment. The drug is also associated with significant ocular side-effects including cataract development (54% after 2 years), raised IOP (44% at 2 years)[90] and sterile uveitis/pseudoendophthalmitis (in up to 13% of eyes) that further limits its clinical use[91].

Dexamethasone intravitreal implant

Dexamethasone intravitreal implant (Ozurdex, Allergan, Inc., Irvine, CA) is a sustained-release biodegradable implant formulation of corticosteroid that has been approved by the FDA for the treatment of macular oedema due to diabetes. In the UK, it has also been approved for this indication but only in pesudophakic eyes. The dexamethasone implant is injected into the vitreous cavity as an outpatient procedure using a 22-gauge injector. The implant provides therapeutic effect for up to 4 months after injection, with peak activity at about 2 months. Several studies have also shown the benefit of dexamethasone implant in treating diabetic macular oedema[92–94].

The MEAD study is a phase-3 randomised controlled trial of patients with DMO that received treatment with dexamethasone implant[94]. Subjects were randomised (1:1:1) to study treatment with a 0.7 mg implant, which is the currently marketed product, a 0.35 mg implant, or a sham procedure. Patients who met retreatment eligibility criteria were retreated no more often than every 6 months. At 3 years, the percentage of patients who gained ≥15 in letter score was 22.2% (0.7 mg group) and 18.4% (0.35 mg), compared with 12% in the sham group. For patients receiving the 0.7 mg implant, IOP was elevated in about one-third of eyes; in most cases it was however possible to control the increase in IOP with topical treatment and only a small proportionate of eyes required glaucoma surgery (0.3%). Cataract surgery was undertaken in nearly 60% of eyes during the 3-year study period in the 0.7 mg implant group compared to 7% in the sham group.

BEVORDEX[92] is a prospective, multicentre, randomised clinical trial that provided direct comparison between intravitreal anti-VEGF (bevacizumab) versus intravitreal sustained steroid therapy (dexamethasone implant) for centre-involving DMO. A total of 86 eyes were included (42 eyes in the bevacizumab arm and 46 in the dexamethasone arm). After baseline treatment, retreatment was considered at each visit as long as treatments were at least 4 weeks apart for bevacizumab and 16 weeks apart for the dexamethasone implant. Twelve-month results showed that improvement of BCVA of ≥10 letters score were similar in both arms, occurring in 40% in bevacizumab arm and 41% in dexamethasone implant arm ($P=0.83$). However, a greater number of bevacizumab treated eyes achieved ≥15 letters gain (31% v. 22%). Mean reduction in central macular thickness was 122 μm in the bevacizumab arm as compared to 187 μm in the dexamethasone implant arm ($P=0.015$). At 24 months, no significant difference between the two groups with respect to 10 letters BCVA gain or mean BCVA gain was also found. However, while central macular thickness at 24 months was not significantly greater for bevacizumab- than dexamethasone-treated eyes, there was greater regression of hard exudates in dexamethasone-treated eyes compared to eyes treated with bevacizumab ($P=0.02$). At 24 months, bevacizumab-treated eyes received a mean of 13.2 injections in comparison to a mean of 5 dexamethasone implants.

Fluocinolone acetonide intravitreal inserts

Fluocinolone acetonide (Iluvein) intravitreal insert is a non-biodegradable cylindrical tube of polymer loaded with 190 μg fluocinolone acetonide (FAc) that is currently available for insertion into the vitreous cavity through a 25-gauge applicator in an outpatient setting (Fig. 7.16). Insert (approximately 3.5 mm in length × 0.37 mm in diameter) provides sustained delivery of FAc in the eye for up to 30–36 months following a single treatment[95].

The FAME study is a controlled trial that investigated the use of FAc in DMO[96]. Subjects with persistent DMO despite at least one macular laser treatment were randomised 1:2:2 to sham injection ($n=185$), 0.2 μg/day insert which is the currently licensed implant dose ($n=375$), or 0.5 μg/day insert ($n=393$). At month 36, the percentage of patients who gained ≥15 letters was 28.7% (low dose) and 27.8% (high dose) in the FAc insert groups compared with 18.9% in the sham group. Almost all phakic patients in the FAc insert groups developed cataract, but their visual benefit after cataract surgery was similar to that in pseudophakic patients. Around 40% of eyes treated with the 0.2 μg/day insert required IOP-lowering medications, and the incidence of glaucoma surgery at month 36 was 4.8% in this group and 8.1% in the high-dose insert group.

Intravitreal FAc was recently granted approval in the UK by NICE, but only for DMO in pseudopakaic eyes that is not responsive to other lines of treatment[97]. It has also been approved in other countries in Europe for treatment of DMO and in the US.

There is increasing evidence for the efficacy intravitreal steroid therapy in treating DMO, which makes it a useful treatment modality for patients with DMO that is refractory to or requires frequent anti-VEGF therapy, particularly if they are pseudophakic. Among the different intravitreal steroid preparations currently available, the dexamethasone implant possibly represents the best treatment option. It allows an extended interval between injections of nearly 4 months and has a more acceptable side-effect profile as compared to either intravitreal triamcinolone injection or fluocinolone acetonide implant.

Diabetic macular oedema

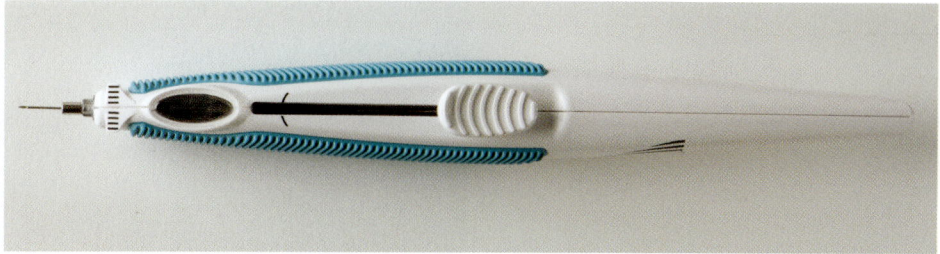

Fig. 7.16 Intravitreal fluocinolone acetonide (Iluvien) applicator

Case History 7.7: Refractory DMO treated with intravitreal intravitreal flucinolone acetonide implant

This is a 61-year-old man with type 2 diabetes diagnosed at the age of 55 and controlled by tablets (metformin 500 mg, twice daily). The colour fundus photograph (Fig. 7.17) of the right eye (top, left) and red-free image (top, right) depicts DMO. The OCT scan and macular thickness map (topographic and numerical) shows DMO involving the foveal centre with significant leakage, particularly nasally (VA = 6/12, CST = 418 μm, nasal subfield thickness = 428 μm) (second row).

Over a period of 3 years he received four sessions of focal macular laser treatment and one intravitreal injection of triamcinolone acetonide, but his DMO was persistent (VA = 6/15, CST = 454 μm, nasal subfield thickness = 454 μm) (third raw).

Poor response was also observed after three intravitreal ranibizumab injections with only marginal improvement of macular oedema (VA = 6/12, CST = 376 μm, nasal subfield thickness = 409 μm) (fourth row). Finally, he was treated with intravitreal flucinolone acetonide implant (iluvien) resulting in morphological improvement of the macular oedema after one month, but this has not translated into better vision (VA = 6/12, CRT = 319 μm, nasal subfield thickness = 374 μm) (fifth row).

COMBINATION THERAPY

There is current interest in combination therapy for treatment of DMO. While treatment with intravitreal anti-VEGF therapy results in excellent anatomical and visual outcomes, repeated injections are usually needed in many patients for a long period of time to maintain such outcomes[50,57]. Combination therapy is mainly aimed to extend the durability of the anti-VEGF effect and decrease the number of injections, which can in turn help decrease the burden of treatment as well as increase patient safety.

Several studies have evaluated combination treatment of anti-VEGF and macular laser v. anti-VEGF monotherapy. While no significant difference in functional and anatomical outcomes was found between monotherapy and combination therapy groups, the latter was associated with a lower number of anti-VEGF injections[46,98,99]. It is possible that using navigating laser in combination with anti-VEGF may provide additional benefits over conventional laser given its higher accuracy in treating microaneurysms, thereby providing faster resolution of macular oedema[99].

When considering combination therapy, it is advisable to use anti-VEGF therapy first and employ subsequent macular laser for areas that have persistent oedema despite anti-VEGF therapy. This is likely to enhance the uptake and reduce the fluency of laser as compared to administering laser with or soon after commencing anti-VEGF treatment when the retina is still markedly oedematous[59]. This view is further supported by results of a DRCR.net study that found combination therapy of anti-VEGF with early macular laser to be ineffective and resulted in worse outcomes than when laser was deferred for ≥24 weeks after anti-VEGF treatment[100].

The PLACID study evaluated combined treatment of dexamethasone implant and modified ETDRS macular laser (n=126) vs. macular laser alone (n=127) in a controlled setting[101]. Macular laser was administered 1 month after dexamethasone implant treatment but retreatment by another dexamethasone implant was not allowed earlier than 6 months. Up to 9 months, more patients in the combination group had better visual outcome (defined as ≥10-letter improvement in BCVA) than in the laser alone group; however, there was no significant difference in visual outcome at 12 months. It is possible that the study protocol limited the clinical effectiveness of the dexamethasone implant and that a more favourable outcome could have been achieved in the combination treatment arm if early retreatment was permitted at a 4-month time point when the effect of the dexamethasone implant was expected to wear off.

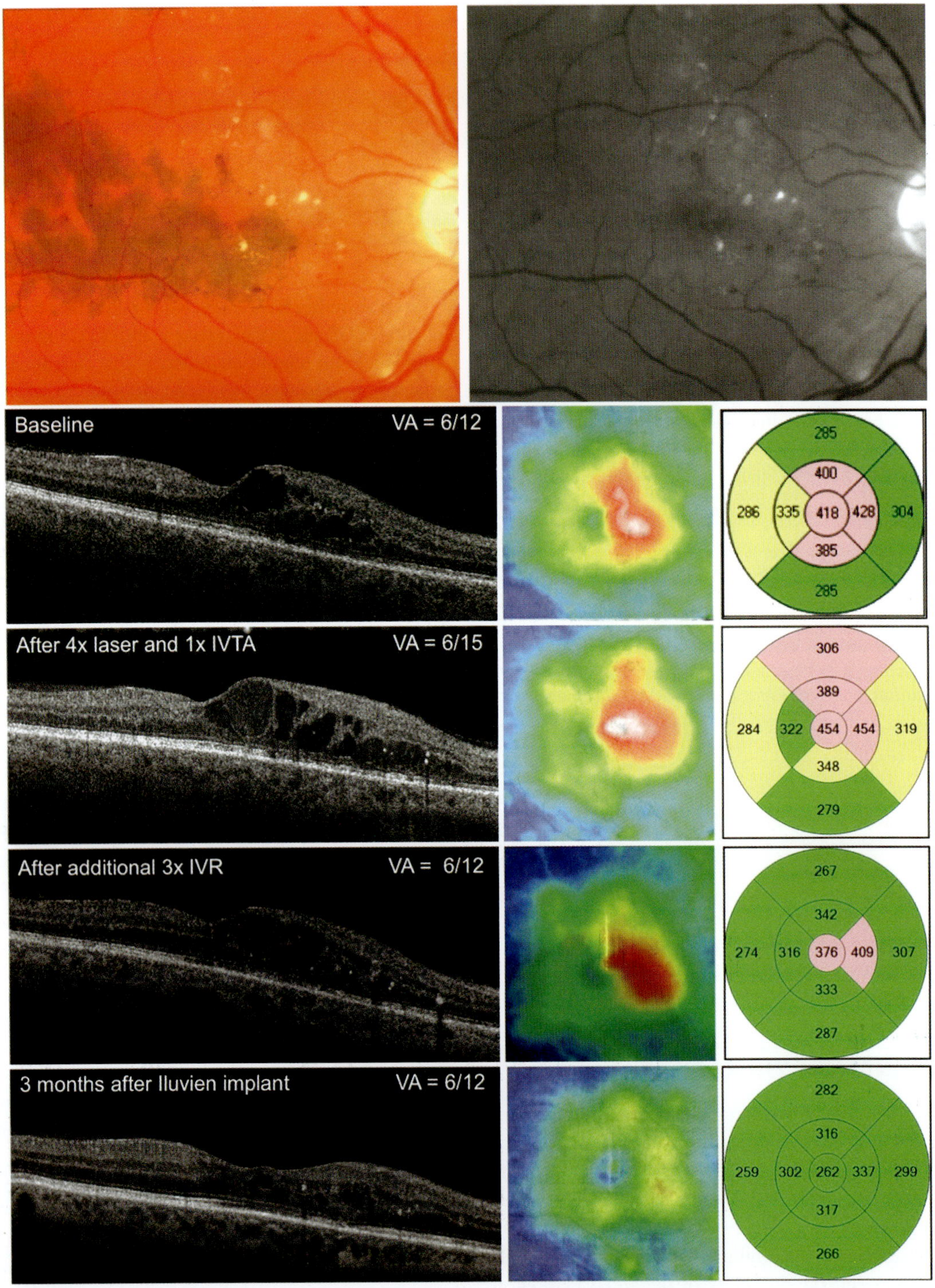

Fig. 7.17 Colour fundus photograph of the right eye (top, left) and red-free image (top, right) depicting DMO. OCT scan and macular thickness map (topographic and numerical) showing DMO (second row), after a period of 3 years, having received four sessions of focal macular laser treatment and one intravitreal injection of triamcinolone acetonide (third row), following three intravitreal ranibizumab injections (fourth row) and following treatment with intravitreal flucinolone acetonide implant (fifth row). CST, central retinal thickness; IVR, intravitreal ranibizumab; VA, visual acuity.

In another study, Maturi et al.[102] evaluated the effect of combining sustained-release intravitreal steroid treatment with anti-VEGF in eyes that were partially responsive to repeat anti-VEGF treatment. Patients in the study were randomised to receive intravitreal bevacizumab plus dexamethasone implant or bevacizumab alone. Eyes in the bevacizumab-only group received monthly treatment if OCT was greater than 250 μm and visual acuity was worse than 6/9. Similarly, the combination treatment group received monthly bevacizumab treatment as required, but in addition dexamethasone implant was also administered at months 1, 5 and 9.

At 1 year, visual acuity improvement was similar in both groups but reduction in retinal thickness was significantly better in the combination therapy group ($P=0.03$). However, no substantial difference in burden of treatment was found between the two groups. While the combination treatment group received three fewer bevacizumab injections than the bevacizumab group over 1 year, they also received two additional dexamethasone implants.

VITRECTOMY

The role of vitrectomy in the treatment of diabetic macular oedema is further discussed in Chapter 13. In brief, we mainly consider vitrectomy for cases of DMO that are associated with vitreomacular traction[103] and achieved no significant response to an initial 3× loading treatment of anti-VEGF therapy. An important practical point to consider when managing DMO patients that have undergone previous vitrectomy surgery is that the vitreous surgery may result in enhanced drug clearance from the vitreous cavity. A recent study demonstrated that while visual outcomes in vitrectomized eyes are not different from those who did not have previous vitrectomy surgery, the rate of anatomical improvement after anti-VEGF treatment may be initially slower with more frequent injections required in the first year of treatment[104].

AUTHORS' TREATMENT RECOMMENDATIONS FOR DMO

Macular (focal/modified grid) laser still has a role in our practice for cases with clinically significant DMO that is non-centre involving. Anti-VEGF therapy is currently our main line of treatment for centre-involving DMO. Our anti-VEGF therapy treatment protocol includes 3× loading injections followed by an as-needed treatment regimen that is based on vision and OCT findings. For patients with persistent fluid despite repeat intravitreal anti-VEGF therapy, particularly when accompanied with reduction of vision, we switch the anti-VEGF agent and closely monitor the anatomical response to the new treatment. Intravitreal corticosteroids are usually considered in those who remain resistant to two successive anti-VEGF agents, particularly in pseudophakic patients or in patients who are averse to repeat injections.

CONCLUSIONS

Anti-VEGF therapy is currently the main line of treatment for centre-involving DMO. Although associated with excellent anatomical and visual outcomes, anti-VEGF therapy has created a significant burden for both patients and healthcare providers with repeat intravitreal injections being needed for long-term maintenance of vision. There is recent interest in combining anti-VEGF therapy with other modalities that have sustained effect on macular oedema such as macular laser or sustained-release steroids in order to help consolidate the effect of anti-VEGF therapy on the retina and thereby reduce the burden of repeat treatment.

PRACTICE POINTS

- Anti-VEGF therapy is currently the treatment of choice for centre-involving DMO. However, repeat treatment for long periods is usually required.
- Macular (focal/modified grid) laser treatment role is now limited to cases with non-centre-involving DMO.
- Pseudophakic patients, particularly those who continue to require repeat anti-VEGF injections or are resistant to anti-VEGF therapy, may be good candidates for intravitreal steroid implants.
- Intravitreal dexamethasone implant appears to be the most attractive steroid option for DMO treatment at present because of its acceptable risk profile.
- Combining laser with anti-VEGF therapy may help reduce the burden of anti-VEGF therapy and repeat treatment, but is not associated with additional visual benefits.

REFERENCE

Please visit www.wiley.com/go/scanlon/diabetic_retinopathy

8 Mild non-proliferative diabetic retinopathy

Peter H. Scanlon

Harris Manchester College, University of Oxford; Medical Ophthalmology, University of Gloucestershire, UK

MILD NPDR (ETDRS AND INTERNATIONAL) AND BACKGROUND DR (UK SCREENING)

Optimum control of glycaemia, hypertension and lipids are recommended for all patients with diabetes. Table 8.1 describes ETDRS grades 20 and 35a–e. The earliest signs of mild non-proliferative diabetic retinopathy (mild NPDR) or background DR are microaneurysms.

Microaneurysms

Patients with no DR and microaneurysms (Fig. 8.1a–e) only were not included in the ETDRS study.

In the Wisconsin Epidemiological Study of Diabetic Retinopathy[2,3], the rate of progression to proliferative retinopathy 4 years after the initial evaluation showed 'no DR' was 0.4% for young insulin-dependent patients <30 years, 0% for older patients ≥30 years with diabetes taking insulin and 0.6% for those not using insulin.

For those with microaneurysms or one haemorrhage in one eye only, the rate of progression to proliferative retinopathy 4 years after the initial evaluation was 3.0% for young (<30 years) insulin-dependent patients, 0% for older patients (≥30 years) with diabetes taking insulin and 1.5% not using insulin. Other studies[4,5] have linked the rate of progression to the number of microaneurysms.

Klein et al.[6] and Wong et al.[7] reported that the rate of progression to proliferative diabetic retinopathy was lower in more recently diagnosed persons, which possibly reflects improvement in care over the period of the study.

A recent study[8] in Gloucestershire demonstrated a much higher rate of progression to proliferative DR if mild changes were found in both eyes than in one alone.

Retinal haemorrhages

In mild NPDR, retinal haemorrhages are usually small dot haemorrhages or flame-shaped haemorrhages (Fig. 8.2a). Because small retinal haemorrhages can be difficult to differentiate from microaneurysms, they are commonly referred to as HMa. Flame-shaped haemorrhages (Fig. 8.2b) are present just under the superficial nerve fibre layer. Blot haemorrhages (Fig. 8.2c) are usually in a deeper retinal layer and denote a sign of ischaemia; multiple blot haemorrhages would therefore not be considered as mild NPDR.

Exudates (or hard exudates)

Exudates (or hard exudates; Fig. 8.3) are a feature of mild NPDR. They are small white or yellowish-white deposits with sharp margins, typically located in the outer layers of the retina. They may however be more superficial, particularly when retinal oedema is present.

Cotton wool spots

Cotton wool spots (Fig. 8.4) are fluffy white opaque areas caused by an accumulation of axoplasm in the nerve fibre layer of the retina. They may be present in mild NPDR or background DR, caused by an arteriolar occlusion in that area of retina. Despite cotton wool spots being the underlying cause, they are not a good sign of increasing retinal ischaemia. They are often associated with hypertension. When several are present, one needs to look closely at the level of blood pressure and for signs of ischaemia that are more closely associated with progression of diabetic retinopathy (e.g. venous beading, intraretinal microvascular abnormalities and multiple blot haemorrhages), which would classify the retinopathy into a more severe grade.

A Practical Manual of Diabetic Retinopathy Management, Second Edition. Edited by Peter Scanlon, Ahmed Sallam, and Peter van Wijngaarden.
© 2017 John Wiley & Sons Ltd. Published 2017 by John Wiley & Sons Ltd.
Companion Website: www.wiley.com/go/scanlon/diabetic_retinopathy

Mild non-proliferative diabetic retinopathy

Table 8.1 ETDRS description of the lesions at the grade of mild non-proliferative diabetic retinopathy

ETDRS final retinopathy severity scale[1]	ETDRS (final) grade	Lesions	Risk of progression to PDR in 1 year(ETDRS interim)	Practical clinic follow-up intervals (not ETDRS)
Mild NPDR	20 35 a b c d e	Microaneurysms only One or more of the following: venous loops ≥ definite in one field; SE, IRMA or VB questionable; retinal haemorrhages present; HE ≥ definite in one field; or SE ≥ definite in one field.	ETDRS level 30 = 6.2%. Risk of progression to proliferative in 1 year	1 year 6–12 months

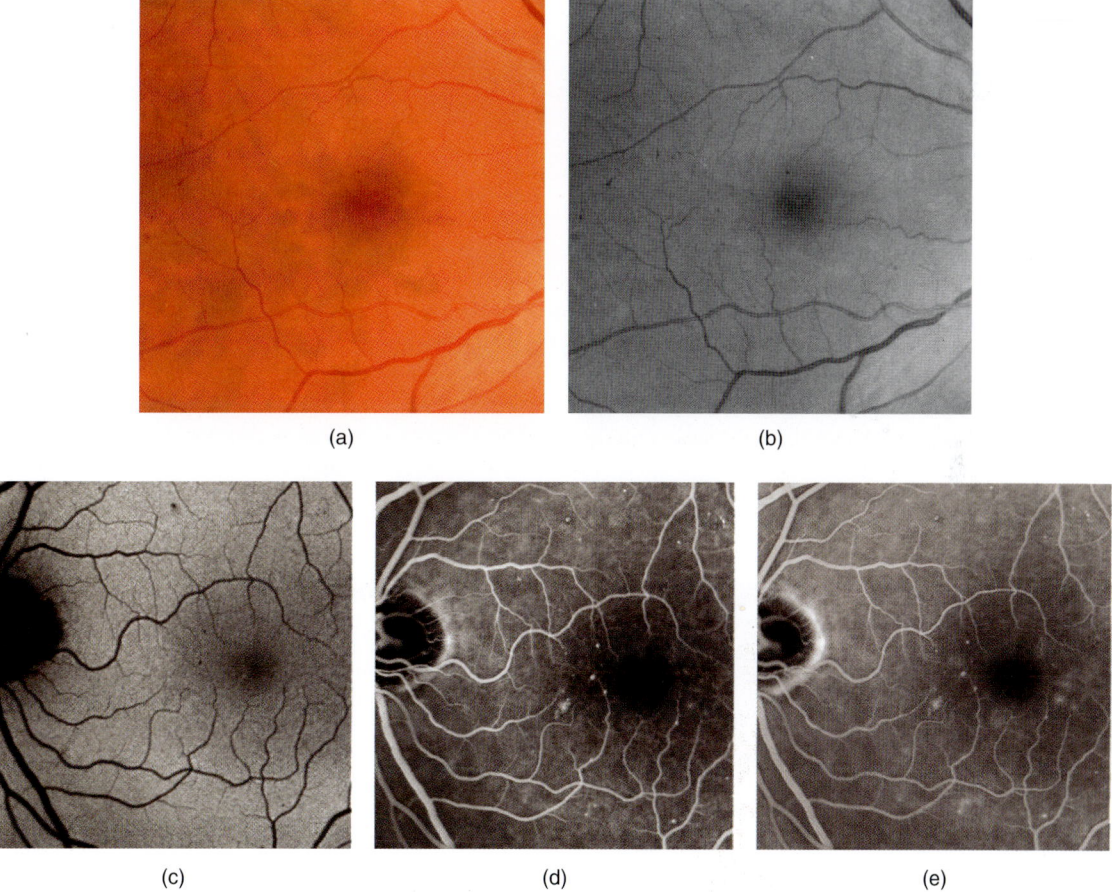

Fig. 8.1 Microaneurysms and fine exudate in mild NPDR: (a) right macula colour and (b) right macula red-free. Microaneurysms in mild NPDR: (c) left macula autofluorescence photo; (d) fluorescein angiogram at 1 min 9 s showing fluorescence from microaneurysms in the left macular area but no signs of leakage and (e) fluorescein angiogram at 5 min 39 s showing a small amount of leakage from microaneurysms in the left macular area.

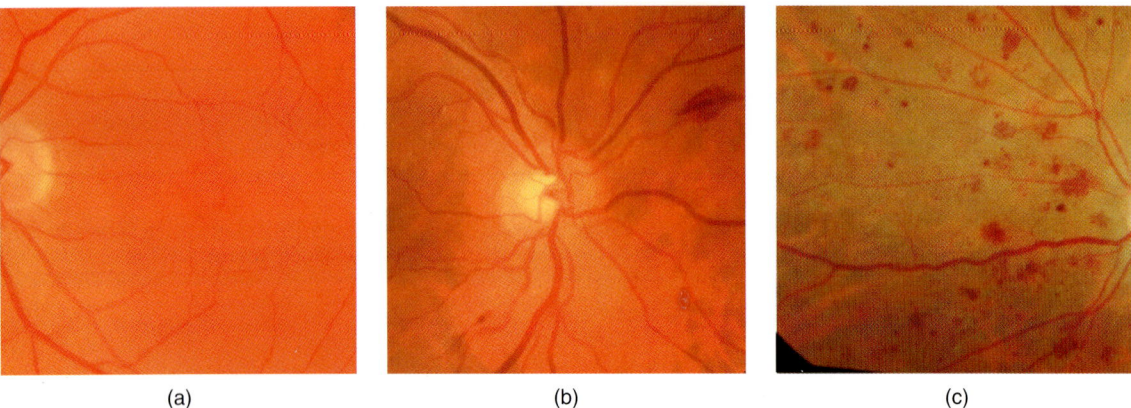

Fig. 8.2 (a) Haemorrhages and microaneurysms in mild NPDR: colour photo left macula. (b) Flame-shaped haemorrhages in mild NPDR: colour photo right disc. (c) Example of blot haemorrhages.

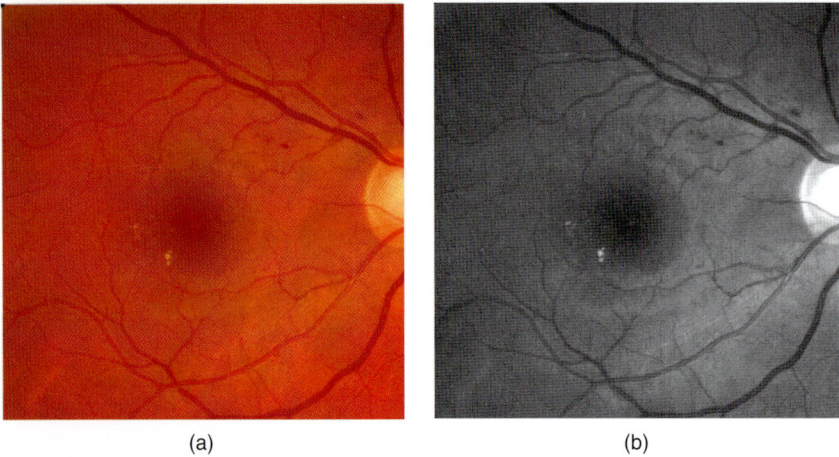

Fig. 8.3 Exudates in mild NPDR developing in right macular area: (a) colour photograph and (b) red-free photograph, both right macula view.

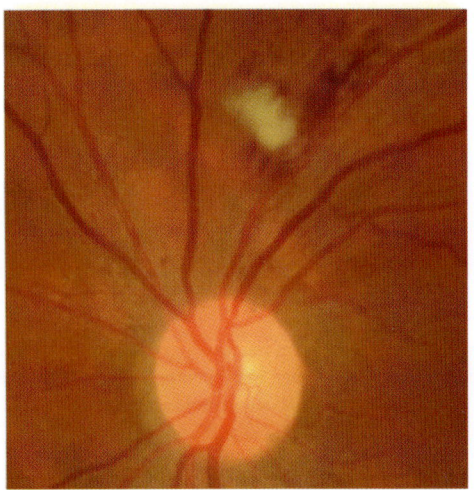

Fig. 8.4 Cotton wool spot in mild NPDR.

A single venous loop

A venous loop (Fig. 8.5) is an abrupt curving deviation of a vein from its normal path, and the ETDRS included a single venous loop in their classification of mild NPDR. This is now also a feature of the UK screening definition of background diabetic retinopathy. Larger venous loops also occur in later ischaemic stages of the disease process.

PRACTICE POINTS

For mild non-proliferative diabetic retinopathy there is a 6.2% risk of progression to proliferative in 1 year.

The International Classification[9] of diabetic retinopathy recommends that anyone who has more than just microaneurysms is referred to an ophthalmologist.

Mild non-proliferative diabetic retinopathy

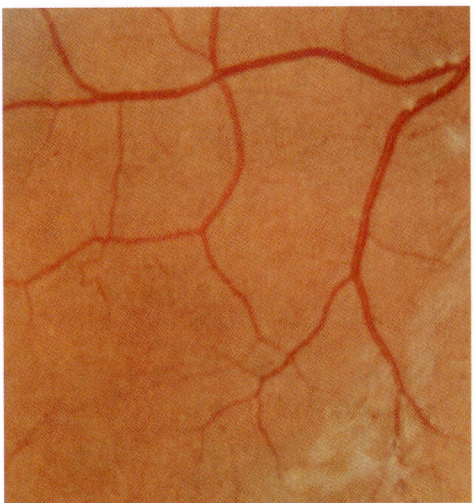

Fig. 8.5 Venous loop in mild NPDR.

In the UK, patients who are screened and who show signs of background diabetic retinopathy only are rescreened annually. For the purposes of the National Screening Programme, background DR is defined[10] by: microaneurysm(s); and retinal haemorrhage(s) with or without any exudates.

REFERENCE

Please visit www.wiley.com/go/scanlon/diabetic_retinopathy

Moderate and severe non-proliferative diabetic retinopathy

Peter H. Scanlon

Harris Manchester College, University of Oxford; Medical Ophthalmology, University of Gloucestershire, UK,

MODERATE AND SEVERE NPDR (ETDRS AND INTERNATIONAL) AND PRE-PROLIFERATIVE DR (UK SCREENING)

Optimum control of glycaemia, hypertension and lipids are recommended for all patients with diabetes. The grades for moderate and severe NPDR (ETDRS and International[1]) and pre-proliferative DR (UK screening[2]) are listed in Table 9.1.

Microaneurysms in increasing numbers have been shown to be an important early measure of progression of diabetic retinopathy[4–6]. Hard exudates (sometimes now just referred to as exudates) are not a good marker of retinal ischaemia. Cotton wool spots (referred to as soft exudates in the ETDRS, a term that is now rarely used) are fluffy white opaque areas caused by an arteriolar occlusion in an area of retina, resulting in an accumulation of axoplasm in the nerve fibre layer. Despite this being the underlying cause, they are not a good sign of increasing retinal ischaemia. They are often associated with hypertension. When several are present one needs to look closely for raised BP and for signs of increasing ischaemia that are more closely associated with progression, such as venous beading, intraretinal microvascular abnormalities and multiple blot haemorrhages, which would classify the retinopathy into moderate or severe diabetic retinopathy.

The main features that warrant classifying a diabetic retinopathy level in the higher levels of moderate and severe NPDR (or pre-proliferative DR) are increasing signs of retinal ischaemia. Lesions associated with increasing retinal ischaemia include: (1) retinal haemorrhages; (2) intraretinal microvascular abnormality; and (3) venous beading.

Retinal haemorrhages

Increasing numbers of haemorrhages, particularly when the pattern of haemorrhages includes an increasing number of blot haemorrhages, denotes increasing retinal ischaemia (Fig. 9.1) and progression of DR. Blot haemorrhages are usually in a deeper retinal layer than more superficial dot haemorrhages and flame haemorrhages.

Intraretinal microvascular abnormality

Intraretinal microvascular abnormalities (IRMA; Fig. 9.2) are defined as tortuous intraretinal vascular segments varying in calibre. By definition, intraretinal microvascular abnormalities are not on the surface of the retina and do not break through the internal limiting membrane. Intraretinal microvascular abnormalities are derived from remodelling of the retinal capillaries and small collateral vessels in areas of microvascular occlusion. They are usually found on the borders of areas of non-perfused retina, and are therefore a sign of retinal ischaemia.

Venous beading

In the ETDRS venous beading was described as a localised increase in calibre of the vein, and the severity was

---

A Practical Manual of Diabetic Retinopathy Management, Second Edition.
Edited by Peter Scanlon, Ahmed Sallam, and Peter van Wijngaarden.
© 2017 John Wiley & Sons Ltd. Published 2017 by John Wiley & Sons Ltd.
Companion Website: www.wiley.com/go/scanlon/diabetic_retinopathy

Moderate and severe non-proliferative diabetic retinopathy

Table 9.1 ETDRS description of the lesions at the grade of moderate and severe non-proliferative diabetic retinopathy

ETDRS final retinopathy severity scale[3]	ETDRS (final) grade	Lesions	Risk of progression to PDR in 1 year (ETDRS interim)	Practical clinic follow-up intervals (not ETDRS)
Moderate NPDR	43a b	H/Ma moderate in 4–5 fields, severe in 1 field or IRMA definite in 1–3 fields	Level 41 = 11.3%	6 months
Moderately severe NPDR	47 a b c d	Both level 43 characteristics: H/Ma moderate in 4–5 fields or severe in 1 field and IRMA definite in 1–3 fields or any one of the following: IRMA in 4–5 fields HMA severe in 2–3 fields VB definite in 1 field	Level 45 = 20.7%	4 months
Severe NPDR	53 a b c d	One or more of the following: ≥ 2 of the 3 level 47 characteristics H/Ma severe in 4–5 fields IRMA $\geq$ moderate in 1 field VB $\geq$ definite in 2–3 fields	Level 51 = 44.2% Level 55 = 54.8%	3 months

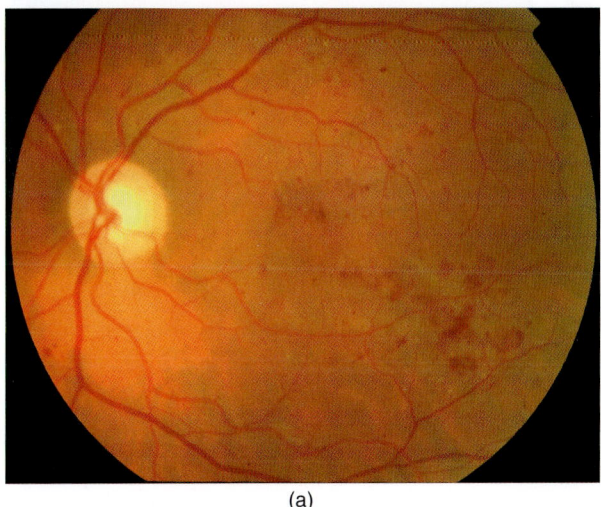 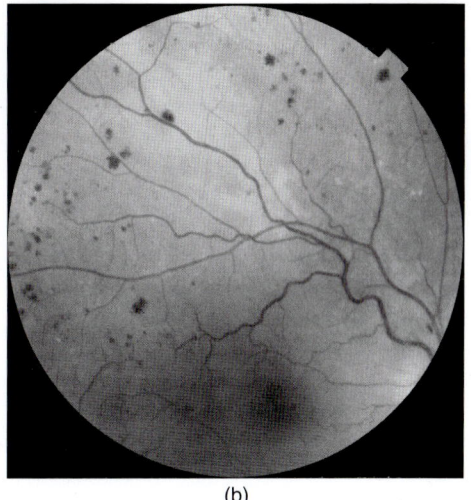

(a)   (b)

Fig. 9.1 (a, b) Retinal haemorrhages.

dependent on the increase in calibre and the length of vein involved. Venous beading (Fig. 9.3) was found to be associated with retinal ischaemia and is used for assessment of severity of diabetic retinopathy.

With increasing ischaemia, there is an increasing risk of progression to proliferative in 1 year. The risk increases from approximately 11.3% in the lower levels of moderate NPDR to 54.8% progression to proliferative in 1 year in the most severe non-proliferative DR level.

ETDRS definitions have been simplified to make them easier for everyday clinical use, both in the International classification and in the UK classification for screening. The ETDRS '4:2:1 rule' indicates that the presence of severe haemorrhages in four quadrants (≥ 20), venous

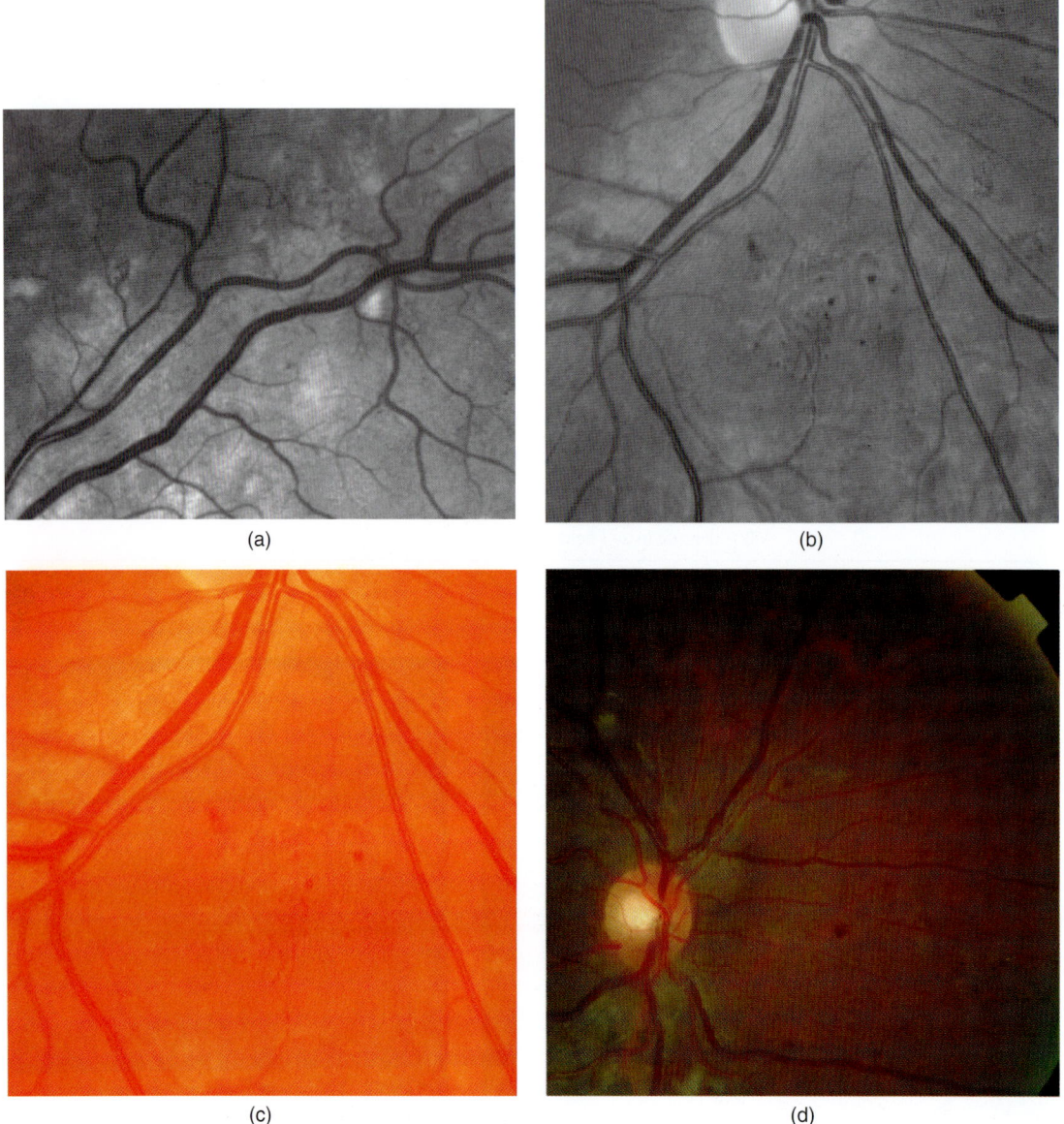

Fig. 9.2 (a) IRMA in superior retina. Example of IRMA below left optic disc: (b) red-free image and (c) colour image. (d) Example of IRMA in superior and nasal retina of right eye.

beading in two quadrants or IRMA in a single quadrant represents severe non-proliferative DR.

In the International classification, severe NPDR is defined by either or (1) extensive intraretinal haemorrhages (>20) in four quadrants; (2) definite venous beading in two or more quadrants; or (3) prominent IRMA in at least one quadrant, *and* no signs of PDR.

Moderate NPDR is classified in the International classification as more than 'microaneurysms only' and less severe than the 4:2:1 rule.

In the UK Screening Classification, pre-proliferative DR is defined by any of: (1) venous beading; (2) venous reduplication; (3) intraretinal microvascular abnormality (IRMA); or (4) multiple deep, round or blot haemorrhages.

Moderate and severe non-proliferative diabetic retinopathy

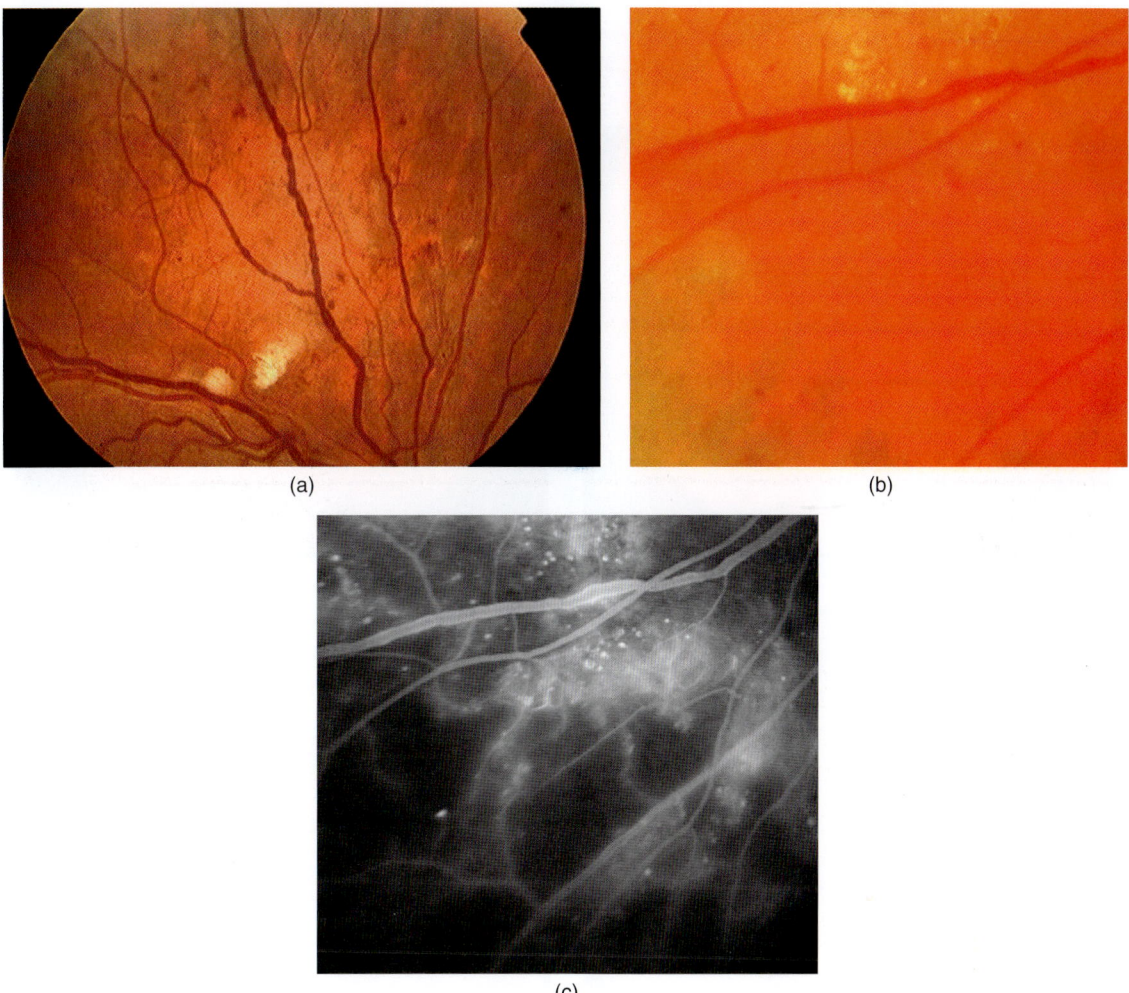

Fig. 9.3 Venous beading in (a) superior retina and (b) infero-nasal retina. (c) Venous beading and ischaemia on fluorescein of the same area as (b).

Case History 9.1: Moderately non-proliferative DR

A 40-year-old lady with type 1 diabetes controlled by insulin since the age of 21 years was referred from retinal screening with intraretinal micravascular abnormalitues (IRMA) in the right temporal area (Fig. 9.4a), which is only seen when the image is enlarged.

Subsequent visits over the next 5 years (Fig. 9.4b–d) showed an increase in signs of ischaemia such as blot haemorrhages, but no treatment was commenced. Her vision has remained good at LogMAR 0.0 (Snellen 20/20) in each eye). The management plan is to treat with laser at a point where neovascularisation develops.

Case History 9.2: Severe non-proliferative DR with maculopathy

A 60-year-old man with type 2 diabetes controlled by Metformin 1000 mg t.d.s. of 19 years duration had never attended screening, but presented to the eye department with reduced vision in both eyes to a level of right Log-MAR 0.62 (Snellen 20/80) and left LogMAR 0.52 (Snellen 20/60). His photographs and fluorescein angiogram showed a combination of severe ischaemia and oedema in both macular areas (Fig. 9.5a–l). No neovascularisation was identified, but the ischaemia is very severe.

He was commeced on intravitreal ranibizumab injections to each eye and panretinal photocoagulation to

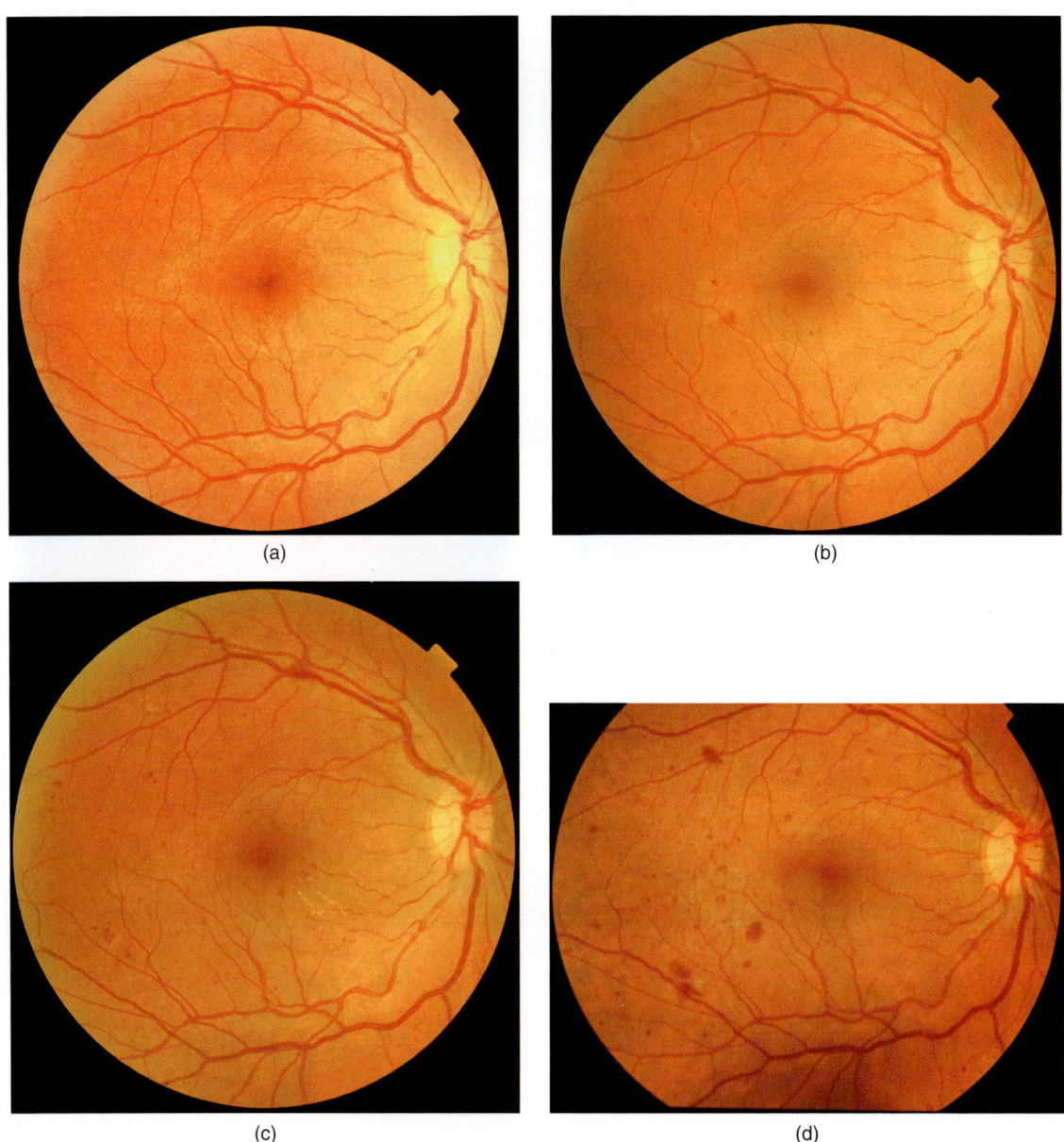

Fig. 9.4 Right macula colour photograph at (a) presentation; (b) 1 year after presentation; (c) 2 years after presentation; and (d) 5 years after presentation.

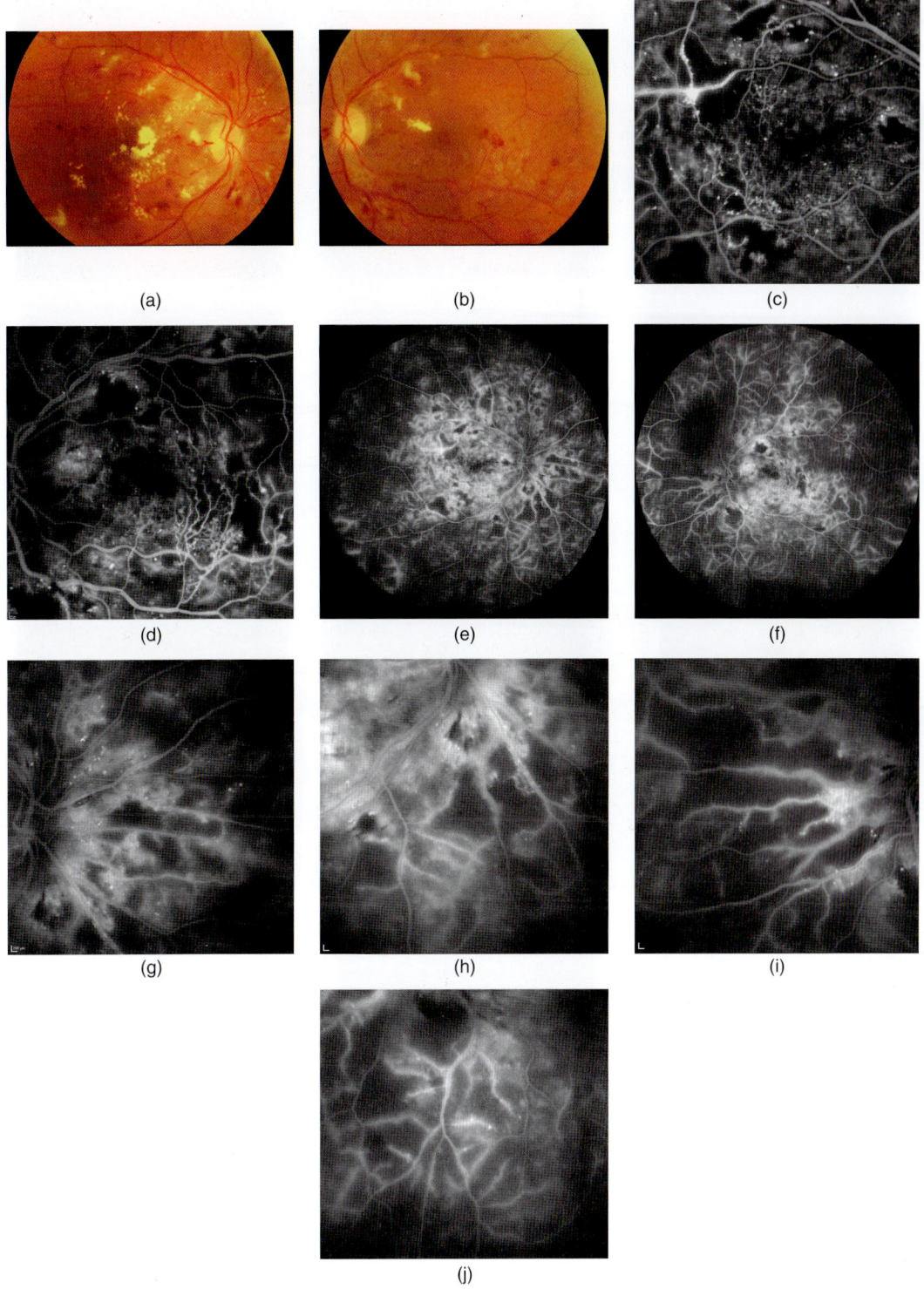

Fig. 9.5 (a) Right macula colour and (b) left macula colour. Fluorescein (c) right eye 56 s and (d) left eye 1 min 31 s. Fluorescein (e) right eye 3 min 14 s and (f) left eye 3 min 28 s. Fluorescein right eye (g) 6 min 17 s and (h) 7 min 34 s. Fluorescein left eye (i) 8 min 19 s and (j) 8 min 44 s. OCT (k) right and (l) left macular area.

126 A practical manual of diabetic retinopathy management

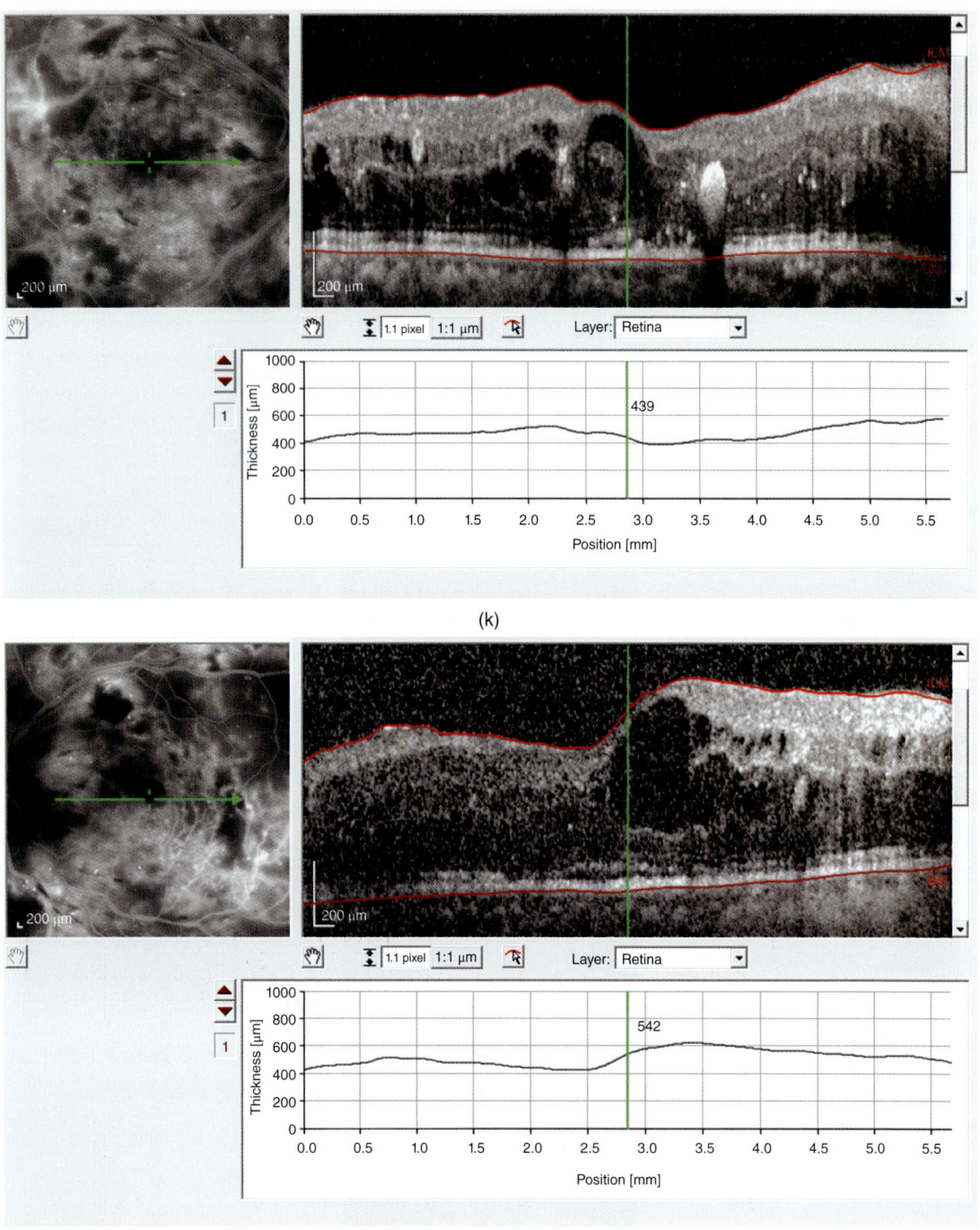

Fig. 9.5 (*Continued*)

each eye. We do not usually treat patients with pan-retinal photocoagulation until they develop proliferative changes, but it was felt that the level of ischaemia warranted early scatter laser treatment. It is too early at present to know how he will respond to treatment.

PRACTICE POINTS

The higher levels of moderate and severe NPDR (or pre-proliferative DR) show increasing signs of retinal ischaemia, which carries an increasing risk of development of proliferative DR.

Treatment of high BP and hyperglycaemia is important to reduce the combined effects, which further increases the risks of progression.

REFERENCE

Please visit www.wiley.com/go/scanlon/diabetic_retinopathy

10 Proliferative and advanced diabetic retinopathy

Ahmed Sallam[1] & Peter H. Scanlon[2]

[1] University of Arkansas for Medical Sciences, USA
[2] Harris Manchester College, University of Oxford; Medical Ophthalmology, University of Gloucestershire, UK

PROLIFERATIVE AND ADVANCED DR

Relevant anatomy

New vessels developing in diabetic retinopathy are characterised according to whether they develop at or near the optic disc (NVD) or elsewhere in the retina (NVE). They can develop from the venous or arterial circulation and grow forwards in the vitreous gel. Over time they may fibrose and retract, causing traction on the underlying retina, or they may haemorrhage. If a patient has a posterior vitreous detachment, this removes the structure that new vessels use to grow forwards into the vitreous gel. Although this may cause a haemorrhage if a patient already has new vessels, subsequent haemorrhages are less common as the base of the vessel has often been sheared off.

New vessels on the disc (NVD, Fig. 10.1a–e) are defined as any new vessel developing at the optic disc or within one disc diameter (1DD) of the edge of the optic disc. New vessels on the disc usually occur as a result of generalised retinal ischaemia. New vessels elsewhere (NVE, Fig. 10.1a–e) are defined as any new vessel developing more than 1DD away from the edge of the optic disc. New vessels elsewhere usually occur on the edge of an area of retinal ischaemia peripheral to the NVE.

Abortive neovascular outgrowths (ANO) is a term that has been used in the past to describe small raspberry-like NVE, which usually lie in an area temporal to the fovea and which, like most NVE, lie adjacent to areas of capillary non-perfusion.

Another consequence of generalised retinal ischaemia can be neovascularisation of the anterior segment. If this neovascularisation involves the angle of the anterior chamber, neovascular glaucoma may result.

Photographic appearance

New vessels appear as fronds either at the disc or elsewhere in the retina. As they develop they grow forwards into the vitreous gel, and this is shown on stereo photographs. On a two-dimensional (2D) photograph the forwards development of these new vessels can be interpreted by the structures that they overlay.

Fluorescein angiographic appearance

The characteristic appearance of new vessels on the fluorescein angiogram (Fig. 10.1b–f), once they have penetrated the internal limiting membrane, is leakage appearing in the arteriovenous phase of the angiogram and increasing through the angiogram. Leakage can be variable, but very little leakage from a small NVE (Fig. 10.2) usually means that these have not yet penetrated the internal limiting membrane.

Presentation

In an ideal world, people with diabetes would receive annual screening for diabetic retinopathy and more frequent assessments once signs of diabetic retinopathy develop and new vessels are detected at an early stage. At the other end of the spectrum, some patients who have not had their eyes examined for years present with a sudden onset of visual loss from a vitreous haemorrhage occurring from bleeding from large new vessels that have developed as a result of advanced diabetic retinopathy. The initial sight loss from a vitreous haemorrhage will depend on the amount of haemorrhage, and the visual prognosis will depend on the level of the underlying diabetic retinopathy and the degree of retinal ischaemia and any associated maculopathy.

A Practical Manual of Diabetic Retinopathy Management, Second Edition. Edited by Peter Scanlon, Ahmed Sallam, and Peter van Wijngaarden.
© 2017 John Wiley & Sons Ltd. Published 2017 by John Wiley & Sons Ltd.
Companion Website: www.wiley.com/go/scanlon/diabetic_retinopathy

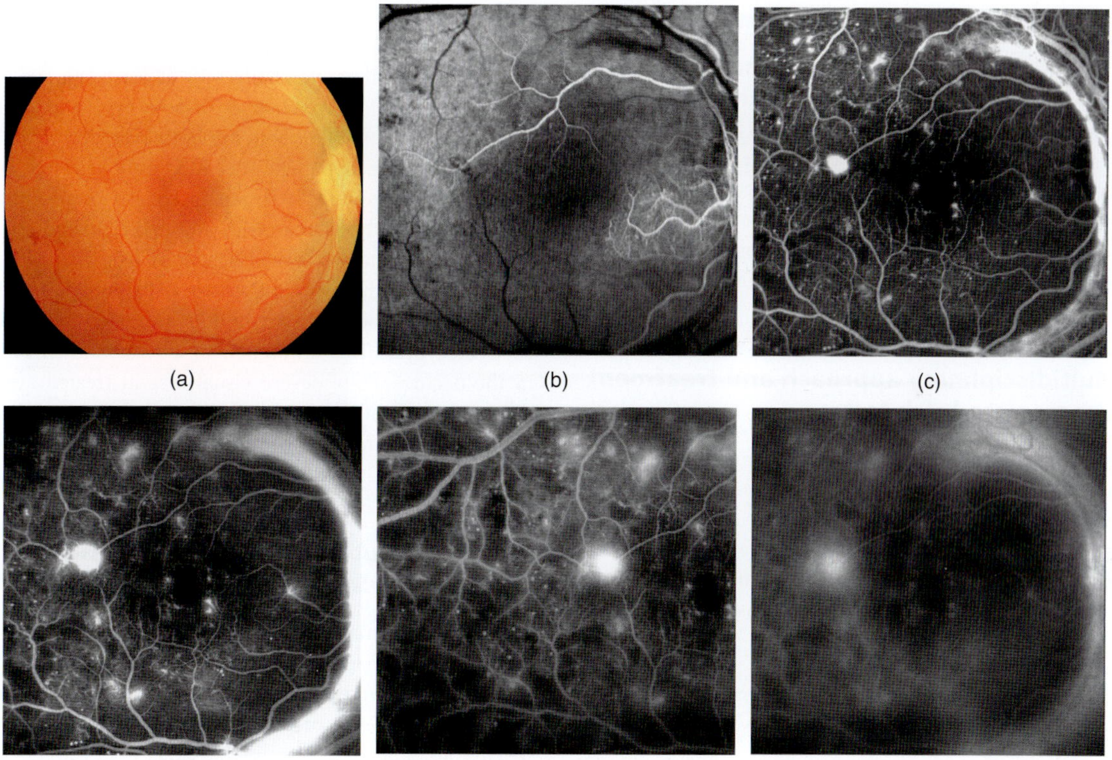

Proliferative and advanced diabetic retinopathy

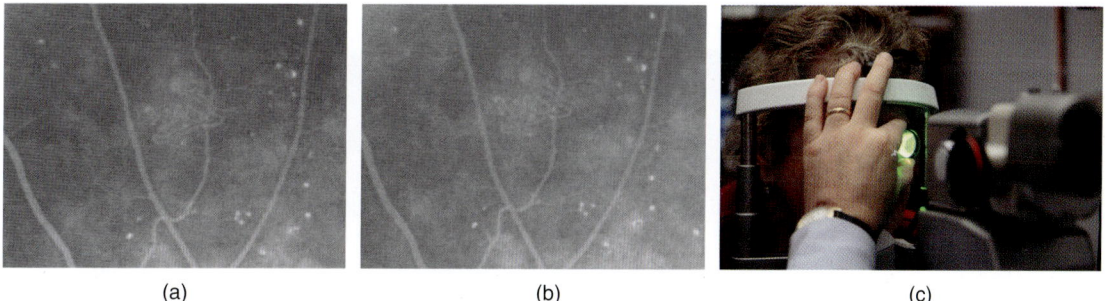

Fig. 10.1 (a) NVD and NVE colour photo. Fluorescein angiogram in early arterial phase: (b) 7 s from patient in (a) showing some early filling in NVD and (c) 12 s showing leakage from NVD and NVE. Fluorescein angiogram in late arteriovenous phase (d) 1 min 8 s showing leakage from NVD and NVE and (e) 1 min 46 s showing areas of ischaemic non-perfusion in temporal retina adjacent to NVE. (f) Fluorescein angiogram in the late venous phase (6 min 34 s) showing leakage from NVD and NVE.

Fig. 10.2 (a, b) NVE showing minimal or no leakage that have not yet penetrated the internal limiting membrane. (c) Laser treatment on a patient with diabetic retinopathy.

The 'early worsening' phenomenon

In 1998 the Diabetes Control and Complications Trial[1] (DCCT) described the effect of early worsening of diabetic retinopathy at the 6- and/or 12-month visit in 13.1% of 711 patients assigned to intensive treatment. Early worsening led to high-risk proliferative retinopathy in two patients in the DCCT. The most important risk factors for early worsening were higher HbA1c level at screening and reduction of this level during the first 6 months after randomisation.

Multidisciplinary approach and treatment of associated risk factors

Many patients who end up with severe diabetic eye disease have suboptimal control of blood glucose, blood pressure and lipid levels. It is important to have a multidisciplinary approach to these patients so that the eye is not treated in isolation and that proper attention is paid to the management of (1) systemic hypertension; (2) glucose control; and (3) blood lipids.

LASER TREATMENT FOR PROLIFERATIVE DR

Figure 10.2c depicts a patient undergoing laser treatment for diabetic retinopathy.

The Diabetic Retinopathy (DRS) Study

In 1976, Diabetic Retinopathy Study (DRS)[2] reported their preliminary results. According to the study protocol, a total of 1727 treatable patients had been enrolled. The eligibility criteria were: (1) diabetic retinopathy in both eyes, either proliferative changes in at least one eye or severe non-proliferative changes in both eyes; and (2) a visual acuity of 20/100 or better in both eyes.

One eye of each patient was randomly selected for treatment with xenon or argon laser and the control eye observed without treatment. The principal endpoint was the occurrence of visual acuity of less than 5/200 at one or more monthly follow-up visits. Visual acuity of less than 5/200 occurred in 129 untreated eyes and 56 treated eyes. This amounted to a reduction in 57% in the occurrence of severe visual loss in treated eyes. The organisers of the DRS[2] modified the trial protocol and recommend treatment for control eyes with high-risk characteristics.

Important outcomes of the Diabetic Retinopathy Study

The DRS[3,4] recommended prompt treatment is the presence of DRS high-risk characteristics, which reduced the 2 year risk of severe visual loss by 50% or more, defined by: (1) the presence of preretinal (Figs 10.3 and 10.4) or vitreous (Fig. 10.5) haemorrhage; (2) eyes with NVD equalling or exceeding one-quarter to one-third disc area in extent with no haemorrhage (Fig. 10.6); or (3) NVE equalling > half disc area with haemorrhage (Fig. 10.7).

Untreated, eyes with high-risk characteristics had a 25.6–36.9% chance of severe visual loss within 2 years, depending on the size and location of the new vessels and whether haemorrhage was present or not.

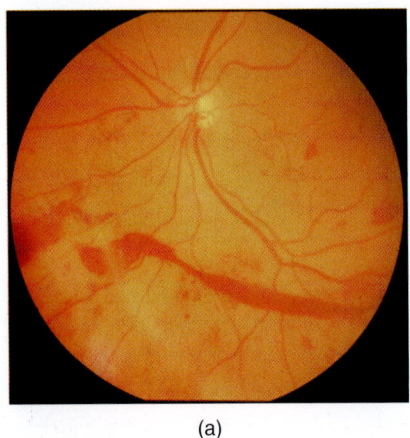
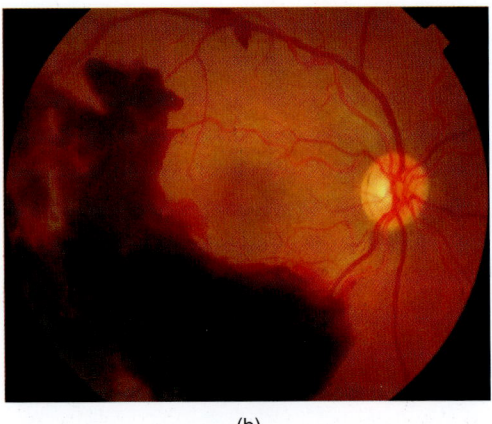

(a)   (b)

Fig. 10.3 (a, b) Example of a preretinal haemorrhage.

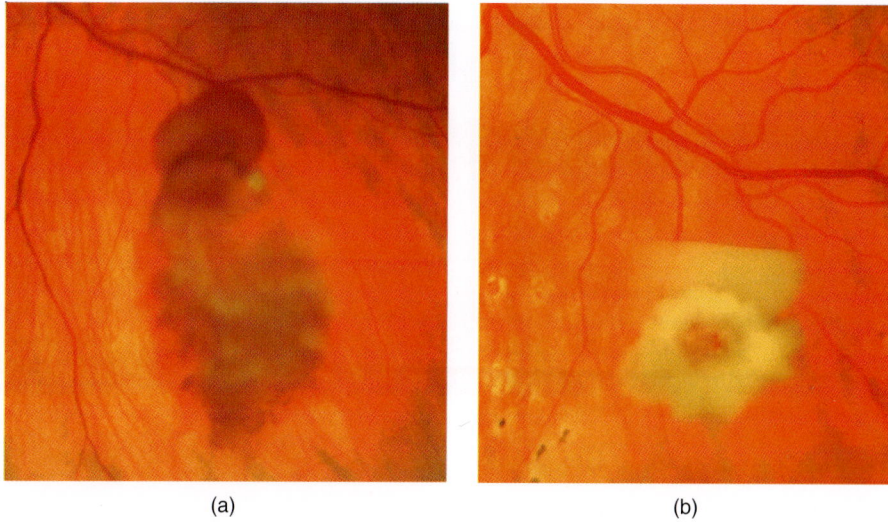

Fig. 10.4 (a) Example of a preretinal haemorrhage and (b) organising.

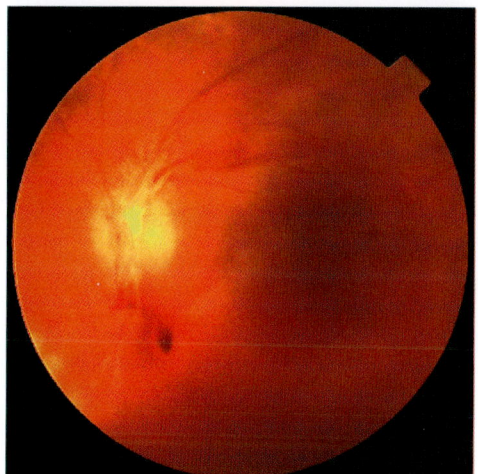

Fig. 10.5 Example of a vitreous haemorrhage

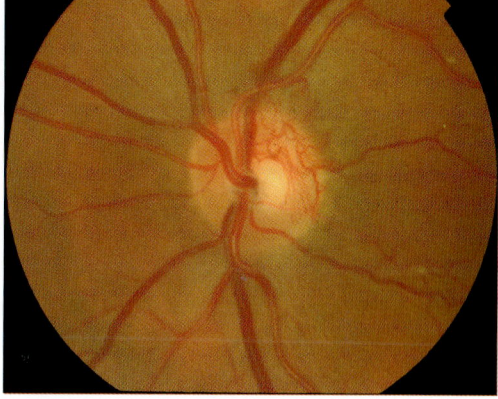

Fig. 10.6 NVD > one-third disc area.

Risks for patients without high-risk characteristics

In eyes with high-risk characteristics, the 2 year risk of severe visual loss (25–35%) clearly outweighed the risks of treatment (small reduction in visual acuity or visual field in approximately 15% of eyes).

The risks of severe visual loss in eyes without high-risk characteristics (Fig. 10.8a, c, d) did show a benefit from treatment but, as the difference was not as great as for those with high-risk characteristics, the risks of harmful effects of treatment need to be taken into consideration.

For patients with proliferative DR without high-risk characteristics and severe NPDR, the DRS findings did not provide a clear choice for these patients between either prompt treatment or careful follow-up with deferral of treatment until high-risk characteristics develop, and other factors need to be considered in these patients.

Eyes with low-risk characteristics had the following risks of severe visual loss:

- non-proliferative control group: untreated 2 year 3.2%, 4 year 12.8%; treated 2 year 2.8%, 4 year 4.3%; and
- proliferative without high-risk characteristics control group: untreated 2 year 7.0%, 4 year 20.9%; treated 2 year 3.2%, 4 year 7.4%.

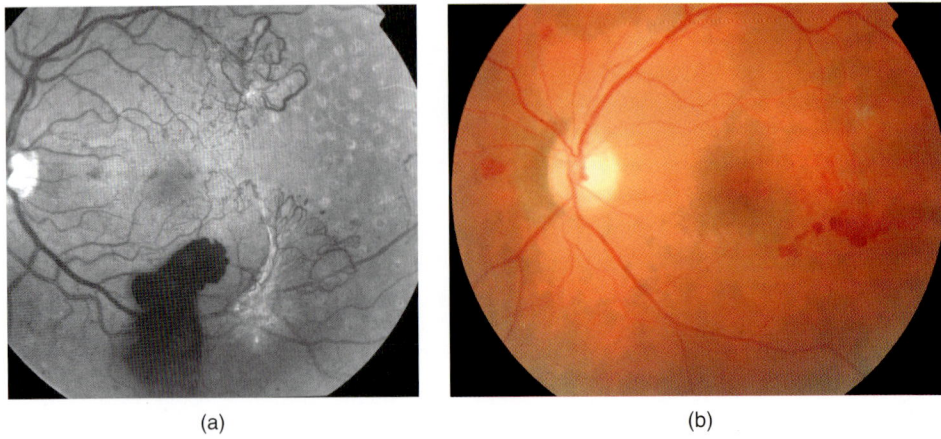

Fig. 10.7 (a, b) NVE equalling > half disc area with haemorrhage.

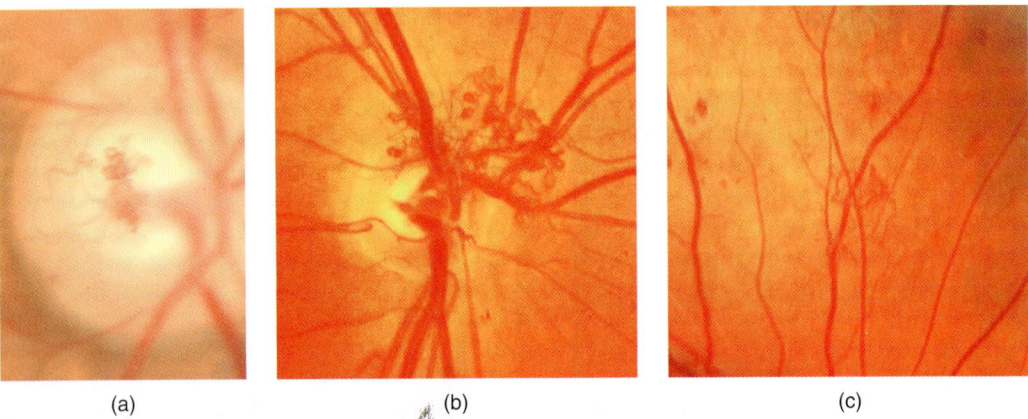

Fig. 10.8 NVD (a) < one-third and (b) > one-third disc area. NVE equalling < half disc area without haemorrhage (c) colour photo.

The ETDRS[5] attempted to alter the treatment protocol to reduce harmful effects (division of scatter treatment between two or more sittings or reduction of the number of burns). In the ETDRS only 50% of eyes assigned to deferral had developed high-risk proliferative retinopathy. For eyes with very severe non-proliferative retinopathy or moderate proliferative retinopathy, the benefits and risks of early photocoagulation were roughly equal. Very few eyes in the ETDRS had more than two disc areas of neovascularisation elsewhere; the possibility that there may be an advantage in prompt scatter photocoagulation for these eyes could not be ruled out. For eyes with macular oedema and more severe retinopathy, the risk of severe visual loss in eyes assigned to deferral of photocoagulation was relatively high (6.5% at the 5 year visit). This risk was reduced to between 3.8% and 4.7% in the eyes assigned to early photocoagulation. The ETDRS did not include evaluation of a strategy that consisted of prompt focal photocoagulation with delayed scatter in eyes with clinically significant macular oedema and eyes that are approaching the high-risk category.

Adverse effects of laser treatment in the DRS and other studies

The potential adverse effects of panretinal photocoagulation treatment were described in 1987 by the DRS[4] Research Group. Loss of peripheral areas of visual field was attributed to argon laser in approximately 10% of eyes, and field loss was nearly three times more common in the xenon-arc-treated group. Visual acuity loss at the 6 week follow-up visit was assumed to be due to treatment.

Among eyes with non-proliferative diabetic retinopathy, 14.3% more argon-treated and 29.7% of xenon-treated eyes than controls had an early persistent loss of one or more lines. For decreases of more than two or five lines, the comparable percentages were 2.5% (argon-treated) and 10.6% (xenon-treated) and 1.3% (argon-treated) and 1.8% (xenon-treated), respectively.

McDonald and Schatz[6] reviewed the results of 175 eyes of 134 patients with proliferative diabetic retinopathy treated with panretinal photocoagulation. A total of 75 (43%) of the treated eyes developed increased macular oedema (Fig. 10.9) 6–10 weeks following laser treatment, with a median follow-up of 15 months. Fluorescein angiography revealed that the post-laser increase in macular oedema persisted in 47 of the 175 eyes (27%). Fourteen eyes (8%) treated with laser developed chronic macular oedema and visual loss of two or more lines. Patients were treated with argon laser photocoagulation (0.05 s, 500 micron spot size, in two or more sessions with an average of 2300 burns). Although 47 eyes developed a persistent increase in macular oedema following treatment, only 16 lost vision. Thirty-one eyes therefore developed increased oedema (demonstrated on fluorescein angiography) and did not lose vision.

Clearly the disease process itself can have an adverse effect on visual acuity and field, and will be more pronounced in those patients with more severe disease. Many studies reported the effect of the disease process, panretinal photocoagulation and vitrectomy on the minimum visual acuity and field for the British driving standard.

In 1994, Mackie et al.[7] reported on the results of the Esterman binocular visual field test and visual acuities in 100 consecutive patients who had received bilateral panretinal photocoagulation (PRP): 4% failed to achieve the VA requirements but met field requirements; 9% failed to achieve the field requirements but met the VA requirements; 17% failed to achieve both the field and the VA requirements; and 74% retained the minimum field for the British driving standard. Of those who failed, it was estimated that approximately one-third were due to

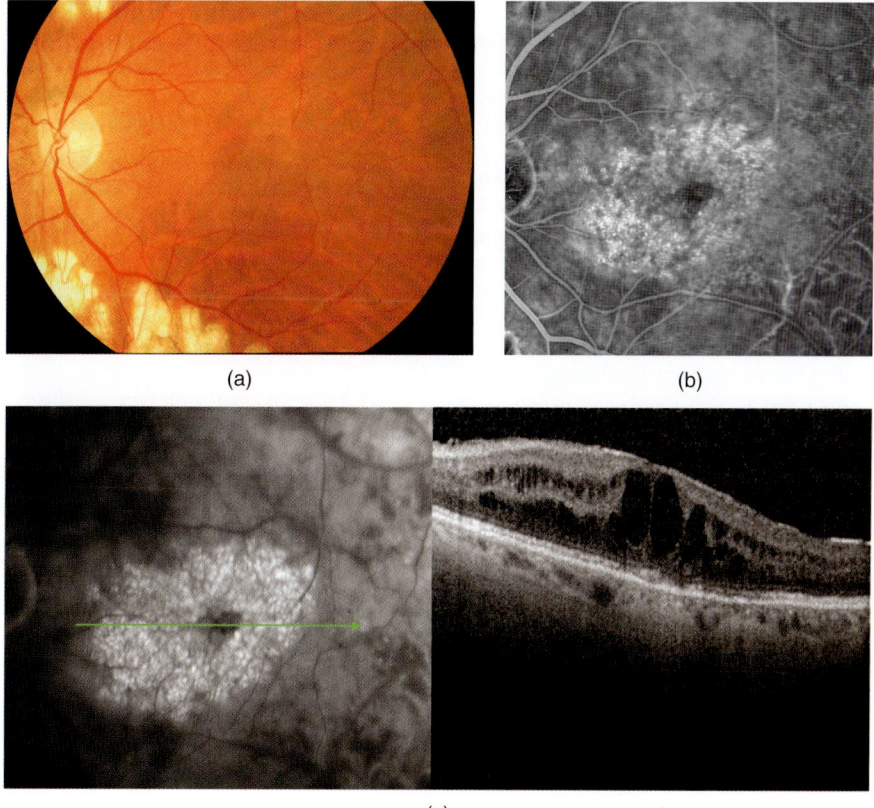

(a)　　　　　　　　　　　　　　(b)

(c)

Fig. 10.9 Persistent cystoid macula following panretinal laser treatment: (a) colour photo; (b) fluorescein photo 1 min 9 s post-injection; and (c) fluorescein and OCT photo 9 min 24 s post-injection.

laser treatment. The remainder failed from a combination of treatment and maculopathy or complications directly related to the disease process.

Compare this to a prospective study in 2006 of ET-DRS acuity and Humphrey binocular Esterman visual field testing by Barsam and Laidlaw[8] in 20 patients who underwent vitrectomy for complications of diabetic retinopathy. A total of 70% of patients had sufficient binocular acuity to drive, and of these 71.4% were shown not to have a minimum visual field for safe driving on binocular Esterman field analysis. Patients who have had a vitrectomy are more likely to have a restricted visual field because their disease is more severe, there is more peripheral retinal ischaemia and they may have received more laser treatment.

Case History 10.1: Driving field difficulties following extensive laser and vitrectomy for very ischaemic retinae

A 48-year-old man with type 2 diabetes (BMI 33) controlled by insulin of 24 years duration had extensive laser to both eyes prior to left pars plana vitrectomy and endolaser. During the period of treatment the HBA1c varied between 7.8 and 8.6 and his BP was well controlled, averaging 125/75. His corrected visual acuity level is right 6/9 (20/30) and left 6/18 (20/60), which would meet the UK visual standard but the Esterman field shown in Figure 10.10a would not. For the Esterman field, one needs to be able to see the points in the area 120 degrees horizontally and 4 degrees vertically, and this field clearly misses many points in this area. Colour (Fig. 10.10b–e) and fluorescein (Fig. 10.10f, g) photographs show the underlying retinal ischaemia that has contributed to the reduced field in this patient.

Other possible adverse effects of panretinal laser treatment include the following.
1. *Unintended laser absorption.* This can occur in the lens of the eye in the presence of lens opacities and in the nerve fibre layer of the retina from intraretinal haemorrhages. In the latter example, uptake of laser from a flame-shaped haemorrhage may result in a burn and destruction of the nerve fibre layer that lies on its surface.
2. *Inadvertent coagulation.* Clearly unintended photocoagulation to the fovea when performing panretinal photocoagulation is the area of most concern and the laser technique employed should allow one to be aware at all times of where the fovea is in relation to area being lasered.
3. *Choroidal detachment.* When a choroidal detachment occurs this is usually as a result of a large dose of laser treatment being applied in a single session. This may result in the precipitation of angle closure glaucoma if a patient has a shallow anterior chamber. The choroidal detachment usually resolves spontaneously within 10 days.
4. *Risks to the ophthalmologist.* There has been some concern in the past that the ophthalmologist is exposed to excessive amounts of reflected light, particularly blue light. However, modern technology with appropriate filters has significantly reduced this risk.
5. *Risks to an observer.* The risk to an observer is extremely small because they are very unlikely to be exposed to a sufficient dose of reflected or direct laser light to produce any adverse consequences. However, as a precaution, it is advised that any observer wears the appropriate spectacle protection.

Factors other than high-risk characteristics influencing the decision to laser

Anterior segment neovascularisation

Extensive neovascularisation in the anterior chamber angle is an urgent indication for scatter laser photocoagulation, if it is feasible, whether or not high-risk characteristics are present.

Case History 10.2: Iris neovascularisation

This 69-year-old man with type 2 diabetes, diagnosed at the age of 42 years and treated with oral gliclazide and metformin, had received panretinal laser treatment to his left eye 5 years previously and his vision had stabilised at 6/18 (20/60). He had been lost to follow-up and presented with a sore eye, which was found to have an intraocular pressure of 58 mm Hg due to a rubeotic glaucoma with extensive neovascularisation on the iris and in the angle of the anterior chamber. The photograph in Figure 10.11a was taken.

He was treated with intravitreal bevacizumab to suppress the iris and retinal neovascularisation. This brought down his intraocular pressure to a level of 14 mm Hg and enabled a sufficiently clear view of his retina to enable further panretinal photocoagulation to be performed to treat the underlying retinal ischaemia, the cause of the iris neovascularisation.

Signs of ischaemia

Venous beading (Fig. 10.11b) in more than one quadrant, extensive retinal haemorrhages and opaque small arteriolar branches are signs suggesting severe retinal ischaemia, which suggest that these eyes are at greater risk of neovascularisation.

Macular oedema

McDonald and Schatz[6] showed that 43% of the treated eyes in their study developed increased macular oedema 6–10 weeks following laser treatment. It was therefore recommended that eyes needing scatter laser treatment and also having macular oedema are less at risk of visual

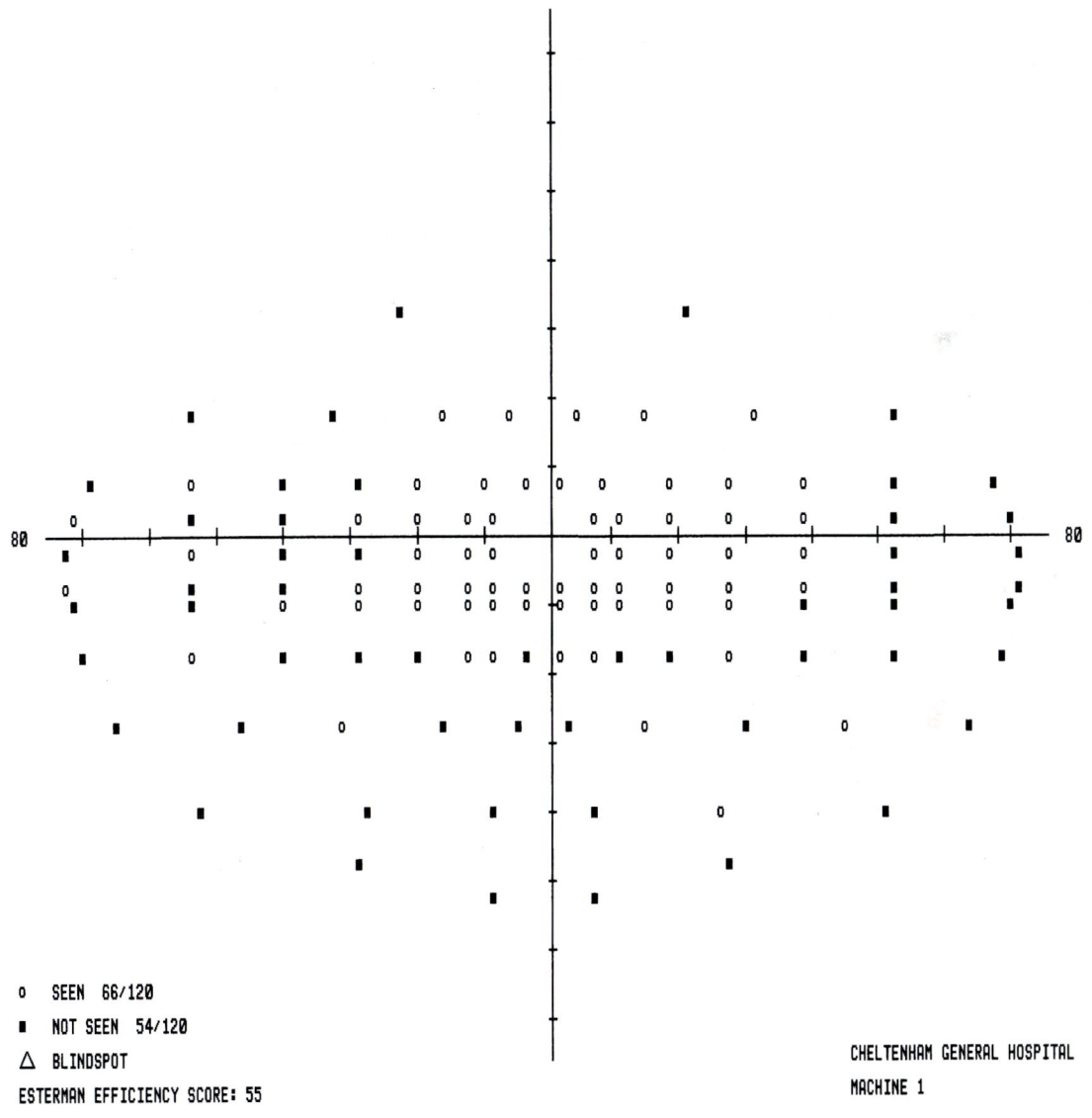

(a)

Fig. 10.10 (a) A restricted Esterman field in a diabetic patient. Colour photo: (b) right macula; (c) right nasal retina; (d) left nasal retina; (e) left macula; and (f) Fluorescein left macular area 45 s after injection, showing ischaemia and IRMA in the area around the left macula. (g) Fluorescein right macular area 1 min 10 s after injection, showing ischaemia and IRMA in the area around the left macula.

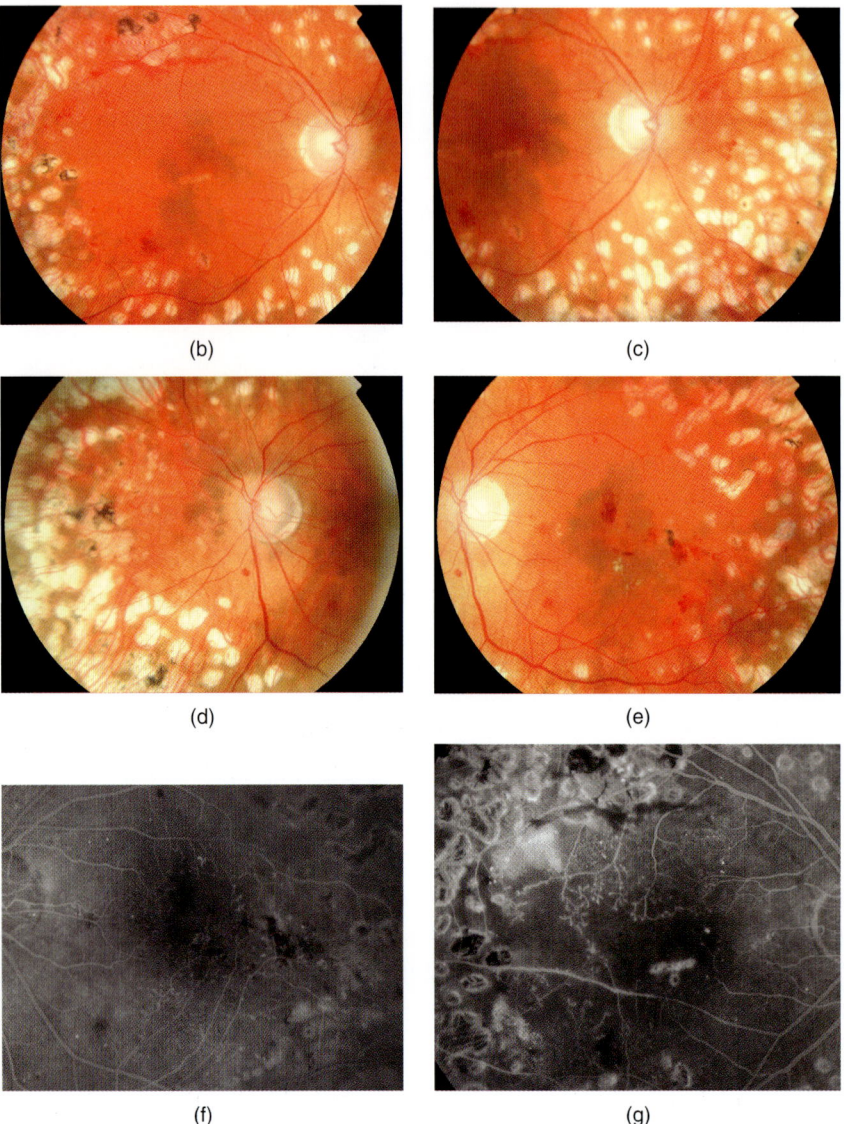

Fig. 10.10 (*Continued*)

acuity loss when focal or grid treatment to reduce the macular oedema precedes scatter laser photocoagulation, where this is possible. If this is not possible, focal or grid laser treatment should be applied at the first scatter laser treatment session.

More recent evidence suggests that eyes with centre-involving DMO and PDR are best treated with a combination therapy of intravitreal anti-VEGF and panretinal photocoagulation treatment. In patients with marked macular oedema, panretinal photocoagulation could be deferred for 2–3 weeks after initiation of intravitreal anti-VEGF therapy. This is further discussed in Chapter 11 on proliferative DR with maculopathy.

Although it could affect its clinical effectiveness, decreasing the fluency of PRP is likely to decrease the risk of macular oedema as shown in a small prospective randomised trial that included 20 eyes treated with reduced fluency laser, by either limiting the extent of laser to only peripheral ischaemic areas (targeted PRP) or decreasing

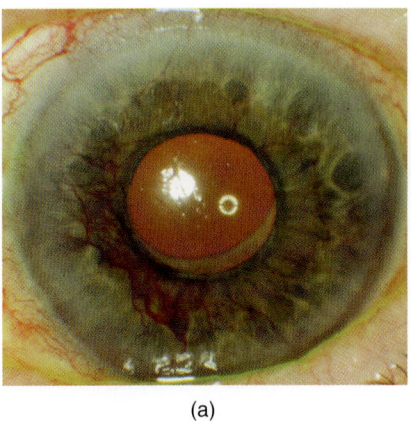 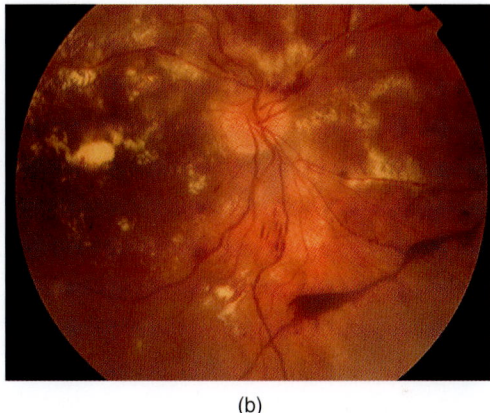

(a) (b)

Fig. 10.11 (a) Iris neovascularisation. (b) Ischaemic eye with venous beading, preretinal haemorrhage, NVE and extensive exudation.

the intensity of PRP treatment by using minimal intensity burns (minimally traumatic PRP).[9]

Pregnancy
See Chapter 15 on pregnancy and diabetic retinopathy.

Renal failure
One needs to coincide treatment with renal dialysis or transplantation. It is also important to control hypertension.

Past history
The past history of retinopathy both in the eye for which scatter laser photocoagulation is being considered and in the fellow eye needs to be considered.

Follow-up after panretinal photocoagulation

In 1991, Blankenship[10] reported the 15 year argon laser and xenon photocoagulation results of Bascom Palmer Eye Institute's patients participating in the Diabetic Retinopathy Study. Fifteen years after panretinal photocoagulation in the DRS, 86 (57%) patients had died, 14 (9%) could not be located and 51 (34%) of 151 patients were examined to determine the long-term treatment effects. Eleven (58%) of the initially argon-treated and 13 (41%) of the initially xenon-treated eyes had 20/40 or better acuity, and 18 (95%) of the initially argon-treated and 26 (82%) of the initially xenon-treated eyes had 20/200 or better acuity. Of the control eyes, 17 (33%) had 20/40 or better and 30 (58%) had 20/200 or better acuity. It was therefore concluded that argon and xenon panretinal photocoagulation for diabetic retinopathy provide good results for at least 15 years.

Quantification of retinal ablation, use of one treatment session and lessons learnt from the UK National Diabetic Laser Treatment Audit

The Diabetic Retinopathy Study (DRS) protocol for panretinal photocoagulation recommended 800–1600 argon laser burns of 500 micron spot size, extending to or beyond the vortex ampullae for eyes with high-risk characteristics. The ETDRS protocol for full scatter laser treatment was developed from this and recommended 1200–1600 argon laser burns of 500 micron spot size. The ETDRS recommended that the treatment should be performed in 2 or more episodes which were no more than 2 weeks apart, and that no more than 900 burns should be applied in one session. An estimate of the area of retina ablated can be described using the standard formula of πr^2 multiplied by the number of burns. According to the DRS protocol the recommended amount of retina treated is equivalent to an area of 157–314 mm^2, while the lower limit for the full panretinal photocoagulation treatment as recommended by the ETDRS is equivalent to an area of 236 mm^2, with the same upper recommended area of 314 mm^2.

In 1998, Bailey et al.[11,12] reported the results of the UK National Diabetic Retinopathy Laser Treatment Audit, which was a prospective survey of laser treatment for diabetic retinopathy throughout the UK. A total of 284 patients who were undergoing their first panretinal photocoagulation for proliferative retinopathy during a 2-month period in 1995 were followed up for a period of 9 months. For eyes with proliferative retinopathy the retinal neovascularisation had regressed fully in 50.8% of cases, while there had been no change or a deterioration in 10.3%. A visual acuity of less than 6/60 at follow-up was present in 8.6% of eyes. There was a poor morphological outcome at follow-up (as defined by rubeosis, new tractional detachment or having had a vitrectomy) in 7.2%. Risk factors for poor morphological outcome were the presence of high-risk characteristics, female sex and the presence of concurrent maculopathy at baseline. Regression of neovascularisation was associated with greater areas of retinal ablation at the initial treatment session. It was considered that the ophthalmologist intended to give the initial panretinal photocoagulation in one sitting in 41.2% of cases and to divide the initial treatment into more than one session in 55.6% of cases; in 3.2% of cases this information was not recorded. For the subgroup with the equivalent of high-risk characteristics who were given their initial treatment in one session (n=65), the median retinal area treated was 104.6 mm^2 (range 10.4–682.5 mm^2) or 377.6 mm^2 (range 37.6–2464 mm^2) if the quadraspheric had been used for all cases.

Unfortunately, UK ophthalmologists had been influenced by a 1992 publication by Hulbert and Vernon[13] which reported on 21 people with proliferative diabetic retinopathy who had received bilateral panretinal photocoagulation. They recommended burns of no larger than 200 micron real spot size and claimed that between 3000 and 3500 burns induced regression in all but severe cases. The reason given for the recommendations was that patients were more likely to pass the standards set for driving in the UK if the smaller spot size was used. This recommendation is considerably less than the recommendation of the DRS and ETDRS. A total of 4997 burns of 200 micron spot size would be required to meet the equivalent area of retinal ablation to 800 burns of 500 micron spot size recommended in the DRS, and 7500 burns of 200 micron spot size would be required to meet the equivalent area of retinal ablation to 1200 burns of 500 micron spot size recommended in the ETDRS.

There is also concern from the UK audit about the percentage that intended to give their panretinal treatment in one session because of the risks of vision loss from macular oedema if large areas of retina were treated in one session, and the apparent under-treatment of the subgroup of patients with high-risk characteristics.

Some eyes do in fact require more treatment than that recommended by the DRS. Reddy et al.[14] studied 294 eyes of 182 patients treated with argon scatter laser treatment and followed up for a minimum of 1 year to quantitate the amount of retinal ablation required for regression of proliferative diabetic retinopathy. Regression was observed in 275 eyes (93%); 19 eyes (7%) failed to regress and eventually required vitrectomy. Panretinal photocoagulation alone successfully led to regression in 229 eyes (77%), whereas 46 eyes (15.6%) required both photocoagulation and peripheral anterior retinal cryotherapy. Low-treatment eyes received an average of 510 mm^2 of retinal ablation (2600 × 500 micron burns), and high treatment eyes received 1280 mm^2 (6500 × 500 micron burns). More extensive treatment was required with more retinopathy risk factors. The authors concluded that the amount of initial treatment required for regression may be considerably more than that recommended by the DRS.

Recommended laser treatment settings using conventional non-pattern argon laser treatment

Following the DRS and ETDRS studies, refinement of scatter laser treatment for proliferative diabetic retinopathy has provided the following recommendations:

1. Argon laser photocoagulation using 1200–2000 burns of 500 micron spot size for an exposure time of 0.1 s.
2. Power is adjusted to obtain mild bleaching that does not spread to be appreciably larger than 500 microns.
3. This number of burns is applied in 2 or more episodes at least 4 days apart (but no less than 2 weeks apart).
4. No more than 900 burns are to be applied in a single setting.
5. The posterior extent of the initial scatter laser treatment is an oval area defined by a line passing 2DD above, temporal to and below the centre of the macula and 500 microns from the nasal half of the disc margin. From this line scatter laser treatment extends peripherally to or beyond the equator, avoiding direct treatment of major vessels (and chorioretinal scars if present).
6. When it is feared that vitreous haemorrhage may occur, it is recommended that the inferior quadrant is treated first.
7. The treatment period should be completed within 6 weeks.

Other factors are described in the following sections.

Retinal dimensions corresponding to different angles of visual field

Davies[15] used a mathematical model of the emmetropic eye to calculate retinal dimensions corresponding to different angles of visual field. He suggested that it is theoretically possible to alter the pattern of PRP to avoid treatment in retinal areas concerned with the driving visual field while leaving the total number of burns constant. This has led many ophthalmologists to extend the area untreated to 1DD or 1500 microns from the nasal half of the disc margin.

Laser spot magnification factor and field of view of lens used

The laser spot magnification factor has a significant influence on the settings on the laser machine used. Many of the modern indirect laser lenses have a magnification factor of 1.9–2.0. Ophthalmologists are commonly using laser spot sizes of 200 microns with these lenses; the effective diameter of the beam is therefore 380–400 microns once it has passed through one of these lenses. If a lower spot size than 500 microns is used, the number of burns needs to be increased as discussed in the section on quantification of retinal ablation.

The field of view of a retinal laser lens alters the area of retina that is available to the operator to treat with that particular lens. Example of the manufacturer's advertised laser spot magnification factors and fields of view (taken from their respective websites) include the following:

- Volk's Superquad 160, 2.0 × laser spot magnification factor, 160° field of view;
- Volk's 130° Quadraspheric lens, 1.92 × laser spot magnification factor, 144° dynamic field of view;
- Volk Transequator, 1.44 × laser spot magnification factor, 132° dynamic field of view;
- Ocular Mainster PRP 165, 1.96 × laser spot magnification factor, 165° static field of view, 180° dynamic field of view; and
- Ocular Mainster Wide Field, 1.5 × laser spot magnification factor, 118° field of view, 127° dynamic field of view.

Duration of the burn

There has been an increasing tendency recently for operators to reduce the duration of the burn and increase the power to produce an apparently similar mild bleaching, because this is more comfortable for the patient. However, it is worth mentioning that the width of the burn may be reduced by this approach and that more burns may therefore be required.[16]

Number of treatment sessions

One of the ways in which the ETDRS[17] attempted to reduce harmful effects was the division of scatter treatment between two or more sittings. This was a direct result of the DRS study in which 14.3% more argon-treated and 29.7% xenon-treated eyes than controls had an early persistent loss of one or more lines. The likely cause of the loss of visual acuity in the xenon-treated group was a persistent increase in macular oedema as a consequence of the increased intensity of treatment[17] in one session in the xenon-treated group. The alternative view suggested in a study by Doft and Blankenship[18] is that there is no major difference in the effect of treatment on visual acuity between groups to whom treatment was administered in a single session as compared with multiple sessions spaced over time. The article stated that exudative retinal detachment, choroidal detachment and angle closure occurred more commonly in single-session-treatment group eyes, but these effects were transient and no long-term difference between treatment groups was found. The view of the current authors is that treatment should be spaced over a minimum of two sessions unless there is a strong suspicion that the individual being treated might not attend for subsequent treatment sessions.

The pattern argon laser and the evidence behind its recommendation

Scatter laser photocoagulation involves the controlled destruction of the peripheral retina using targeted laser pulses. A full course of treatment typically requires two or more sessions, each lasting approximately 15 min (or longer with less-experienced operators).

With conventional methods of retinal laser photocoagulation, the ophthalmologist uses a mechanical joystick and foot pedal to deliver single 100 ms laser pulses to the peripheral retina.

Optimedia Corporation introduced the Pascal (pattern scan laser) Photocoagulator in June 2006, which is a frequency-doubled Nd: YAG diode-pumped solid-state laser producing a wavelength of 532 nm. With the patterned scanning laser photocoagulation the laser pulse time is reduced from 100 ms to just 10–20 ms, and automated multiple spots are produced with each depression of the foot pedal. Relatively higher power is required for the shorter burns. From the main control panel, an LCD display with a touch screen control is used to select from pre-determined pattern types and administer up to 25 spots at a time for scatter laser treatment. The operator can select different arcs, circular grid patterns or sectors of grids for treatment, or use a rectangular array. Once the pattern is selected, a separate red beam is used for aiming and visualisation of the placement before delivery. The touch screen interface is also used for selecting various parameters, such as aim beam intensity, treatment laser power, exposure time, system status and shut down.

Blumenkranz et al.[19] conducted pre-clinical experiments with reduced pulse duration (1–100 ms) to determine retinal burn characteristics associated with these rapidly delivered light pulses. The histological appearance of light burns at 10–100 ms demonstrated that the damage is confined to the outer retina and retinal pigment epithelium. However, at pulse durations of >20 ms, significant diffusion of heat occurred with less localised homogenous lesions histopathologically. The reduced pulse duration burns appear to produce less inner retinal (e.g. choroidal) injury, and this may be the reason for the observation of less patient discomfort.

The potential advantages over conventional single spot laser include: (1) increased uniformity and precision of spot placement with less chance of overlap (a potential safety benefit); (2) reduced discomfort felt by the patient has been widely reported; and (3) reduced overall treatment duration/procedure time (thereby reducing costs).[20,21]

However, some aspects relating to the use of Pascal require attention. First, while it was initially suggested that the availability of a retinal photocoagulator capable of the rapid sequential application of a large number of spots makes single-session PRP practically feasible, and was later advocated by the findings of a small prospective study that demonstrated significant reduction in neovascularisation after single-session treatment,[22] data from other studies indicate that, in clinical practice, most clinicians would deliver treatment over at least two sessions.[20,23] As mentioned in the section on number of treatment sessions above, the view of the current authors is that treatment should be spaced over a minimum of two sessions unless there is a strong suspicion that the individual being treated might not attend for subsequent treatment sessions.

Second, there is concern that the use of short pulses in Pascal could be associated with decreased clinical efficacy and an increased need for re-treatment compared to conventional long-pulse (100 ms or more) laser. In a retrospective study that compared 41 eyes of high-risk PDR treated with Pascal and a similar number of eyes treated with conventional argon laser, persistence or recurrence of neovascularisation within 6 months of initial treatment was significantly higher in the Pascal-treated eyes (73% v. 34%; $P=0.0008$), although a comparable number of laser spots were used in both treatment groups.[23] This could be related to smaller zones of retinal photocoagulation with short-pulse laser spots. As shown in an OCT-based study which demonstrated that, in order to achieve a total treatment area of 1000 standard ETDRS burn (100 ms, moderate intensity) with a 20 ms short-pulsed laser, the number of laser shots need to be increased by a factor of approximately 1.4 × for the 400 mm spot size and 1.9 × for the 200 mm.[16]

Third, while using a large number multiple spot array appears to be time efficient, in our experience it is difficult to achieve well-focused spots when using arrays of more than 5×5 even when laser is applied in non-peripheral retinal areas.

Finally, caution is required when using short-pulse laser due to an increased risk of Bruch's membrane rupture with increasing burn intensity as compared to conventional (long) pulse laser.[24]

Targeted PRP

The concept of targeted PRP laser was reported recently by Muqit et al. from Manchester, UK in order to decrease the risk of PRP-associated complications such as macular oedema.[9,25] In this strategy, widefield fluorescein angiogram-guided laser treatment was employed to only cover areas of capillary non-perfusion from the ora serrata, extending up to 1DD into perfused retina. While significant reductions in central retinal thickness at the fovea after targeted laser treatment versus standard short-pulse PRP were achieved at 12 weeks with no statistically significant difference in regression of neovascularisation,[9] this study included only a small number of eyes (10 in each arm) which makes it difficult to draw any firm conclusion on the efficacy of this strategy for PRP or on its advantages over conventional Pascal treatment. It does, however, appear logical to be targeting areas of capillary non-perfusion if results of widefield fluorescein angiography are available to the operator.

Navigating laser treatment

Navilas is a new technology for delivering retinal laser with integrated imaging and navigation systems. The technology is further discussed in Chapter 6 under laser treatment for DMO.

For PRP, navigating pattern laser has a few advantages over Pascal; the most important is its ability to deliver multiple spots of both long- and short-pulse laser. In contrast to Pascal where only short-pulse laser could be delivered when using multiple spot patterns, the eye-tracking system in Navilas compensates for the eye movements and it is therefore possible to deliver multiple spot ETDRS-standard long-pulse laser. Second, navigated laser treatment also achieves more uniform laser burns with less variation in spot size.[26] Finally, a recent randomised study found that treatment duration is significantly shorter when performing PRP with a median time per 100 spots in navigated 30 ms laser of 34 s, compared with 60 s for Pascal 30 ms laser.[27]

Case History 10.3: Severe NVD in both eyes

This 28-year-old man with type 1 diabetes (BMI 24) since the age of 6 years had been referred after a visit to his optometrist with a diagnosis of proliferative diabetic retinopathy but failed to attend four clinic appointments that were sent to him. His recent HbA1c result had been 9.4 and his BP 115/84.

At the age of 29 years he presented with a sudden onset of blurred patch in the vision of his right eye due to a vitreous haemorrhage from NVD, and he showed signs of proliferative diabetic retinopathy in both eyes.

Laser treatment was commenced to each eye:
- Right eye 1531 burns in 2 sessions, 710 of 350 micron size, 170 mW, 0.1 s, Transequator lens (magnification factor 1.44), and 821 burns 200 micron size, 180 mW, 0.1 secs, Superquad lens lens (magnification factor 2), argon laser.
- Left eye 1442 burns in 2 sessions, 700 of 350 micron size, 190 mW, 0.1 s, Transequator lens (magnification factor 1.44), and 742 burns 200 micron size, 190 mW, 0.1 secs, Superquad lens (magnification factor 2), argon laser.

He then failed to attend five follow-up appointments. Photographs of his eyes when he attended again 18 months later are shown in Figure 10.12a–c. He was then given further treatment to both eyes at the first attendance:
- Right eye 850 burns, 200 micron size, 250 mW, 0.03 s, Transequator lens (magnification factor 1.44), Pascal laser.
- Left eye 875 burns, 200 micron size, 190 mW, 0.1 s, Transequator lens (magnification factor 1.44), Pascal laser.

Photographs of his eyes immediately after laser treatment are shown in Figure 10.12d and e.

Case History 10.4: NVE in superotemporal retina with some macular ischaemia

This 44-year-old lady with type 1 diabetes for 26 years (BMI 41) was being followed up for moderate non-proliferative diabetic retinopathy. She developed an increasing right cataract reducing her preoperative VA to 6/18 (20/60), but post-operatively her vision was noted to be worse at a level of 6/36 (20/180). A fluorescein angiogram (Fig. 10.13) demonstrated the presence of large NVE in her right superotemporal retina and a degree of macular ischaemia.

Her BP readings had averaged 132/70 and her HbA1c results had improved from 12.3 to 10.6 over the previous 6 years. Her right retina was treated with panretinal photocoagulation using 1933 burns of 200 micron spot size using the Superquad 160 lens (magnification factor 2.0). The NVE gradually fibrosed over the subsequent 5 months and the vision has gradually improved to a level of 6/9 (20/30) over a 6 month period; it has fortunately remained at this level.

Case History 10.5: NVD treated with panretinal photocoagulation (attendance intermittent)

This 42-year-old man, controlled by insulin (diagnosed at the age of 30 years), was referred by the retinal screening service with proliferative diabetic retinopathy in both eyes as can be seen in the colour and red-free photographs in Figure 10.14. His attendance record over the last 2 years since these photographs were taken has made it very difficult to control the neovascularisation with laser treatment.

Case History 10.6: Undertreated proliferative retinopathy

This 73-year-old female with type 2 DM (diagnosed at the age of 40 years), previously treated for bilateral diabetic macular oedema and right proliferative diabetic retinopathy with macular laser (Fig. 10.15a) and PRP, was found to have active PDR in the left eye with preretinal haemorrhage (Fig. 10.15b) and multiple areas of NVE during routine hospital follow-up. Fluorescein angiogram showed multiple areas of NVE in the left eye (Fig. 10.15c and d). The right eye also had areas of active NVE and was felt to be under-treated with laser (Fig. 10.15e). Left PRP laser was commenced and right fill in laser was undertaken. Vison remained good at 6/9 in both eyes.

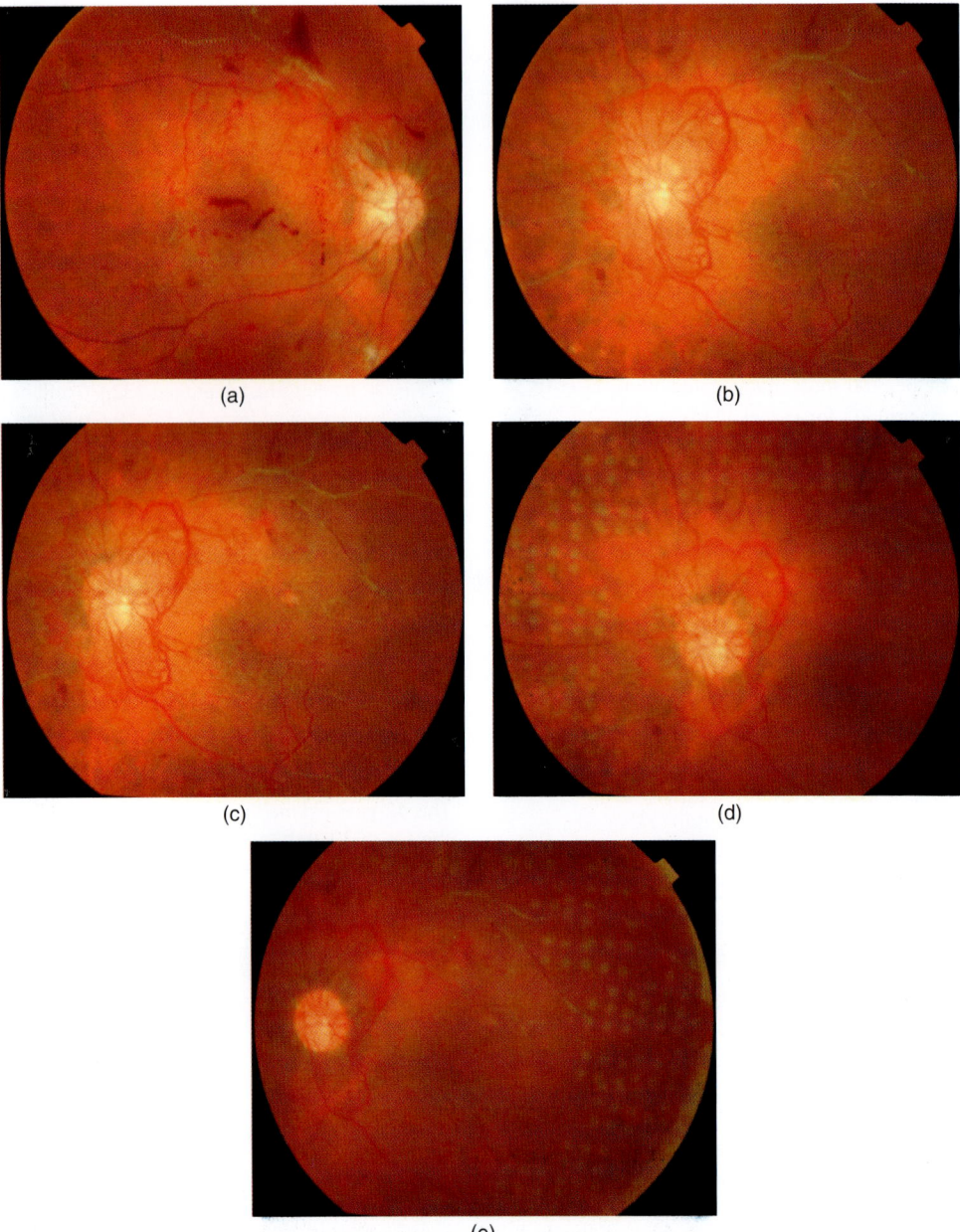

Fig. 10.12 (a) Right macula colour pre-treatment; (b) left disc colour pre-treatment; and (c) left macula colour pre-treatment. Left (d) disc and (e) macula colour immediately post-treatment.

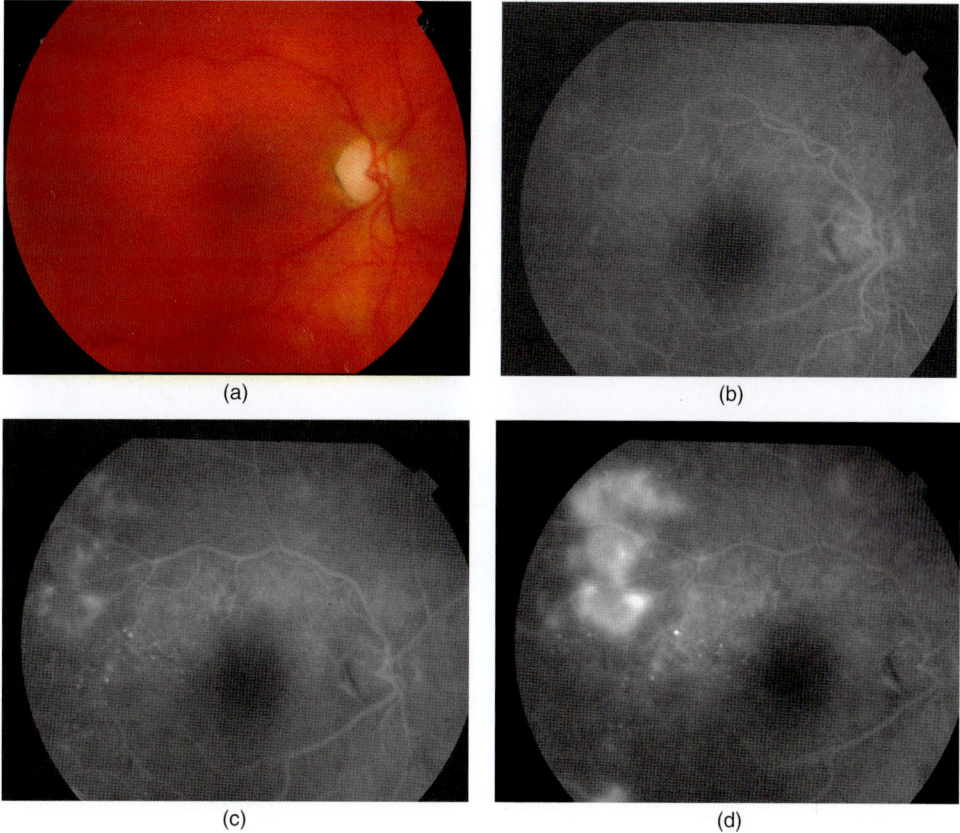

Fig. 10.13 (a) Colour right macular area. Fluorescein right macular area: (b) 35 s, (c) 52 s and (c) 1 min 45 s after injection.

Case History 10.7: Posterior vitreous detachment with horseshoe-shaped tear at the site of NVE

A 62-year-old lady with type 1 diabetes (BMI 20) of 11 years duration had been treated with panretinal photocoagulation to her left eye for NVE and changes of severe NPDR 4 years before her current presentation. Her HBA1c had improved from 9.4 to 7.0 and her BP from 153/77 to 136/68 over the previous 8 years. On this occasion she presented with a sudden onset of a 'blob' in the centre of the vision of her left eye and a greyish haze. The VA was 6/6 (20/20) and on examination a small haemorrhagic PVD was noted. One month later, an increase in blurriness was accompanied by occasional yellow flashes noted in half-light conditions. At that time the VA was 6/9 (20/30) and the source of the bleeding was noted to be a small patch of NVE in the left temporal retina. Some scatter laser treatment was given to some gaps in the previous panretinal laser treatment in the left temporal retina. At a subsequent follow-up visit 6 weeks later, an operculated tear was noted (see Fig. 10.16a–c).

Argon laser treatment to encircle the retinal tear was undertaken with 126 burns, 210 mW, 100 micron size, argon laser, Area Centralis lens (see Fig. 10.16d).

PATIENT EXPERIENCES OF LASER

Many patients are very anxious about the possibility of having to receive laser treatment. Their experience can often be much improved by adequate explanations being given of the reasons for the laser treatment and what is involved with the treatment. If the patient remains very anxious following adequate explanation, this can make laser treatment more difficult for the patient and the ophthalmologist.

Anaesthesia for retinal laser

The vast majority of macular and panretinal laser treatments are performed without difficulty using a

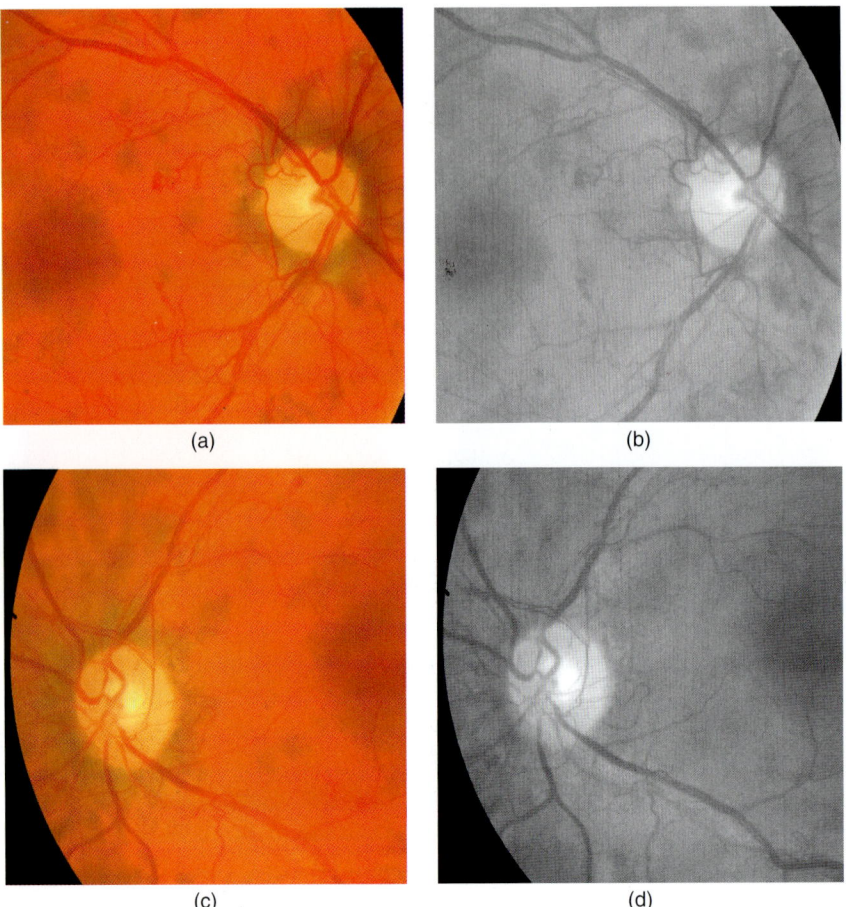

Fig. 10.14 (a) Colour and (b) red-free photograph of NVD at right disc; (c) colour and (d) red-free photograph of NVD at left disc.

contact lens under topical anaesthesia. Macular laser usually causes little or no discomfort but panretinal laser can cause pain, particularly during prolonged treatments sessions or when using high-power settings in lightly pigmented eyes. Pain is often worse during re-treatment sessions using a 'fill-in' pattern or when using long-wavelength diode lasers. Most patients characterise the pain associated with laser as brief, intermittent, sharp or piercing. As previously mentioned, the use of short-pulse laser is associated with less pain than conventional ETDRS standard laser. Randomised trials have found no benefit from oral[28] or intramuscular analgesics[29] prior to panretinal photocoagulation compared with placebo, but peribulbar anaesthesia was very effective[29] at reducing pain. Sub-Tenon injection of local anaesthetic is also effective[30] at reducing discomfort, and eliminates the risk of globe perforation or damage to the orbital structures that sometimes occur with sharp-needle techniques.

General anaesthesia is only very rarely required, but can be useful when thorough bilateral treatment is urgently required or when treating patients with learning difficulties or those who, for whatever reason, cannot cope with laser under local anaesthesia.

ANTI-VEGF TREATMENTS

Panretinal photocoagulation laser continues to be the gold standard for treatment of PDR. However, there remains an unmet need for additional treatment strategies in eyes with florid neovascularisation despite adequate laser treatment. Ocular neovascularisation and increased vascular permeability have been associated with increased vitreous levels of vascular endothelial

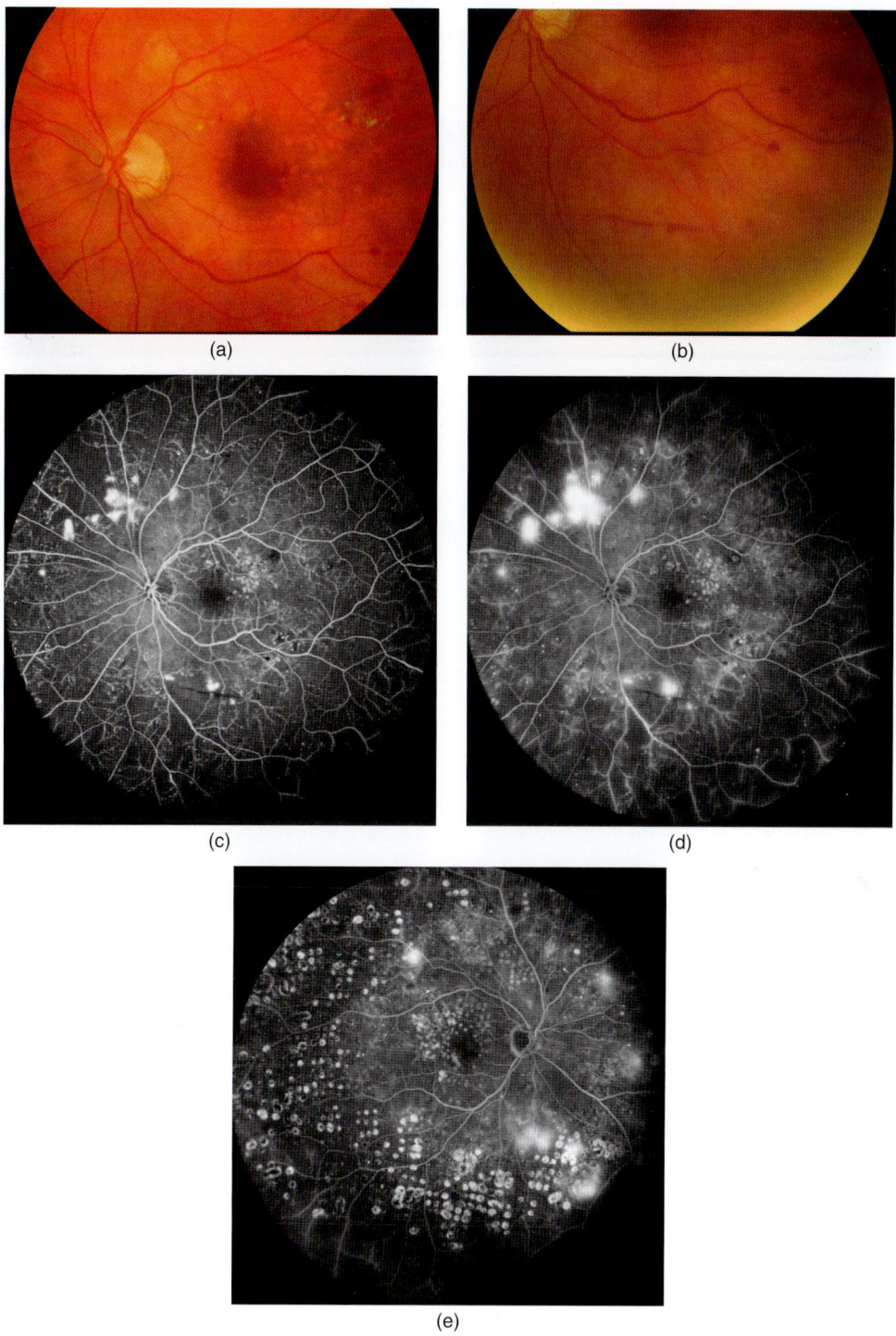

Fig. 10.15 Colour image of the left eye showing (a) macular laser scars and (b) preretinal haemorrhage. Photograph of the left eye in the (c) arteriovenous phase of the fluorescein angiogram, showing darker areas of non-perfusion and leakage from NVE and (d) venous phase of the angiogram, showing areas of non-perfusion and leakage from NVE. (e) Photograph of the right eye in the venous phase of the angiogram showing incomplete coverage of panretinal laser scars, areas of non-perfusion and leakage from NVE.

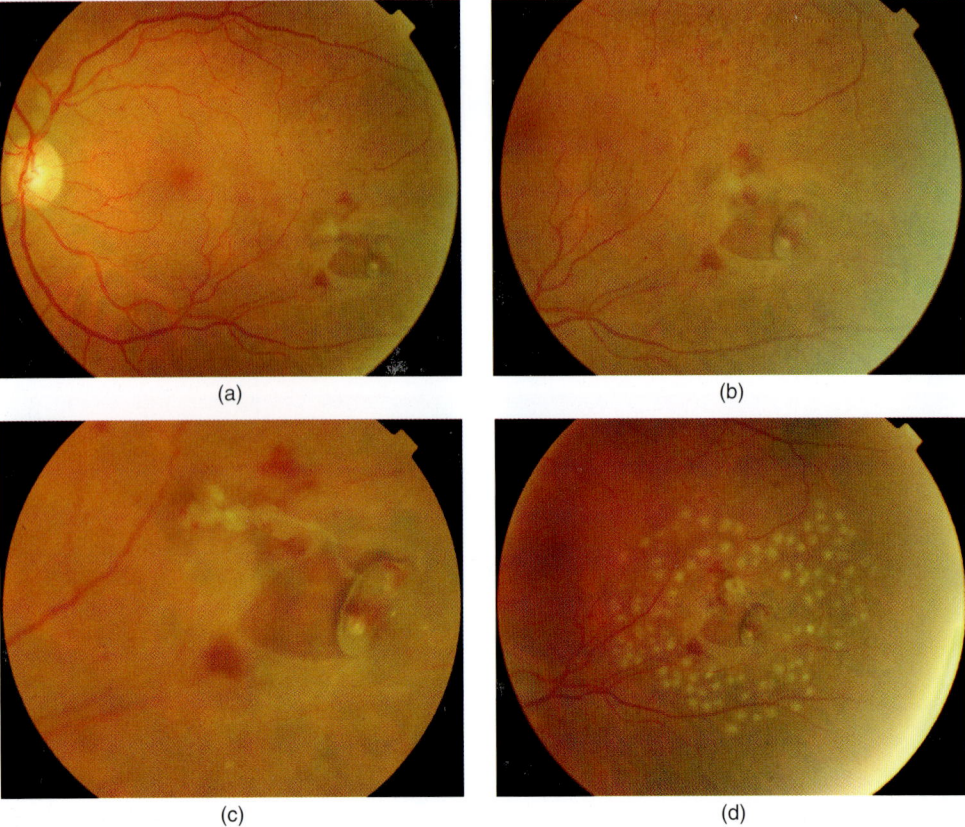

Fig. 10.16 Avulsion of NVE leaving horseshoe tear: (a) colour photograph; and (b, c) magnified. (d) Colour photograph taken immediately after laser treatment to encircle horseshoe tear.

growth factor. Neovascularisation is dependent on the presence of VEGF; expression of VEGF in animal models is sufficient to induce neovascularisation, whereas inhibition reduces this effect. In humans, ocular VEGF levels have been shown to rise with the growth and leakage of new vessels. This provides a therapeutic rationale for the targeting of VEGF in diabetic retinopathy.

VEGF inhibitors have been used for treatment of proliferative retinopathy in recent years. Favourable results have been reported with some regression of neovascularisation and reduction in fluorescein leakage in studies by Arevalo et al.[31], Jorge et al.[32], Avery et al.[33], Mason et al.[34] and Spaide and Fisher[35] using bevacizumab, and Adamis et al.[36] using pegaptanib. Avery et al.[33] reported that recurrent leakage was seen as early as 2 weeks after intravitreal injection in one case, whereas in other cases no recurrent leakage was noted at last follow-up of 11 weeks. Arevalo et al.[31] reported total regression of retinal neovascularisation on fundus examination with absence of fluorescein leakage in 61.4% (27 eyes) after a mean of 28.4 weeks (range 24–40 weeks). Adamis et al.[36] reported that, in 3 of 8 eyes with regression, neovascularisation progressed at week 52 after cessation of pegaptanib at week 30. Exploratory analysis from randomised trials of DMO treatment with ranibizumab also supports the role of anti-VEGF in decreasing the progression of diabetic retinopathy.[37,38] A DRCR network study evaluating macular laser, ranibizumab and triamcinolone for treatment of DMO showed a significant reduction in the probability of worsening in PDR eyes with a lower need for having PRP, occurrence of vitreous haemorrhage, or requiring vitrectomy in study arms that utilised ranibizumab (18–21%) compared to sham laser treatment (40%) at 3 years.[38]

In general, available data indicate a rapid and consistent beneficial effect of anti-VEGF agents in eyes with florid neovascularisation that have not responded to PRP and also as an adjunctive treatment to PRP to decrease the risk of laser-associated side-effects as macular oedema and visual field loss. However, because of its short-lived effect, anti-VEGF treatment as a replacement for laser is debatable. In addition to other risks of intravitreal anti-VEGF use such as endophthalmitis, there is also some concern about increased risk of fibrosis and exaggerated tractional detachment when used in patients with PDR.[39] Few randomised trials have specifically researched the role of anti-VEGF therapy vs. PRP for the treatment of PDR. Of these studies, the DRCR network study (protocol S) showed that mean visual acuity letter improvement at 2 years vision in PDR eyes treated with ranibizuamb was non inferior to eyes treated with PRP (difference, +2.2; 95% CI, −0.5 to +5.0; P < .001 for non inferiority) and was associated with significantly less peripheral visual field sensitivity loss (difference, 372 dB; 95% CI, 213–531 dB; P < .001) as well as a lower risk of DMO. However, cost of anti-VEGF treatment and its non durable effect are barriers to its routine use for treatment of PDR particularly in patients who are not fully compliant with their follow up visits.[40]

VITREOUS HAEMORRHAGE OBSCURING THE RETINAL VIEW

Vitrectomy surgery is currently the main line of treatment for persistent vitreous haemorrhage that is dense enough to cause vision impairment and preclude PRP treatment. The timing, technique and complications of vitrectomy in vitreous haemorrhage are discussed in detail in Chapter 13.

There is no role for anti-VEGF in the treatment of vitreous haemorrhage once it has occurred in eyes with PDR. While previously thought of having a role in accelerating the clearance of vitreous haemorrhage without the need to perform vitrectomy, a DRCR network randomised study (protocol N) showed a non-significant difference between intravitreal ranibizumab and saline on the rate of vitrectomy surgery in PDR-related vitreous haemorrhage.[41]

Case History 10.8: Optic disc neovascularisation treated with PRP laser and intravitreal anti-VEGF

This is 54-year-old male with type I DM (diagnosed at the age of 24 years) was treated for left proliferative retinopathy (Fig. 10.17a) with combined intravitreal ranibizumab (3×) and 20 ms PRP laser (2 sessions, 3000 burns, power 300–375 mW, size 200 microns, Transequator lens, magnification factor 1.44) as part of a clinical study. Optic disc neovascularisation completely disappeared 4 months after his combined treatment (Fig. 10.17b).

Case History 10.9: NVE with vitreous haemorrhage

This 43-year-old man with type 1 diabetes for 31 years had treatment for right clinically significant macular oedema at the age of 31 years. At the age of 35 years he subsequently received panretinal photocoagulation to his right eye when small NVE were found in his right temporal retina, right infero-nasal retina and right superior and supero-nasal retina. The treatment given was 2022 burns, power 170–200 mW, size 350 microns, Transequator lens (magnification factor 1.44), argon laser, spread over 3 sessions 1 week apart.

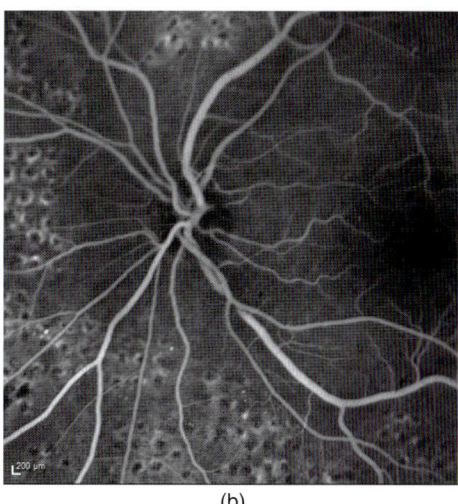

(a)   (b)

Fig. 10.17 (a) Leakage from neovascularisation at the optic disc (NVD) before treatment. (b) Regression to normal disc vessels after treatment.

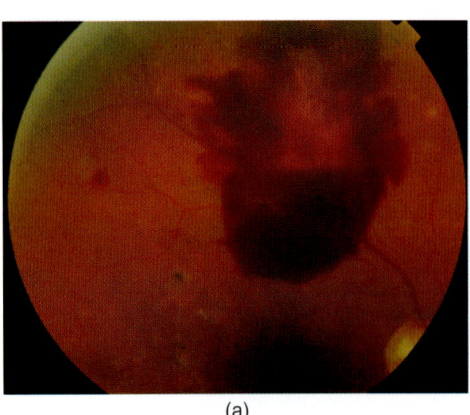
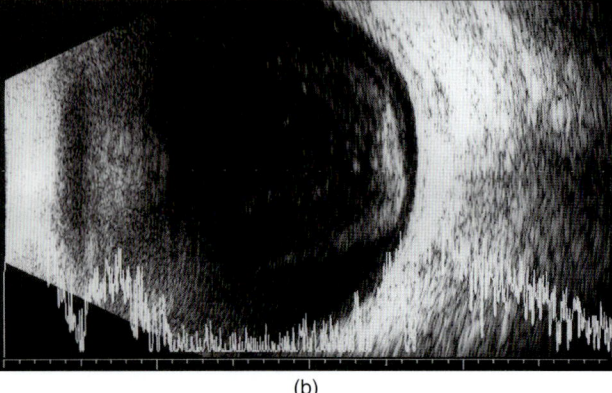

Fig. 10.18 (a) Preretinal haemorrhage. (b) B-scan showing intragel haemorrhage. The retina is flat in all quadrants.

At the age of 39 years, he noticed a spot in the inferior vision of his right eye; clinical examination demonstrated the presence of a preretinal haemorrhage as shown in Figure 10.18. This vitreous haemorrhage then broke through into the vitreous 6 weeks later reducing the right VA to 6/24 (20/80). Clinically, the vitreous haemorrhage interfered with the retinal view on slit-lamp biomicroscopy and an ultrasound B-scan was therefore undertaken (Fig. 10.18b). A right pars plana vitrectomy was performed with a good post-operative visual result of 6/6 (20/20).

It is important to perform a B-scan on patients whose retina cannot be viewed due to a vitreous haemorrhage to exclude an underlying retinal detachment as shown in the B-scan in Figure 10.19.

Fig. 10.19 Vitreous haemorrhage with underlying retinal detachment: B-scan.

Our views on the treatment of NVD less than one-quarter disc area

If signs of severe ischaemia are present, we would recommend panretinal photocoagulation. Venous beading in more than one quadrant, extensive retinal haemorrhages and opaque small arteriolar branches are signs suggesting severe retinal ischaemia and eyes at greater risk of neovascularisation. Treatment is also undertaken for these cases if future cataract surgery is contemplated.

If signs of severe ischaemia were not present, we would perform a fluorescein angiogram to check that the NVD were definitely leaking. We would also ask for peripheral retinal views in order to identify the extent of peripheral retinal ischaemia.

In the past we have watched some of these small NVD; in time they have become bigger or bled and become high risk. We have never seen one that has spontaneously resolved. We therefore have a low threshold for performing panretinal photocoagulation, especially as the complication rate with modern laser machines is considerably less than that reported in the DRS. This is because the extent of whitening (intensity of the burn) that is currently used with the recommended panretinal laser treatment is less than in the argon laser arm of the DRS study; the other arm of the DRS study used xenon-arc laser which caused considerably more damage to the peripheral retina.

Our views on the treatment of NVE that have not haemorrhaged

There is no clear-cut answer to this because each patient presents a different picture. However, if signs of severe ischaemia are present, we would recommend panretinal photocoagulation. Venous beading in more than one quadrant, extensive retinal haemorrhages and opaque small arteriolar branches suggest severe retinal ischaemia and eyes at greater risk of neovascularisation.

If there are no signs of severe retinal ischaemia, we would perform a fluorescein angiogram asking for peripheral retinal views, and we would identify the extent of peripheral retinal ischaemia. There are usually ischaemic signs peripheral to the NVE in the quadrant in which the NVE have occurred. If the ischaemia was localised to this quadrant, we would perform segmental lase treatment to the area of ischaemia peripheral to the NVE in this quadrant (this was recommended by Hamilton et al.[42] and would now extend by 1DD into the perfused retina as recommended by Muqit et al.[9] for a targeted PRP technique). If the ischaemia was more extensive, we would consider which segments of ischaemic retina might require laser treatment.

PRACTICE POINTS

In the treatment of neovascularisation, involution of neovascularisation is dependent upon a sufficient area of retinal ablation[3,11].

Panretinal laser treatment should be spaced over a minimum of two sessions unless there is a strong suspicion that the individual being treated might not attend for subsequent treatment sessions.

At least 2000 PRP laser spots are required when using Pascal to match the ETDRS treatment protocol.

Early use of intravitreal anti-VEGF in treatment in the management of iris neovascularisation helps early regression of iris and retinal neovascularisations, providing a 'window of opportunity' of 2–3 weeks until definitive treatment with PRP could be employed.

Patients with florid PDR despite adequate laser may benefit from anti-VEGF treatment, but close monitoring for risks such as exaggerated retinal fibrosis is required.

Though short term results of anti-VEGF treatment for PDR are not inferior to PRP, drug cost and short-lived effect are barriers to its routine use particularly in patients who are not fully compliant with their follow up visits.

REFERENCE

Please visit www.wiley.com/go/scanlon/diabetic_retinopathy

11 Proliferative diabetic retinopathy with maculopathy

Ahmed Sallam[1] & Peter H. Scanlon[2]

[1] University of Arkansas for Medical Sciences, USA
[2] Harris Manchester College, University of Oxford; Medical Ophthalmology, University of Gloucestershire, UK

While there has been a paradigm shift from macular laser to intravitreal anti-VEGF pharmacotherapy for treatment of macular oedema in the last 6–8 years, panretinal photocoagulation laser continues to be the 'gold standard' treatment for PDR.

LASER FOR PROLIFERATIVE DR AND CONCURRENT MACULOPATHY

In the past when laser was the only modality available to treat macular oedema, cases with PDR and concurrent macular oedema posed a management challenge for the retina specialist. Results from the Diabetic Retinopathy Study[1] (DRS) demonstrated that scatter photocoagulation is associated with some loss of visual acuity soon after treatment, and this was more common in eyes with pre-existing macular oedema. In addition, increased macular oedema following panretinal photocoagulation was demonstrated by Meyers[2] and McDonald and Schatz[3].

A report from the DRS[4] suggested that 'reducing macular oedema by focal photocoagulation before initiating scatter treatment and dividing scatter treatment into multiple sessions with less intense burns may decrease the risk of the visual loss associated with photocoagulation'.

Lee et al.[5] combined treatment in two sessions consisting of initial modified grid to the macula and panretinal photocoagulation to the inferior half of the peripheral retina, followed 2–4 weeks later by panretinal photocoagulation to the superior half. The study evaluated 52 patients and found that macular oedema resolved in 43 of 46 eyes (93%), and proliferative retinopathy was reduced in 25 of 29 eyes (86%) at the last examination.

The ETDRS[6] compared giving immediate panretinal photocoagulation with either simultaneous or delayed focal treatment. For eyes with DMO and more severe retinopathy, the risk of severe visual loss in eyes assigned to deferral of photocoagulation was relatively high (6.5% at the 5 year visit). This risk was reduced to between 3.8% and 4.7% in the eyes assigned to early photocoagulation. The strategy associated with the least visual loss (both moderate and severe) was immediate mild scatter combined with immediate focal photocoagulation. The ETDRS did not include evaluation of a strategy that consisted of prompt focal photocoagulation with delayed scatter in eyes with clinically significant macular oedema and eyes that are approaching the high-risk category.

It was therefore recommended that eyes needing scatter laser treatment and also having macular oedema are less at risk of visual acuity loss when focal/grid treatment to reduce the macular oedema precedes scatter laser photocoagulation. If this is not possible, as in eyes with high-risk PDR, vitreous haemorrhage or neovascular glaucoma, focal/grid laser treatment should be applied at the first scatter laser treatment session.

Hamilton et al.[7] recommended an exception to this approach for young patients with insulin-dependent diabetes mellitus (IDDM) who have rapidly accelerating peripheral ischaemia associated with macular oedema that may resolve following panretinal photocoagulation.

Case History 11.1: New vessels at the disc and new vessels elsewhere with maculopathy

A 41-year-old man with type 1 diabetes (BMI 28) of 30 years duration was referred from the retinal screening programme when the photographs showed signs of proliferative diabetic retinopathy in both eyes and maculopathy in the left (Fig. 11.1).

A Practical Manual of Diabetic Retinopathy Management, Second Edition. Edited by Peter Scanlon, Ahmed Sallam, and Peter van Wijngaarden.
© 2017 John Wiley & Sons Ltd. Published 2017 by John Wiley & Sons Ltd.
Companion Website: www.wiley.com/go/scanlon/diabetic_retinopathy

Proliferative diabetic retinopathy with maculopathy

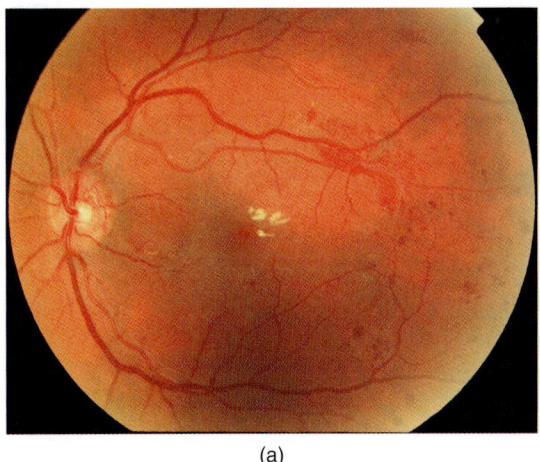
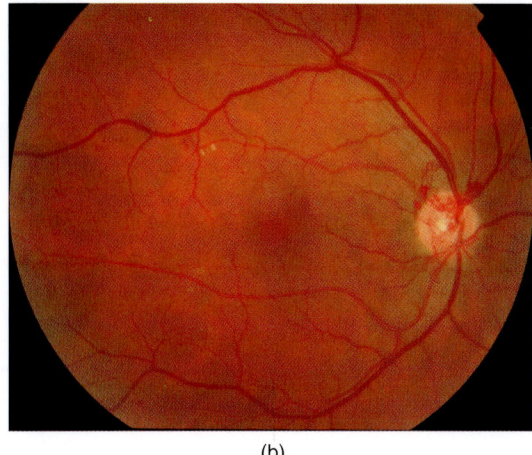

(a)   (b)

Fig. 11.1 (a) Proliferative DR with maculopathy: left macula colour photo. (b) Proliferative DR: right macula colour photo.

The left macular area was treated first with 23 burns of 100 micron size 260 mW, 0.1 s using an Area Centralis lens and argon laser.

Panretinal photocoagulation was commenced to both eyes at the first treatment session. In total, 4010 burns, 2550 using the Transequator lens (magnification factor 1.44) and 350 micron spot size and 1460 of 200 micron spot size using the Superquad 160 lens (magnification factor of 2.0) of average power 220 mW, were required to control the neovascularization in his right eye. In total 4847 burns, 2303 using the Transequator lens (magnification factor 1.44) and 350 micron spot size and 2544 of 200 micron spot size using the Superquad 160 lens (magnification factor of 2.0) of average power 220mW, were required to control the neovascularization in the left eye.

His HbA1c has gradually improved from 10.1 to 8.1 over the last 5 years and his BP was consistently satisfactory at 122/86, but has recently elevated to 153/92. The exudates and CSMO in the left macular area cleared with one course of focal laser treatment.

Focal laser treatment was commenced to the area of retinal thickening on the temporal side of the left macula with 31 burns 100 micron size, 170 mW, 100 ms, Area Centralis lens, argon laser and panretinal photocoagulation was commenced at the same appointment following the macular laser treatment.

Panretinal photocoagulation was given over three sessions giving a total of 2425 burns, which included 1620 burns of 350 micron spot size (average power 330 mW spot size 200 microns) using the Transequator lens with a magnification factor of 1.44, and 805 burns of 200 micron spot size using the Superquad 160 lens with a magnification factor of 2.0.

With this treatment the VA improved over the next 5 months to a level of 6/9 (20/30) but there remained some activity of the NVD and NVE, which required two further scatter laser treatments requiring a total of a further 1745 burns of 200 micron spot size using the Superquad 160 lens to control the neovascularisation. His left VA subsequently stabilised at 6/12 (20/40). Over the 5 years, his HbA1c varied between 8.4 and 8.1 and his BP varied between 195/78 and 138/83.

Case History 11.2: New vessels at the disc and new vessels elsewhere with maculopathy

This 59-year-old man with type 2 diabetes controlled on metformin 850 mg b.d. presented with a sudden onset of blurring of vision in his left eye (VA reduced to 6/24, 20/120; Fig. 11.2a). As the haemorrhage started to clear, a fluorescein angiogram (see Fig. 11.2b, c) showed NVD, NVE, severe ischaemia in the temporal retina and clinically significant macular oedema in the macular area.

LASER FOR PROLIFERATIVE DR AND INTRAVITREAL ANTI-VEGF THERAPY FOR MACULOPATHY

The introduction of anti-VEGF therapy for treatment of DMO has simplified the management of cases with combined proliferative retinopathy and maculopathy.

In addition to its favourable functional and anatomical effects on DMO, available data on anti-VEGF therapy

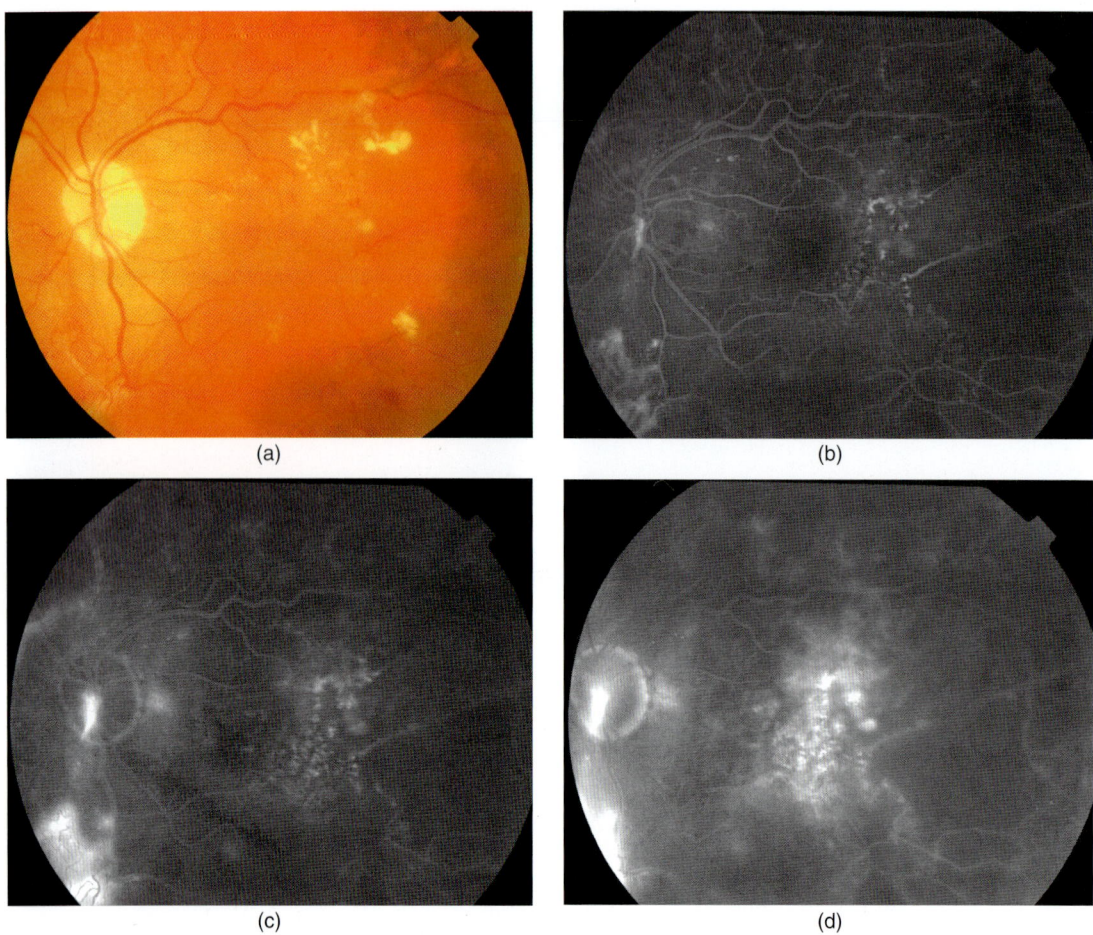

Fig. 11.2 Left macular area: (a) colour; (b) fluorescein image 29 s; (c) 57 s; and (c) 4 min 15 s after injection.

indicate a rapid and consistent beneficial effect on florid retinal and iris neovascularisations. Regression of neovascularisation and reduction in fluorescein leakage have been reported in studies by Arevalo et al.[8], Jorge et al.[9], Avery et al.[10], Mason et al.[11] and Spaide and Fisher[12] using bevacizumab, and Adamis et al.[13] using pergaptanib. Exploratory analysis from a study evaluating macular laser, ranibizumab and triamcinolone for treatment of DMO also showed a significant reduction in the probability of worsening of PDR eyes with a lower need for PRP, occurrence of vitreous haemorrhage or vitrectomy surgery in study arms that utilised ranibizumab (18–21%) compared to sham (40%) at 3 years.[14]

It is therefore recommended that eyes requiring scatter laser treatment that also have macular oedema are treated with a combination therapy of intravitreal anti-VEGF and panretinal photocoagulation. Because of the beneficial effect of anti-VEGF on retinal neovacularisation, it is possible to initiate treatment with intravitreal anti-VEGF and defer the panretinal photocoagulation treatment for 2–3 weeks in eyes with significant macular oedema to allow time for the macular oedema to subside, thereby reducing the risk of visual loss with subsequent panretinal photocoagulation laser treatment.

Case History 11.3: Proliferative diabetic retinopathy and macular oedema

This 28-year-old female patient with type 1 DM controlled by insulin and tablets noted reduction of vision in her

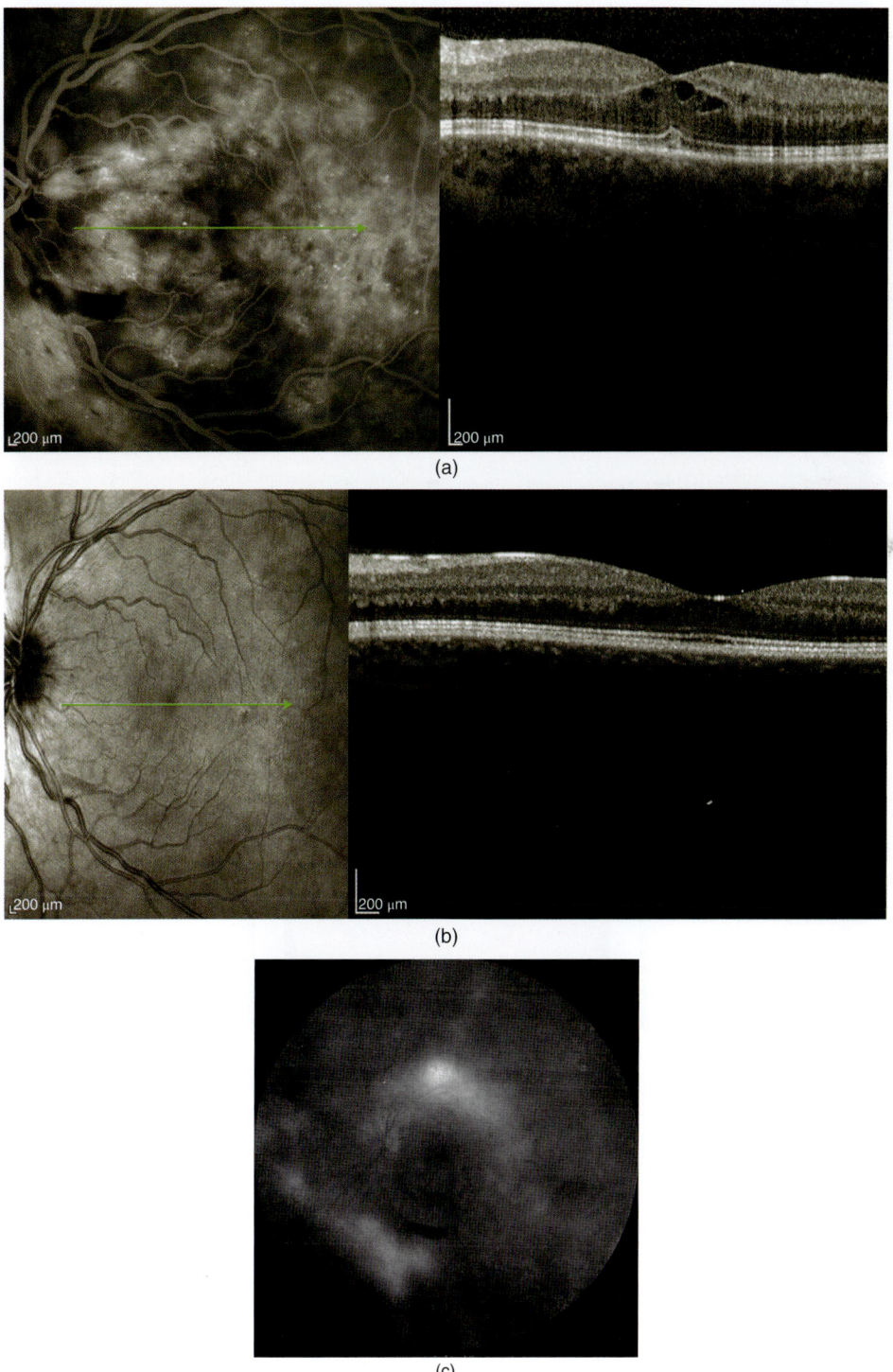

Fig. 11.3 (a) Late fundus fluorescein frame of the left eye with OCT scan of the centre of the fovea. (b) Infrared photograph of the same eye and OCT of the fovea after treatment with intravitreal ranibizumab. (c) Late fundus fluorescein frame of the left eye after scatter laser treatment.

left eye. The vision in the left eye was measured as 6/18, although 6 months previously it was recorded as 6/6 in this eye. Late fundus fluorescein image shows preretinal haemorrhage inferior to the disc and diffuse macular oedema with corresponding multiple cystoid spaces on the OCT scan (Fig. 11.3a, left). The OCT shows multiple cystoid spaces in the foveal and parafoveal region. She was treated by intravitreal ranibizumab (x3) with good resolution of the macular oedema and improvement of the vision back to 6/6 (Fig. 11.3b) followed by panretinal laser photocoagulation for the proliferative retinopathy. Note vascular leakage from persistent NVE after laser treatment along the superior arcade and below the preretinal haemorrhage on the widefield late fundus fluorescein image (Fig. 11.3c).

Case History 11.4: **Proliferative diabetic retinopathy and macular oedema**

This 59-year-old man has type 2 diabetes, which has been controlled with tablets since it was diagnosed at the age of 36 years.

He was referred from retinal screening at the age of 43 years with exudate in his left macular area. Attendance in clinic was poor and was lost to follow-up. He presented with a shower of floaters in his right eye at the age of 52 years when he was found to have extensive neovascularisation of both optic discs, a preretinal haemorrhage in his right nasal retina (Fig. 11.4b) with some haemorrhage in his right vitreous, making the photograph slightly blurred. Leakage in both macular areas was indicated by the exudate present in both macular areas (Fig. 11.4a, c, d).

He was treated with panretinal photocoagulation to both eyes. A total of 3100 burns, 200 micron size, 350–500 mW, 0.02 s were given to the right eye and 2956 to the left eye over three sessions, and 2953 burns to the left eye over three sessions with similar settings on the Pascal laser. Macular laser treatment was given at the first treatment session to both eyes. Despite this treatment, a large preretinal haemorrhage formed in the right eye after 3 months (Fig. 11.4e). There was incomplete regression of the neovascularisation at both discs and he developed a non-clearing vitreous haemorrhage in his right eye.

He was treated with indirect laser to his right eye and required a pars plana vitrectomy operation to his left eye with delamination and endolaser.

His left eye became more stable, but he then developed some further leakage in both macular areas (Fig. 11.4f, h). We obtained permission to treat the right eye with intravitreal anti-VEGF and treated the left eye with focal

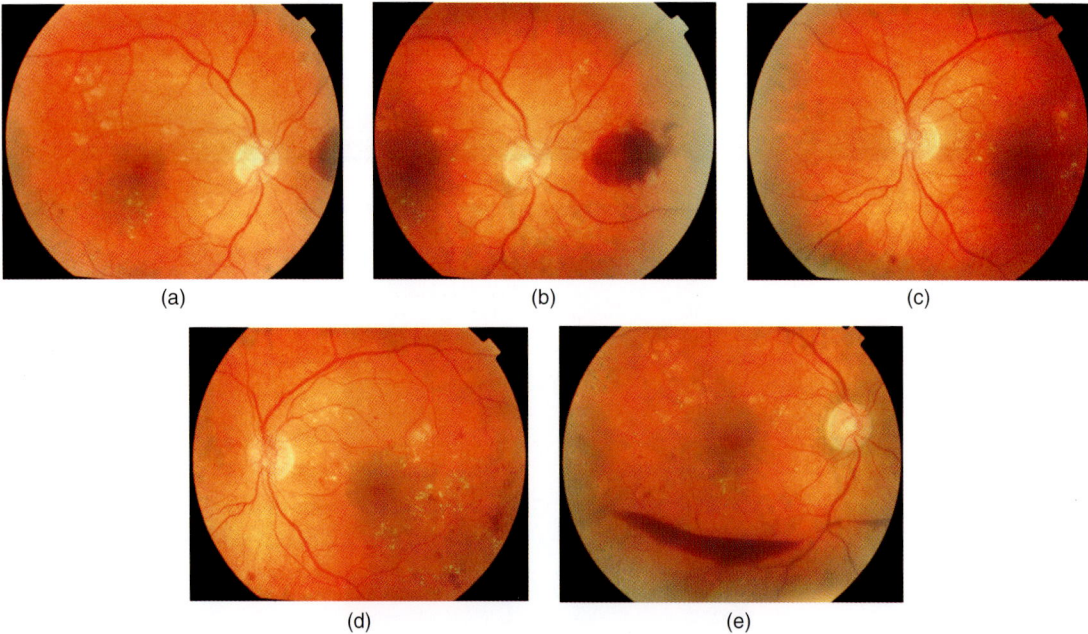

Fig. 11.4 Colour photographs showing (a) exudate in the right macular area; (b) preretinal haemorrhage in right nasal retina; (c, d) exudate in the left macular area; and (e) preretinal haemorrhage below the right macula over the right infero-temporal arcade. OCTs showing diabetic macular oedema pre-treatment in (f) right eye and (h) left eye and post-treatment in (g) right eye and (i) left eye.

Proliferative diabetic retinopathy with maculopathy

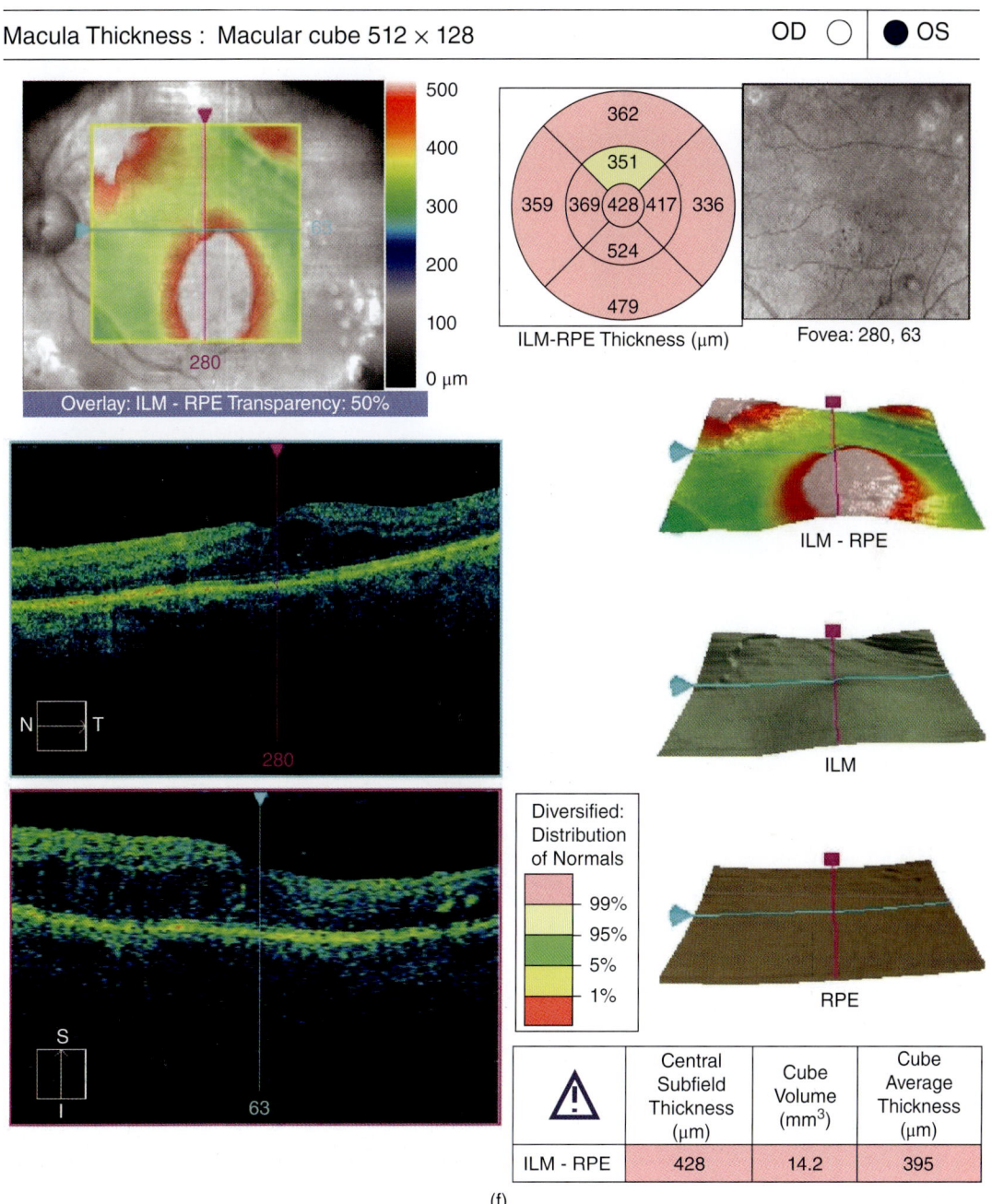

(f)

Fig. 11.4 (*Continued*)

156 A practical manual of diabetic retinopathy management

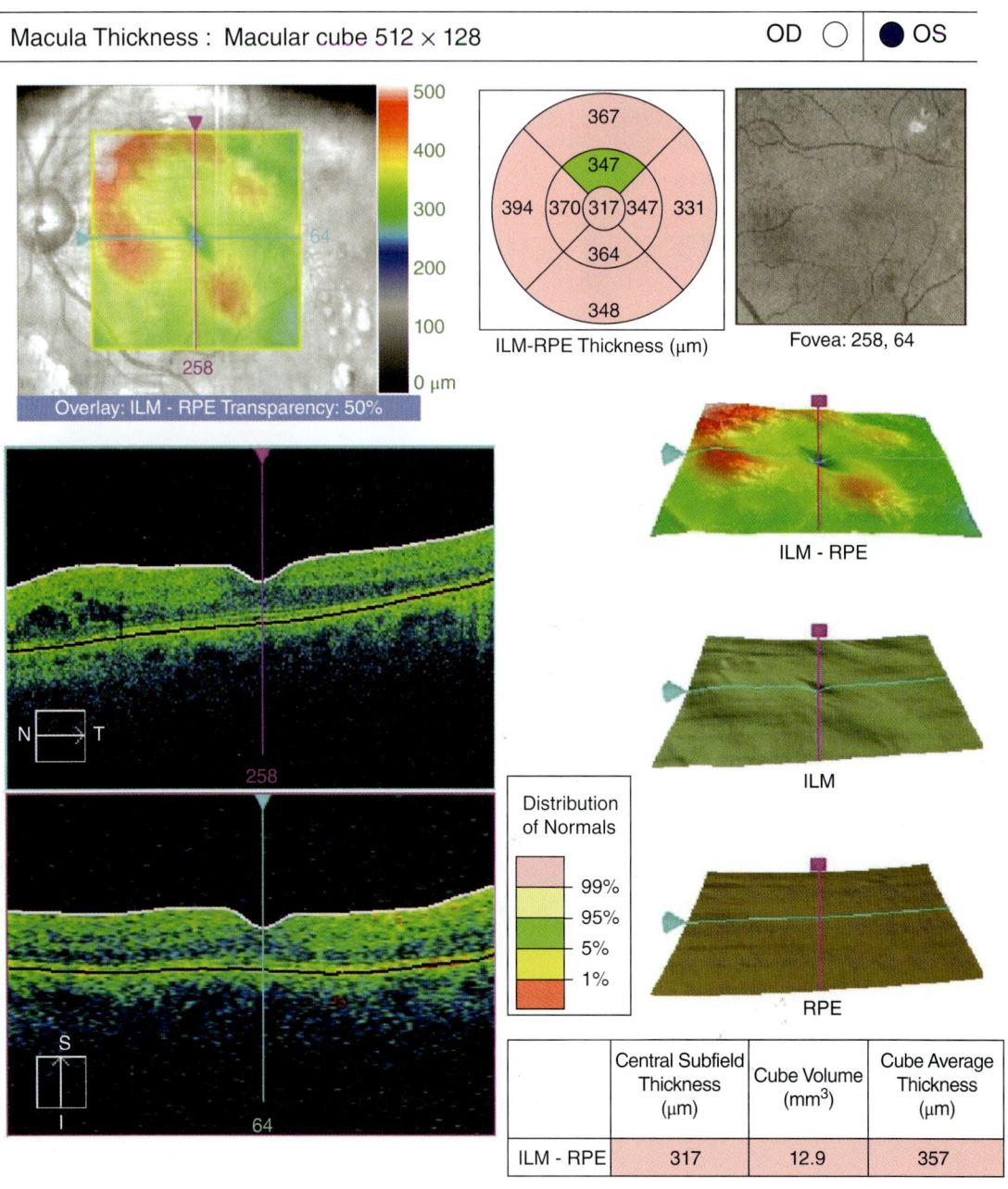

Fig. 11.4 (Continued)

Proliferative diabetic retinopathy with maculopathy 157

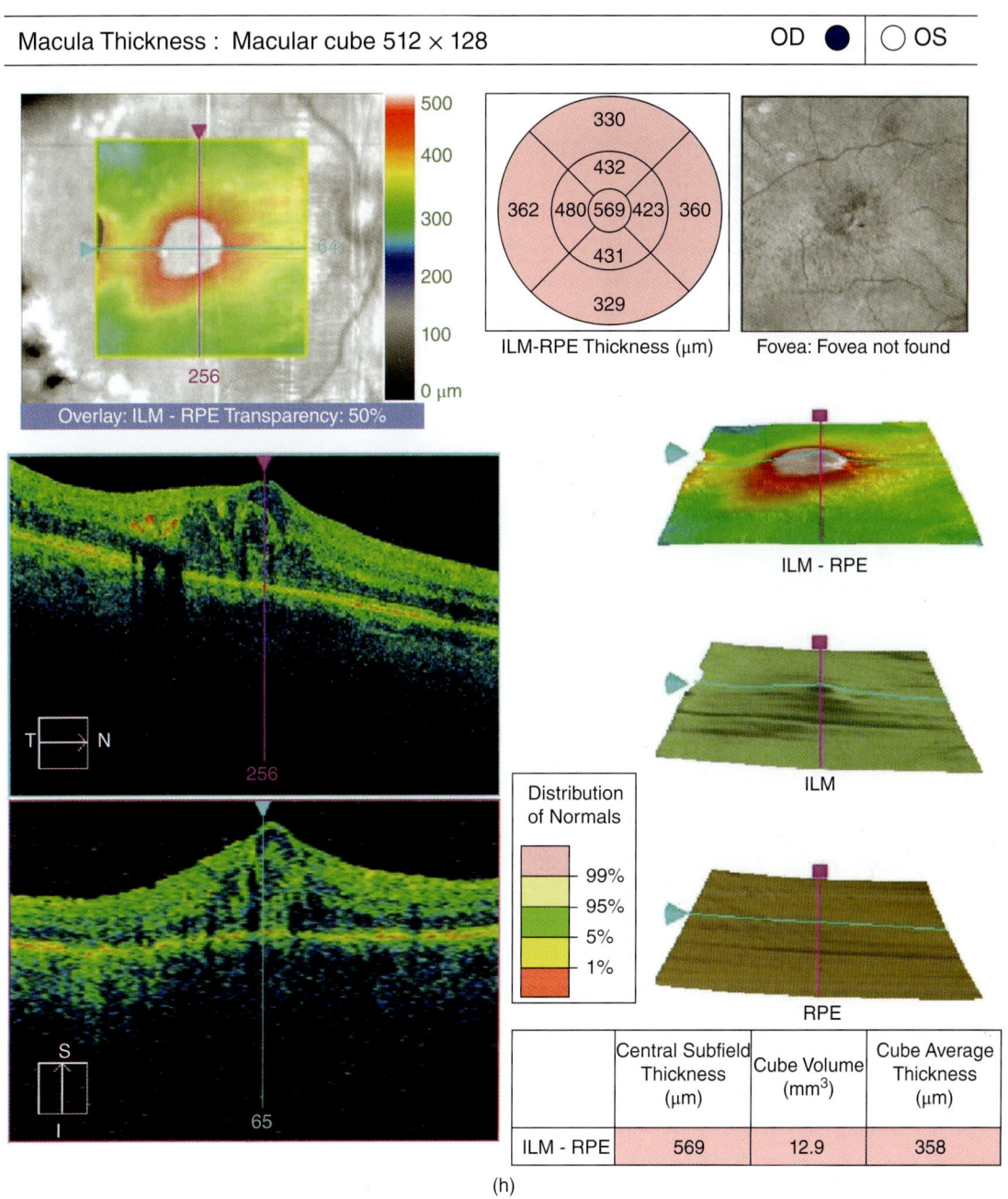

Fig. 11.4 (Continued)

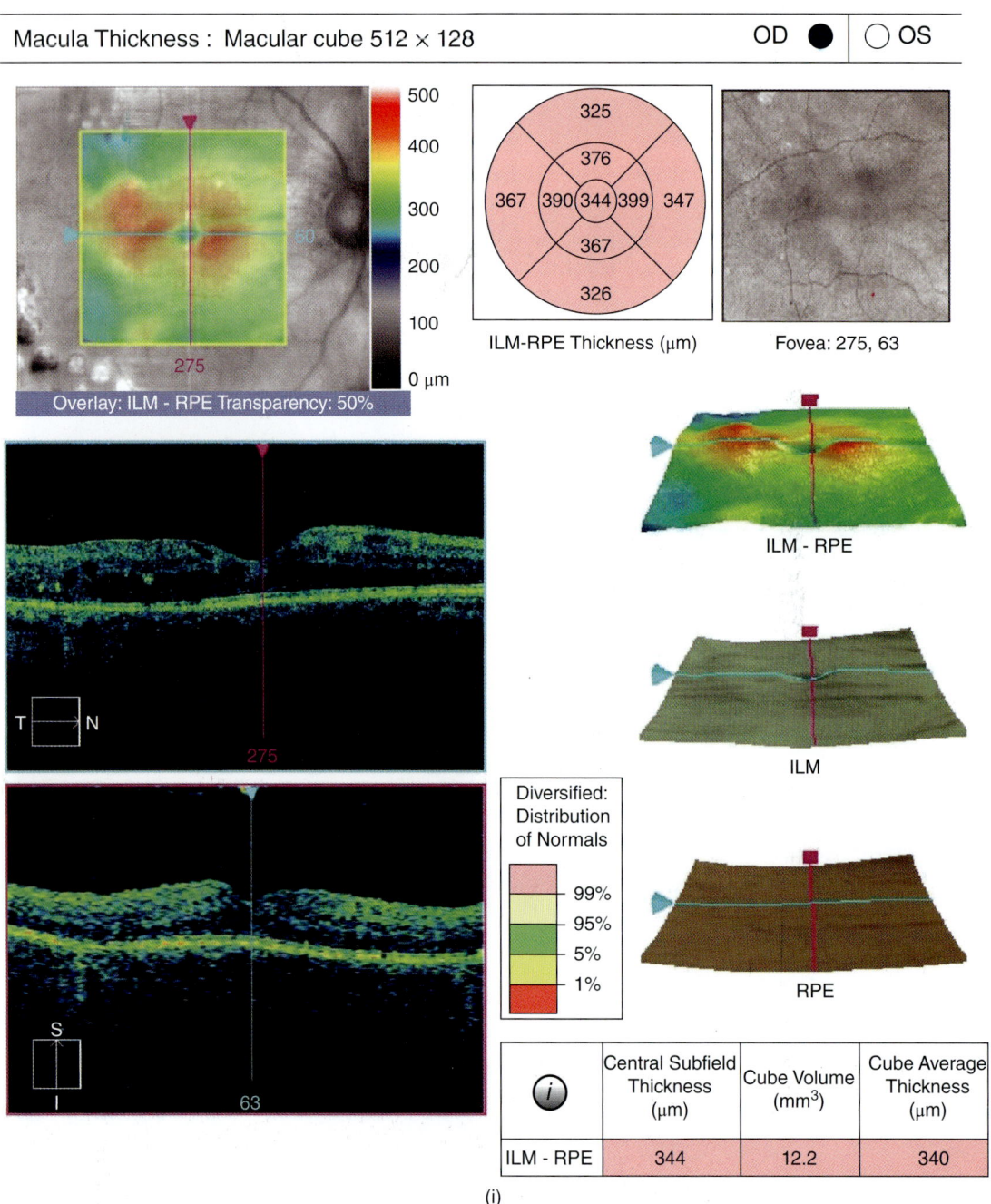

Fig. 11.4 (*Continued*)

laser treatment. The right eye was given 9 injections of ranibizumab in the first year and 3 injections of ranibizumab in the second year.

The current visual acuity levels are right eye LogMAR 0.40 20/60 best corrected, left eye LogMAR 0.38 20/40 best corrected. The most recent OCTs are shown in Figure 11.4g and i.

PRACTICE POINTS

Eyes with centre-involving DMO and PDR are best treated with a combination therapy of intravitreal anti-VEGF and panretinal photocoagulation treatment.

In patients with macular oedema, panretinal photocoagulation treatment could be deferred for 2–3 weeks after initiation of intravitreal anti-VEGF therapy.

In young patients with IDDM who have aggressive peripheral ischaemia associated with diffuse or cystoid macular oedema, panretinal photocoagulation may help resolution of macular oedema by decreasing the VEGF drive.

REFERENCES

Please visit www.wiley.com/go/scanlon/diabetic_retinopathy

12 The stable treated eye

Peter H. Scanlon

Harris Manchester College, University of Oxford; Medical Ophthalmology, University of Gloucestershire, UK

FOLLOWING MACULOPATHY TREATMENT

Treatment of centre-involving or diffuse diabetic macular oedema

A good result following treatment of centre-involving or diffuse diabetic macular oedema with VEGF inhibitor injections is resolution of the oedema with improvement in visual acuity. For those people who do respond to treatment, there appears to be a reducing need for intravitreal injections in second and subsequent years[1]. For those who respond to treatment, the average number of treatments required during the first year to provide resolution of the oedema is 7–9 treatments, with 3–4 treatments being required in the second year to maintain this. If it is not possible to clear the oedema, chronic oedema tends to cause pigment epithelial changes relating to damage to the photoreceptors in the central fovea and permanent loss of vision. If VEGF inhibitor injections are not available, treatment with laser is generally much more difficult[2] and less effective [3].

> **Case History 12.1:** Treated centre-involving diabetic macular oedema with VEGF inhibitors
>
> A 55-year-old man with type 2 diabetes controlled by tablets and insulin developed centre-involving macular oedema in his right eye (Fig. 12.1a), reducing his right vision to a level of 0.8 LogMAR.
>
> He was given monthly injections of a VEGF inhibitor for 5 months when his oedema had resolved (Fig. 12.1b). He was given 2 further injections of a VEGF inhibitor (months 7 and 9) when a small amount of oedema recurred. He has not yet needed any injections in the second year (month 16; Fig. 12.1c) and is now being monitored at 2 monthly intervals.

Treatment of focal exudative or focal/multifocal oedema

A good result following treatment of focal exudative or focal/multifocal oedema with laser[4] is clearing of the areas of exudates and oedema. There are usually signs of clearing at the 3 month follow-up appointment, but clearing may continue for a further 3–6 months. Providing clearing has commenced by the first 3-month appointment, a decision does not need to be made at that appointment regarding further focal laser treatment until no further clearing is apparent.

Subsequent prognosis for the eye and vision will depend on control of systemic factors such as glucose[5,6], hypertension[7] and lipids[8]. It is not uncommon to successfully treat one area of leakage and subsequently find leakage appearing in a completely different area around the fovea of the same eye.

> **Case History 12.2:** Treated non-centre-involving diabetic macular oedema with focal laser
>
> A 53-year-old man with type 2 diabetes, controlled with insulin from 6 months after diagnosis (at the age of 33 years), was referred from the retinal screening service and was found to have oedema in his left macular area (Fig. 12.2a). His left vision was good at LogMAR 0.1.
>
> He was given focal laser treatment to the area of oedema in the left macular area using a Pascal laser (15 burns, 100 micron size, 240 mW, 0.05 s, Area Centralis lens).
>
> His VA remained stable at 6/6 (20/20). The thickening and exudates cleared over the next 12 months. After 3 months there was still some thickening (Fig. 12.2b). The oedema continued to clear over the next 6 months (Fig. 12.2c).

A Practical Manual of Diabetic Retinopathy Management, Second Edition.
Edited by Peter Scanlon, Ahmed Sallam, and Peter van Wijngaarden.
© 2017 John Wiley & Sons Ltd. Published 2017 by John Wiley & Sons Ltd.
Companion Website: www.wiley.com/go/scanlon/diabetic_retinopathy

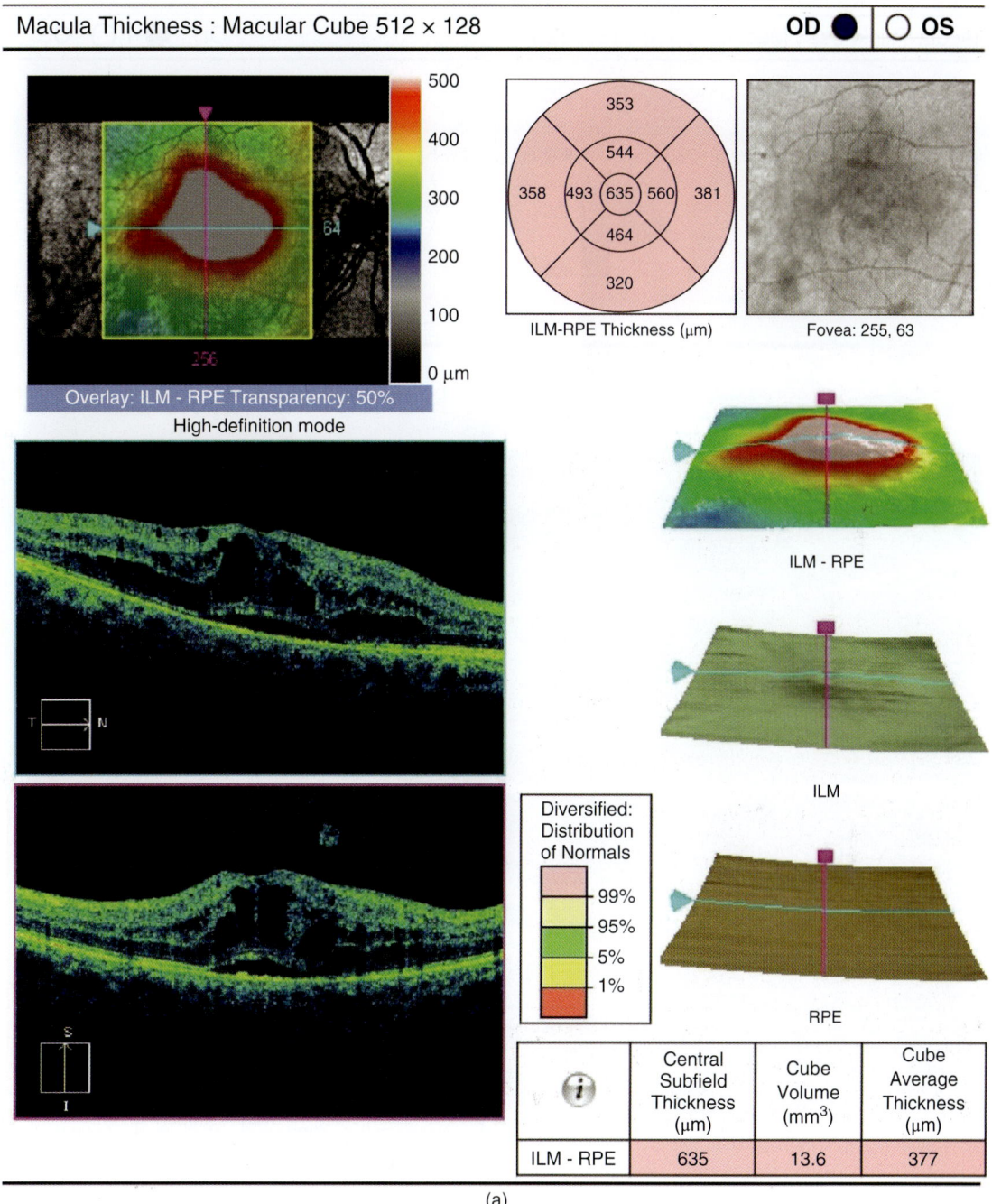

(a)

Fig. 12.1 OCT right macular area (a) before treatment with VEGF inhibitor; (b) after 5 months of treatment with VEGF inhibitor; and (c) at month 16.

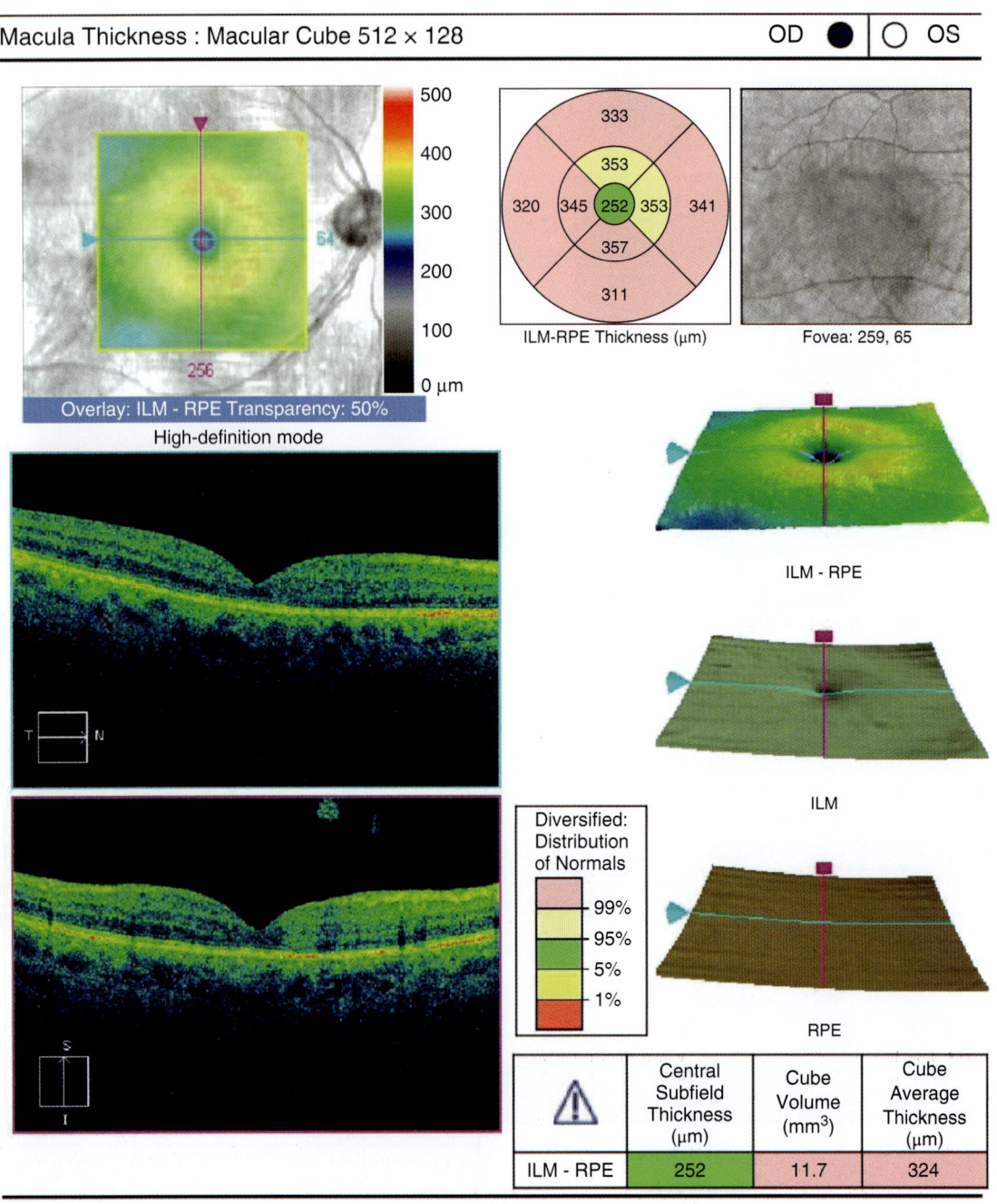

Fig. 12.1 (*Continued*)

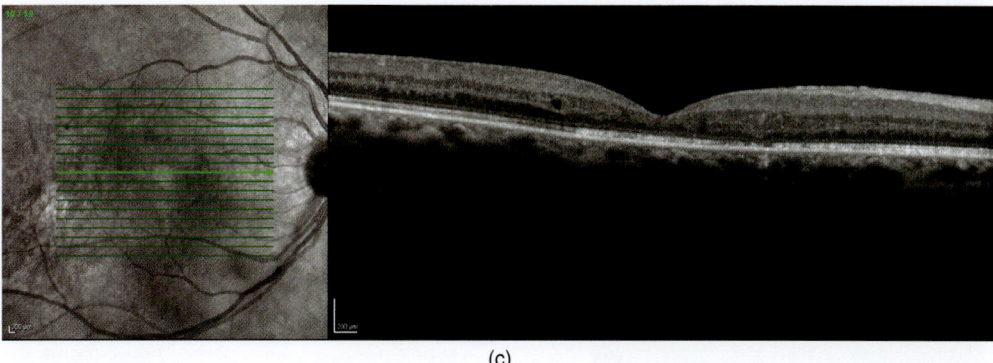
(c)

Fig. 12.1 (Continued)

Ischaemic maculopathy

The recommendations that were a modification of the Early Treatment Diabetic Retinopathy study technique were to apply laser to all areas of diffuse leakage or non-perfusion (providing there is retinal thickening) within the area considered for grid treatment, but not within 500 microns of the foveal centre. However, if there is ischaemia that involves the central fovea, laser treatment in isolation is unlikely to improve the vision. Treatment of systemic hypertension does, in some patients, lead to an improvement or a stabilisation of vision. It is therefore important that an ophthalmologist pays careful attention to the BP in this group of patients. A good result in this group of patients is stabilisation of the vision at a reasonable level.

An example of a patient with diabetes and hypertension whose maculopathy improved following treatment of his hypertension is described in the maculopathy section (Chapter 7, Case history 7.1).

FOLLOWING NVD OR NVE TREATMENT

NVD and NVE usually respond well to laser treatment. If involution of the vessels does not occur after a full panretinal photocoagulation, further scatter laser treatment is the recommended first approach. Involution of neovascularisation is dependent upon a sufficient area of retinal ablation[9,10], which depends on the extent of the retinal ischaemia. NVD are more likely to show signs of complete involution following laser treatment than NVE.

NVD or NVE may persist as thin fine vessels or 'ghost vessels' where no red blood corpuscles appear to pass through these vessels. If NVD or NVE persist, varying degrees of fibrosis surrounding the new vessel complex often occur. 'Ghost vessels' rarely progress or haemorrhage except when a posterior vitreous attachment occurs, and this usually results in avulsion of the vessels from their stem. Once the haemorrhage clears, the vessels have been avulsed and recurrent haemorrhage does not therefore occur.

Vitreous haemorrhage may occur following scatter laser treatment and may be asymptomatic. If small and asymptomatic, the haemorrhage often lies in the inferior vitreous cavity. A careful search needs to be made of the retina to determine the source of the haemorrhage to determine whether there is recurrent neovascularisation, a partial or complete posterior vitreous detachment (resulting in avulsion of new vessel complexes) or whether another source such as a retinal tear is the cause.

Successful scatter laser treatment is indicated by the following:

1. signs of adequate scatter laser photocoagulation scars;
2. signs of involution and finally disappearance of the new vessels where possible;
3. signs of lack of activity of the new vessel complex in the form of (a) no further growth (and preferably involution as above); (b) no red blood cells in the tips of the frond-like ends of the new vessels; or (c) fibrosis around the new vessel complex;
4. signs of the overall venous calibre returning from a dilated and possibly beaded calibre back to a narrower width or the absence of venous beading;
5. the absence of recurrent vitreous haemorrhages;
6. no new areas of neovascularisation developing; and/or
7. no signs of rubeosis iridis or neovascular glaucoma developing.

A good result following treatment of neovascularisation is complete involution of the new vessels. It is more common to achieve this goal of complete involution in patients with NVD than NVE.

The second-best result is incomplete involution of the new vessels with signs of lack of activity as described above, often associated with a degree of fibrosis.

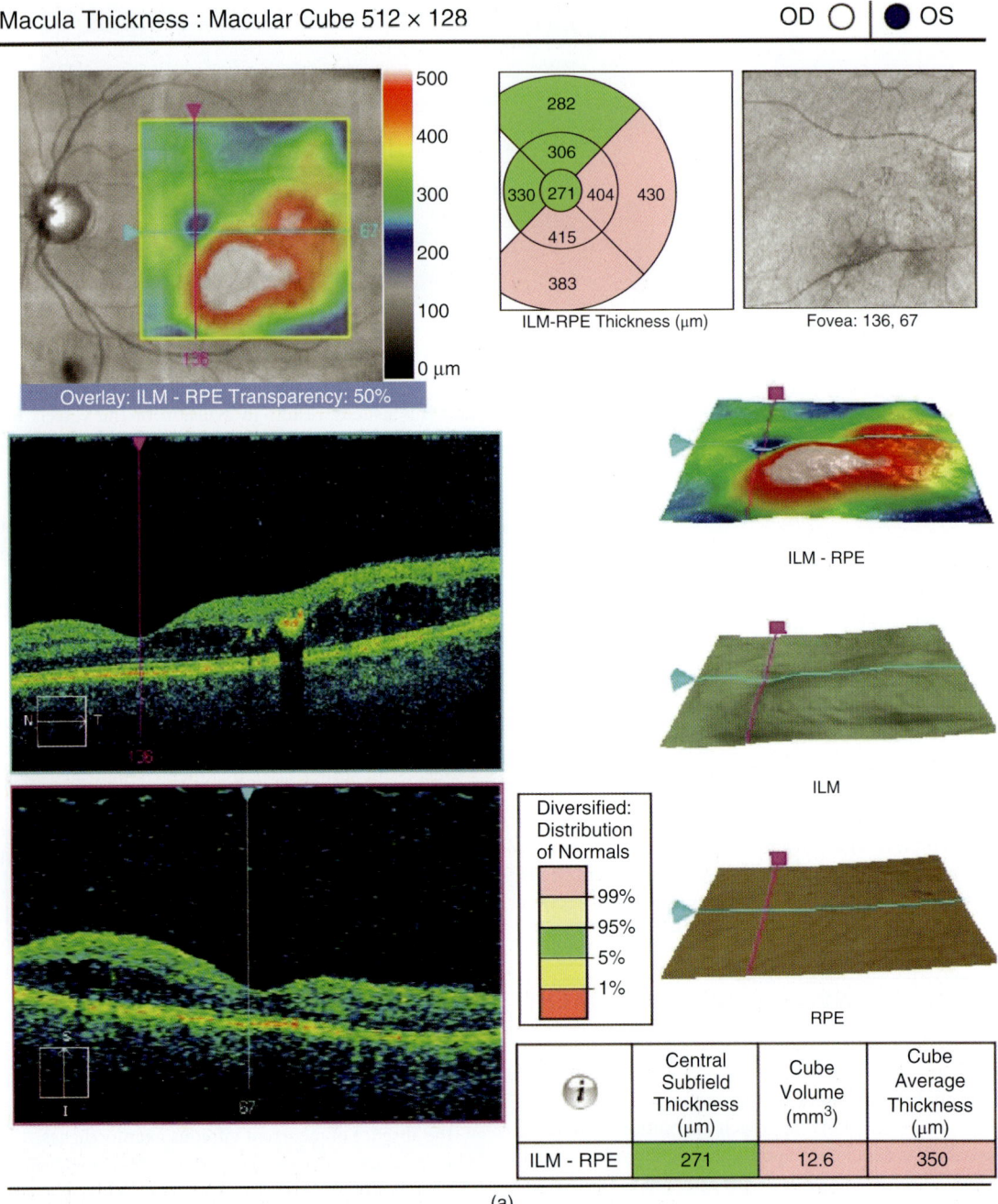

(a)

Fig. 12.2 OCT left macular area (a) before treatment with laser and (b) 3 months and (c) 9 months after treatment with laser.

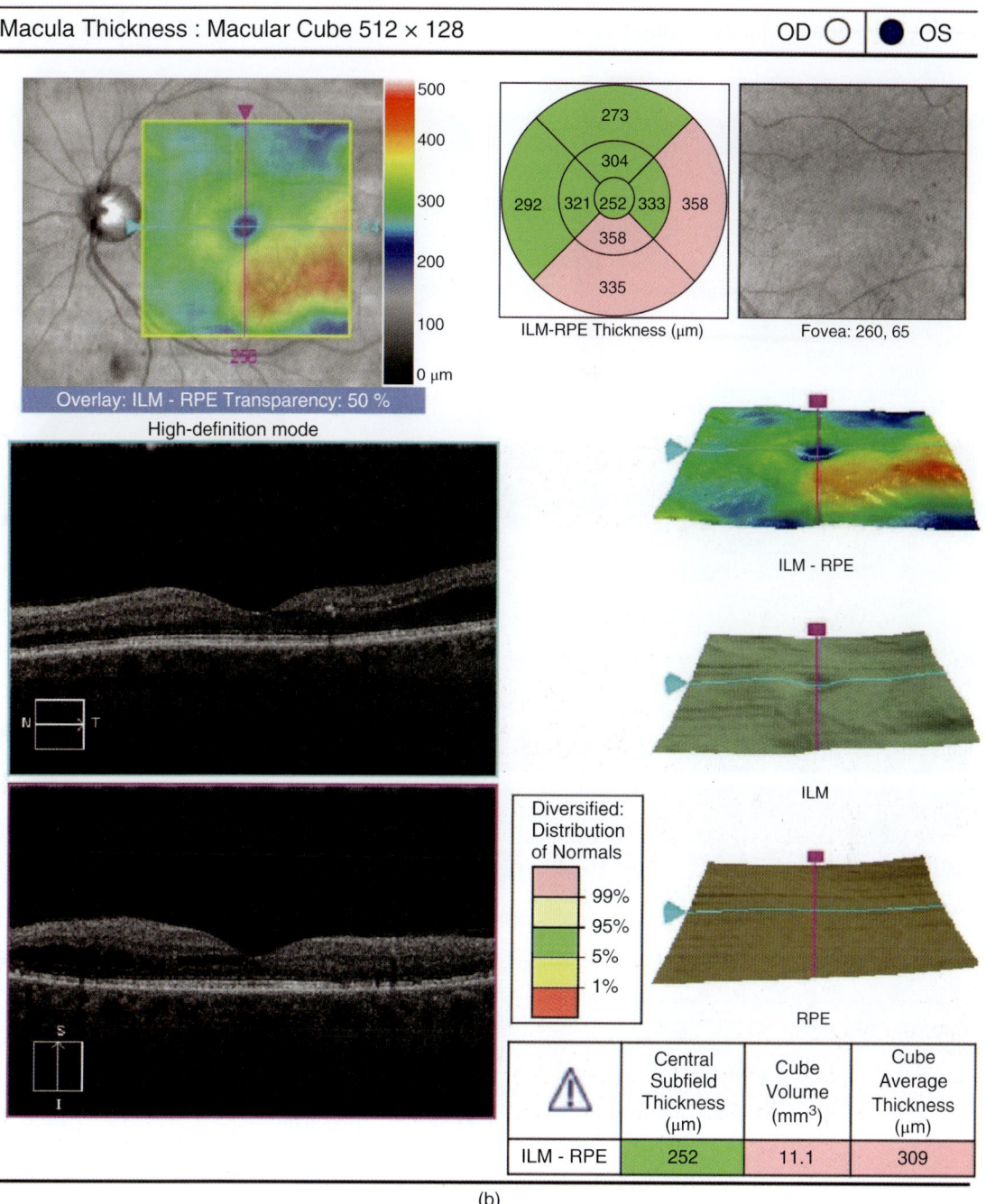

Fig. 12.2 (*Continued*)

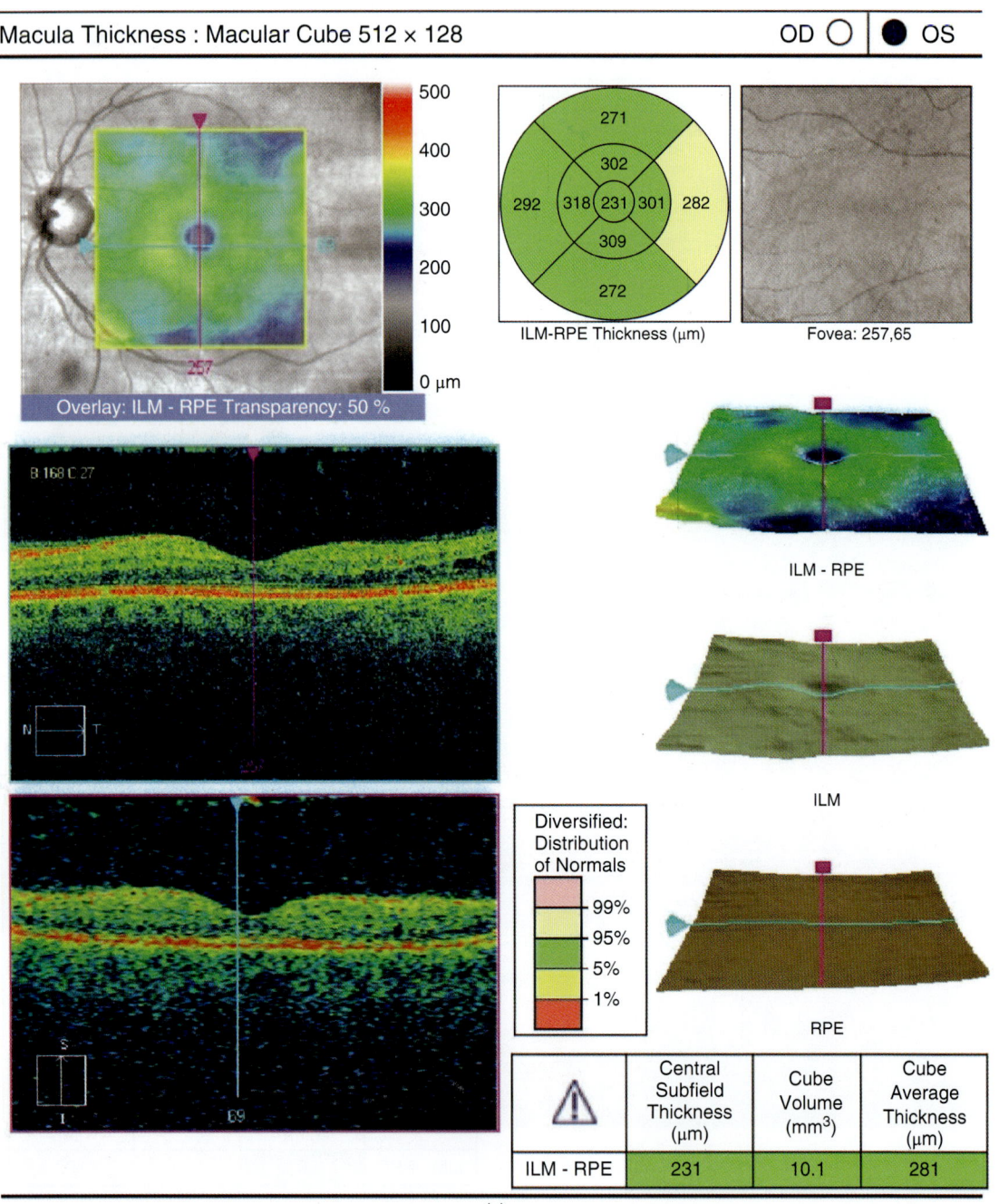

Fig. 12.2 (*Continued*)

It is important to note that treatment with VEGF inhibitors for diabetic maculopathy will suppress any neovascularisation; when the intravitreal treatment for maculopathy is ceased, there may be a rebound progression of neovascularisation requiring treatment.

Case History 12.3: Treated NVD proliferative DR

A 25-year-old woman with type 1 diabetes of 18 years duration was referred by her optometrist and was found to have proliferative diabetic retinopathy in her left eye with small NVD (>one-third disc area) and NVE (<half disc area) in the superior and nasal retina.

Treatment was given to the left eye with 1684 burns over 2 sessions, 500 micron size, 0.1 s, 230–280 mW, Karickhoff 4 mirror lens. The NVD regressed over the following 6 months and the NVE partially regressed and fibrosed.

Six years after the initial presentation, proliferative diabetic retinopathy developed in the right eye with small NVD (>one-third disc area) and NVE (<half disc area) in the temporal retina. Treatment was given to the left eye with 2419 burns over 3 sessions, 200 micron size, 0.02 s, 350–400 mW, Superquad lens, Pascal laser.

The NVD regressed over the following 6 months and the NVE partially regressed and fibrosed. Five years after the initial presentation, this lady had a successful pregnancy with no deterioration in her stable treated retinae. Her visual acuities have remained good at 6/6 (20/20) in each eye, her HbA1c results have been good at levels of between 6.7 and 7.3 and her BP has remained at an average of 125/81. Photographs of her left retina are shown in Figure 12.3.

Case History 12.4: Treated NVE proliferative DR

A 23-year-old man with type 1 diabetes (BMI 26) of 22 years duration was referred from retinal screening with possible new vessels in the superior retina of his left eye. Over the previous 2 years, his HbA1c result had varied between 9 and 10.5 and his BP had averaged 139/80. A fluorescein angiogram confirmed that he had neovascularisation in the superior retina. He also showed signs of extensive retinal ischaemia with severe IRMA in two other quadrants and venous beading in two quadrants. Panretinal photocoagulation was therefore commenced but, despite extensive treatment, he required a vitrectomy for his left eye.

At the age of 26, the photographs in Figure 12.4a, b were taken of his right eye. The photographs show venous beading in an ischaemic area of right superior retina. New vessels formed at the right disc and superotemporal retina, and panretinal photocoagulation was commenced to the right eye.

Treatment was given to the right peripheral retina of 3345 burns in 4 treatment sessions, 1895 using the Transequator lens (magnification factor 1.44), 350 micron size, 250 mW, 0.1 s, and 1895 using the Superquad 160 lens (magnification factor 2), 200 micron size, 230 mW, 0.1 s, argon laser. Indirect laser was later given in theatre of right 1469 burns, 260–300 mW, 0.2 s. This resulted in regression of the neovascularisation, as shown in Figure 12.4c–e. The photograph of the superior retina after regression of the neovascularisation demonstrates that the venous calibre that was dilated and beaded has returned to a more normal calibre.

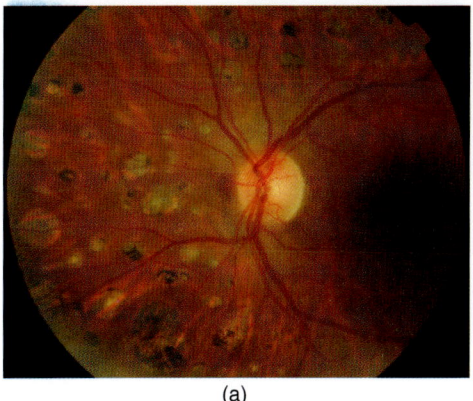
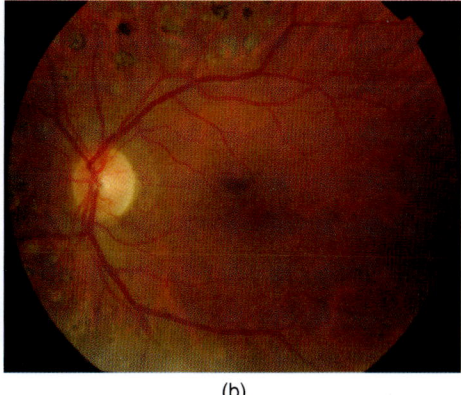

(a)   (b)

Fig. 12.3 Treated NVD proliferative DR: (a) left disc colour photo and (b) left macula colour photo.

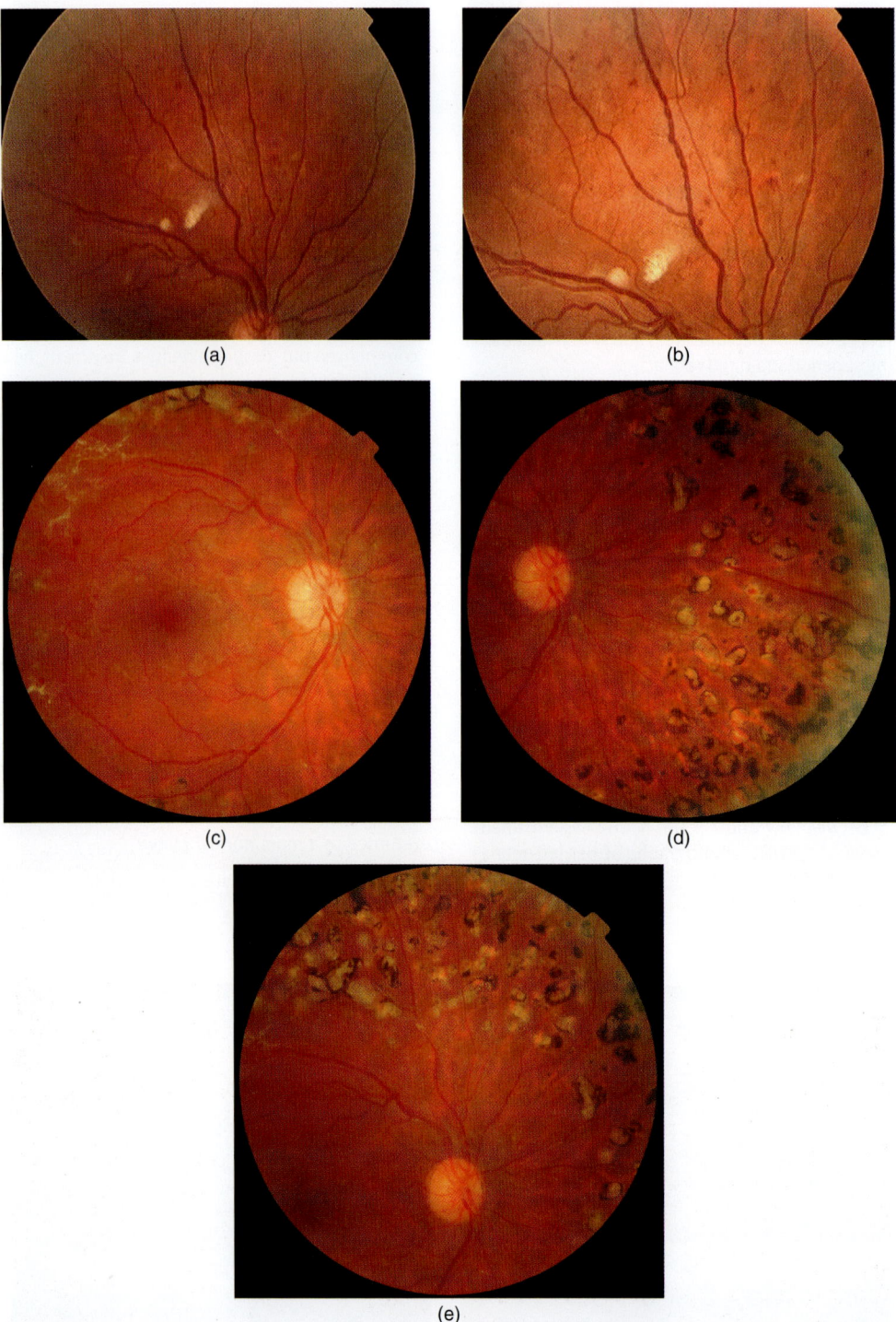

Fig. 12.4 (a, b) Right superior colour showing ischaemia before NVE developed. Treated NVE proliferative DR: (c) right macula colour; (d) right nasal colour; and (e) right superior colour.

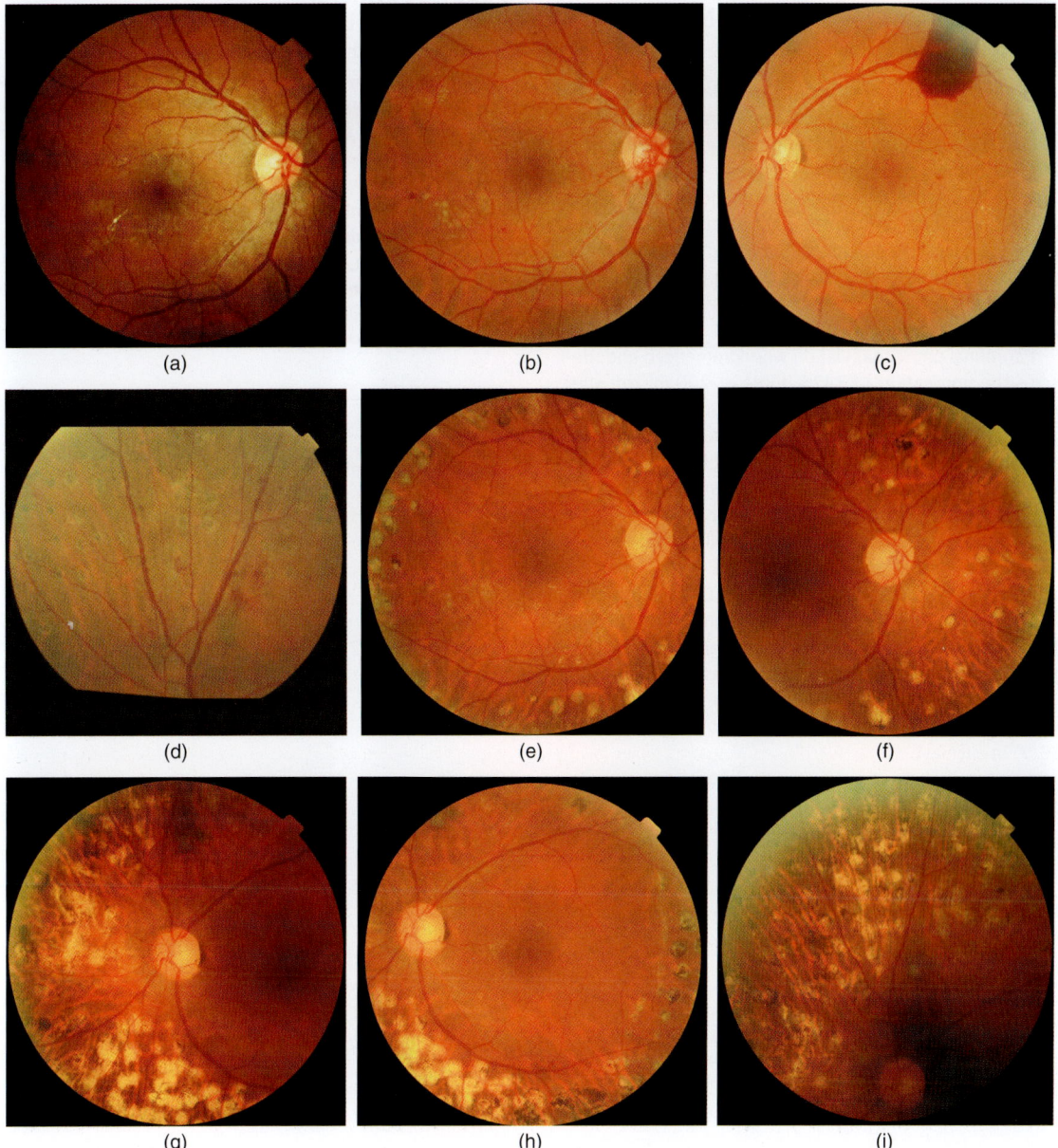

Fig. 12.5 Right macula showing (a) exudate infero-temporal to right fovea and (b) old macular laser scars and NVD developing at the right optic disc. (c) Left macula showing NVD developing at the left optic disc and a preretinal haemorrhage over the left supero-temporal arcade of vessels. (d) Left superior retina: venous beading present between laser scars. Stable treated: (e) right macular area; (f) right disc area; (g) left disc area; (h) left macular area; and (i) left superior retina with no further signs of venous beading.

Case History 12.5: Treated NVD proliferative DR

A 47-year-old man with type 1 diabetes since the age of 17 years was referred from retinal screening at the age of 33 years with exudate in the right macular area (Fig. 12.5a). No treatment was required on presentation, but the leak in the right macular area increased and was treated with focal laser to the right macular area 4 years after the initial presentation. Ten years after the initial presentation, neovascularisation developed at both optic discs and a preretinal haemorrhage formed in the left upper temporal retina (Fig. 12.5b and c).

Panretinal photocoagulation was commenced and, despite the application of 3420 burns of 200 micron spot size (0.02 s duration, 300–450 mW, Pascal laser and Superquad lens) over four sessions to the left eye, there was still venous beading present in the left superior retina (Fig. 12.5d), suggesting that this area was still ischaemic and the neovascularisation had not resolved.

A similar amount of laser was applied to the right eye. Three further sessions were then given, applying approximately 2800 burns to each eye. Despite this both continued to show signs of activity and continued to have episodes of vitreous haemorrhage; a pars plana vitrectomy with delamination and endolaser was therefore performed to each eye. This resulted in stability to each eye (Fig. 12.5e–i) with visual acuities of LogMAR 0.10 (6/9) in each eye.

PRACTICE POINTS

In the treatment of maculopathy, one aims to stabilise the vision by clearing the oedema with VEGF inhibitor treatment for centre-involving diabetic macular oedema and laser treatment for non-centre-involving oedema, and then paying careful attention to systemic factors such as glucose[5,6], hypertension[7] and lipids[8], recognising that the treatment of diffuse maculopathy is usually more difficult[2].

In the treatment of neovascularisation, involution of neovascularisation is dependent upon a sufficient area of retinal ablation[9,10]. When deciding how much laser to undertake in an individual patient, the calibre of the venous circulation is an important determining factor as well as regression/fibrosis of any neovascularisation.

REFERENCE

Please visit www.wiley.com/go/scanlon/diabetic_retinopathy

13 Vitrectomy surgery in diabetic retinopathy

Charles P. Wilkinson

Johns Hopkins University; Greater Baltimore Medical Center, USA

INTRODUCTION

This chapter is limited to a discussion of vitrectomy[1–3], an intraocular procedure specifically aimed at the pathological features of diabetic retinopathy, as well as its complications. Other types of surgery such as cataract surgery (Chapter 14), laser (Chapters 7 and 10) as well as anti-vascular endothelial growth factor (VEGF) and corticosteroid injection treatment for diabetic retinopathy (Chapter 7) are discussed in relevant chapters.

VITREOUS SURGERY (VITRECTOMY)

The vitreous gel is a vital structural component in the pathogenesis of proliferative diabetic retinopathy (PDR) and some selected cases of diabetic macular oedema (DMO). The critical variable in these situations is the relationship between the posterior cortical surface (PCS) of the vitreous gel and the inner surface of the retina.

In PDR, extraretinal neovascular and fibrovascular tissue grows almost exclusively along the PCS on the optic nerve head and elsewhere, which is identical to the legend in figure 13.1. If the PCS has separated from the retina prior to the threat of neovascularisation, literal PDR almost never occurs. In DMO many cases are probably not significantly influenced by the PCS, although there are a substantial percentage of cases in which it may be an important factor. In many of these, the PCS appears as a 'taught posterior hyaloid' which exerts tangential traction upon the retinal surface. In other cases, antero-posterior vitreoretinal traction may play a role, even though it cannot be visualised clinically. In addition, a relatively uncommon syndrome occurs when a partially detached PCS remains adherent to the macula and the resultant traction disturbs the permeability of central capillaries (Fig. 13.2). Finally, both an attached and detached PCS may be associated with the formation of fibrocellular epiretinal membranes that contract the inner surface of the macula and cause macular oedema and/or distortion.

Indications of vitrectomy in diabetic retinopathy

The most common indication for diabetic vitrectomy surgery is persistent or recurrent vitreous haemorrhage. In general, the timing for vitrectomy surgery usually ranges from 1 to 3 months from the onset of bleeding, with most surgeons operating earlier on patients with type 1 DM compared to type 2, based on the recommendations

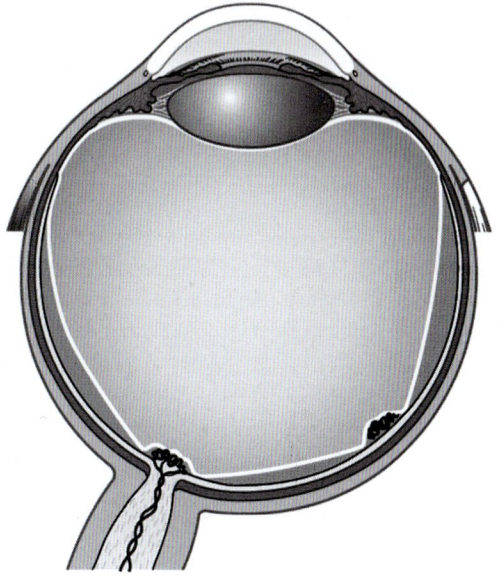

Fig. 13.1 Neovascularisation on the optic nerve and elsewhere occurs at locations at which there are vitreoretinal interfaces.

A Practical Manual of Diabetic Retinopathy Management, Second Edition.
Edited by Peter Scanlon, Ahmed Sallam, and Peter van Wijngaarden.
© 2017 John Wiley & Sons Ltd. Published 2017 by John Wiley & Sons Ltd.
Companion Website: www.wiley.com/go/scanlon/diabetic_retinopathy

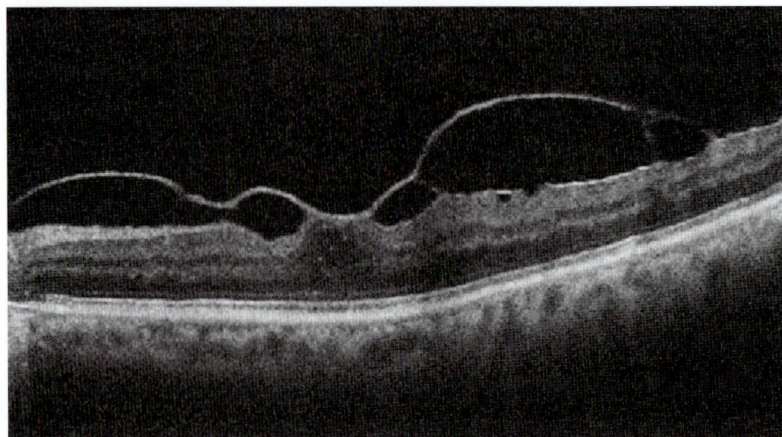

Fig. 13.2 OCT studies provide a means of more accurately identifying vitreoretinal traction forces that are occasionally responsible for DMO. In this case a partial vitreous detachment is causing persistent traction upon the macula.

of the Diabetic Vitrectomy Study[4] which showed benefit from early vitrectomy surgery in patients with type 1 DM but not type 2. Regardless of the type of diabetes and the duration of vitreous haemorrhage, the timing of vitrectomy surgery is also influenced by the state of the diabetic retinopathy before the bleeding including whether previous PRP treatment was applied, the severity and the location of the bleeding and also the condition of the fellow eye. Early surgical intervention is therefore usually considered in patients who did not receive sufficient PPR laser before the occurrence of bleeding, in cases with dense premacular haemorrhages due to possible toxicity of blood to the macula and also for monocular patients. Furthermore, patients with co-existing rubeosis iridis or rhegmatogenous retinal detachment are at risk of severe irreversible visual loss and need to be urgently operated upon.

Retinal detachment is the second most common indication for vitrectomy in patients with diabetic retinopathy. This includes tractional retinal detachment that threatens or involves the fovea and cases with combined traction and rhegmatogenous retinal detachment, even if the detachment is still away from the fovea. Other less common indications for vitrectomy in diabetic patients include florid PDR despite adequate laser, and some cases of DMO where vitreomacular traction exists.

Preoperative use of intravitreal anti-VEGF treatment

In recent years, the preoperative use of intravitreal anti-VEGF before vitrectomy in patients with active diabetic fibrovascular membranes has come into play. Data from several randomised controlled trials[5] looking at the use of bevacizumab before PPV surgery have demonstrated a beneficial effect with decreased risk of intraoperative bleeding and hence shorter surgery duration, as well as lower rates of early post-operative bleeding in comparison to vitrectomy alone. However, caution need to be exercised when using anti-VEGF in patients with diabetic fibrovascular membranes, as its use could be associated with an increased risk of fibrosis and exaggerated tractional detachment. This risk could be lessened by operating early, within 5–7 days from the time of anti-VEGF administration.

TREATMENT TECHNIQUES FOR PDR

Contemporary vitrectomy techniques provide a means of removing vitreous haemorrhage and the PCS in a relatively safe and effective fashion. Most systems employ three small (20–27-gauge) entry 'ports' into the eye, and a cutting/suction device, an intraocular light source and an infusion cannula are inserted through these trans-scleral incisions (Fig. 13.3). In a right eye, the cutting instrument and light pipe are typically inserted 3–4 mm posterior to the limbus at approximately 10:30 and 2:15 respectively, with the infusion device inserted at approximately 8:30. Additional equipment, such as picks, scissors and forceps, are frequently substituted temporarily to replace the routine cutting device if required. Cataract surgery can be combined with vitrectomy if the lens opacity prevents an optimal view and in other selected cases.

Vitrectomy surgery in diabetic retinopathy

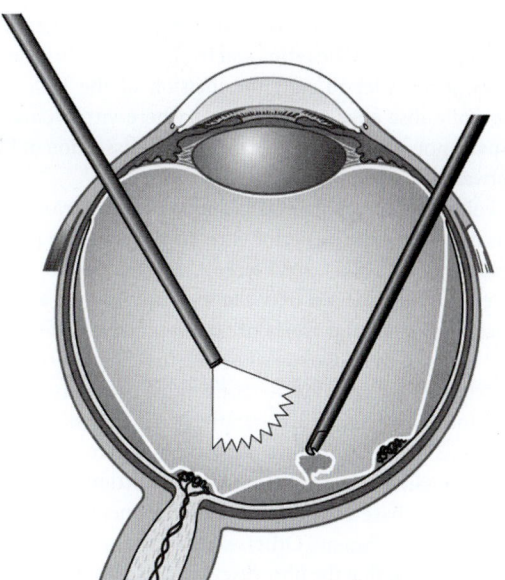

Fig. 13.3 Vitreous surgery usually includes three incisions for a cutting/aspiration device, an illumination system and a continuous infusion site (not pictured). Vitreous haemorrhage in the gel is easily removed if the posterior vitreous cortical face is separated from the surface of the retina.

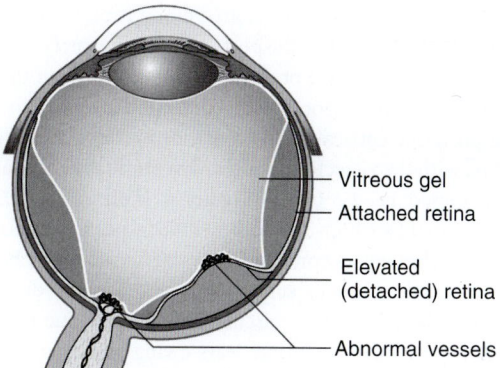

Fig. 13.4 Fibrovascular tissue growth and secondary changes in the vitreous gel cause traction at sites of vitreovascular attachments, resulting in haemorrhage and traction retinal detachment. Retinal breaks and rhegmatogenous detachments can also occur.

The primary goals of vitreous surgery for PDR include removal of vitreous haemorrhage, wide excision of the PCS and associated neovascular tissue, and the elimination of epiretinal tissue and traction forces affecting macular function. In PDR, extraretinal neovascular and fibrovascular tissue grows almost exclusively along the posterior vitreous surface, as noted earlier. This proliferation often causes changes in the vitreous gel that result in separation of some of the cortical vitreous from the retina. The vitreous always remains attached to the anterior retina at the vitreous base, and frequently exhibits a funnel-shaped configuration that extends between the vitreous base anteriorly and posterior areas of neovascular proliferation. Variable portions of the posterior cortical vitreous remain near the plane of the retinal surface and bridge from one area of retinal neovascularisation to another (Fig. 13.4). When little or no posterior vitreous detachment occurs the proliferative tissue grows along the interface of the PCS and the inner retinal surface, and widespread adhesions to the retina may develop. This fibrovascular tissue can contract, causing tangential traction on the retina and visual loss from swelling, distortion or displacement of the macula. Fibrovascular tissue growth and secondary changes in the vitreous gel cause traction resulting in further complications including haemorrhage, traction retinal detachment, retinal breaks, and rhegmatogenous retinal detachment.

If complete removal of vitreous haemorrhage and the posterior cortical vitreous with all attached fibrovascular tissue is accomplished without complications, further vasoproliferation on the posterior retina can usually be prevented and reattachment of a detached retina can usually be accomplished. Removal of vitreous haemorrhage is relatively easily performed, and the most difficult surgical step in most vitrectomies for diabetic retinopathy is the removal of fibrovascular tissue from the surface of the underlying retina, a manoeuvre that is particularly difficult if the retina is also detached. These steps are usually performed with a variety of microsurgical vitrectomy instruments including picks, forceps and scissors. However, with today's smaller gauge vitreous cutters and ability to control fluidics including vacuum and cutting rates, the vitreous cutter could be used as a multifunctional instrument to segment and even delaminate epiretinal membranes. Following successful vitreous surgery, scatter laser photocoagulation is usually applied before the end of the procedure if this was not completed before the surgery.

Removal of vitreous haemorrhage and vitreous gel

The posterior vitreous surface is frequently incised initially in an area of partial vitreous detachment and away from vitreoretinal attachments and/or areas of underlying retinal detachment. If non-clotted blood is present in the preretinal space behind the posterior vitreous surface, it is evacuated using active or passive aspiration. When there is little or no posterior vitreous detachment, portions of the posterior cortical vitreous can be elevated from the retina with the vitrectomy cutter, vitreoretinal pick, sharp bent-tipped needle or myringotomy knife (Fig. 13.5). Employment of high suction to induce posterior vitreous detachment, as conventionally used in macular hole or retinal detachment surgery, is not recommended in cases with diabetic fibrovascular membranes due to the high risk of inducing retinal tears owing to strong adhesions between the PCS and the retina. Non-vascularised posterior hyaloid and immature proliferative membranes can frequently be bluntly dissected from the surface of the retina. Recently proliferating tissue is characterised by neovascularisation with little or only translucent fibrous tissue. Older fibrovascular tissue becomes more white and opaque and more firmly adherent to the retina, and sharp dissection may be required. It is also worth noting that vitreoschisis as a consequence of anomalous PVD is not uncommonly encountered in patients with PDR-related traction. This phenomenon could make identification of the plane between the retina and the PCS difficult; in some cases, it is easier to start the incision of the PCS over the optic disc edge or the macula where vitreoschisis is usually not present, and then extend the dissection of PCS outwards.

Following the controlled induction of posterior vitreous dissection, the posterior vitreous surface is frequently excised around the circumference of its cone-like structure to relieve traction between the vitreous base and the posterior retina and zones of fibrovascular proliferation. The edges of the posterior vitreous surface often separate widely after the gel is cut, demonstrating that considerable traction was present preoperatively. At this stage some surgeons prefer to remove as much of the cortical vitreous as possible, except for the anterior portion adjacent to the vitreous base and posterior remnants near areas of vitreoretinal attachment. Others remove the avascular gel at the same time that the fibrovascular tissue itself is excised.

Removal of fibrovascular tissue

'Delamination' and 'en bloc' are terms used to describe methods of dissecting epiretinal fibrovascular tissue from the surface of the retina. Using the delamination technique, surgeons initially remove all elevated cortical vitreous that is producing antero-posterior traction on posterior fibrovascular tissue. Identification of the proper plane between the PCS and the retina is crucial and greatly facilitates membrane dissection. Vitreoretinal picks and scissors are then used to elevate and divide avascular portions of the more organised posterior vitreous cortex until only islands of tightly adherent fibrovascular tissue remain. Bimanual techniques are used to delaminate those focal membranes that appear to be excisable without major structural damage to the retina (Fig. 13.6). Other surgeons prefer the 'en bloc' technique, leaving portions of anterior vitreous gel intact so that the residual antero-posterior traction will assist in the dissection of epiretinal tissue by elevating its edges (Fig. 13.7), which is subsequently removed after removal of the membranes.

Removing all fibrovascular 'islands' is believed to reduce the frequency of post-operative bleeding, contraction of residual epiretinal membranes, recurrence of epiretinal proliferation and missed small retinal breaks. 'Segmentation' techniques, in which localised islands of epiretinal fibrovascular tissue are left following vitrectomy, have therefore become much less popular. Still, segmentation techniques are useful when the combination of relatively mature epiretinal tissue

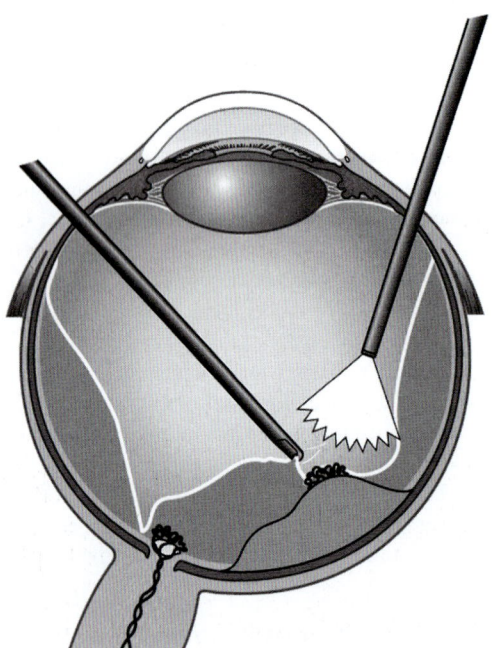

Fig. 13.5 The major surgical goal in vitrectomy for PDR is to separate and excise the posterior cortical vitreous surface and associated areas of fibrovascular proliferation from the retinal surface.

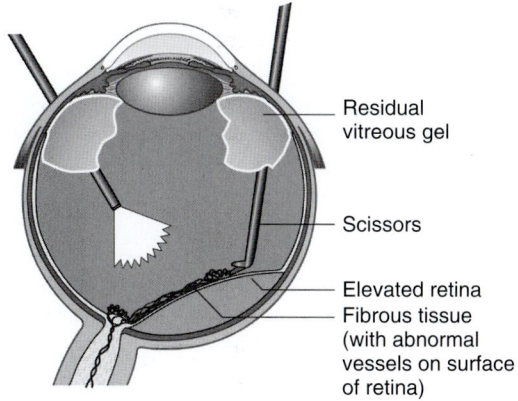

Fig. 13.6 Segmentation 'delamination' techniques can be employed to remove fibrovascular proliferation from the surface of the retina.

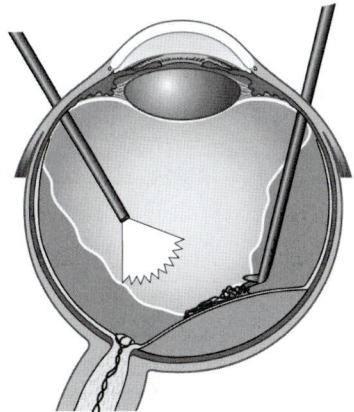

Fig. 13.7 Some surgeons prefer to employ 'en bloc' excision ('delamination') of fibrovascular tissue from the retinal surface. Vitreous traction can assist in elevating the abnormal vessels from portions of the retina.

and atrophic retina results in a significant increase in risk of retinal breaks associated with complete epiretinal membrane dissection, or when vascular membranes are located anteriorly and are difficult to remove safely. If no segmentation has been performed, the entire organised posterior cortical vitreous is usually removed in a single piece. Peeling of diabetic fibrovascular membranes in diabetic vitrectomy is generally not advisable due to strong attachment of retina and membranes; however, fibrovascular tissue attached to the optic nerve head could gently be avulsed or excised from the nerve after all surrounding attachments to the retina have been eliminated. If retinal mobility associated with retinal detachment interferes with dissecting epiretinal tissue, a small amount of heavy perfluorocarbon liquid can be injected onto the posterior retina. This stabilises the retina and makes delamination easier. Combinations of techniques are frequently employed, but the goal to remove the posterior cortical surface out to the vitreous base along with all fibrovascular membranes is always the same in these cases.

Intraoperative haemorrhage during segmentation and delamination is unfortunately not uncommon. Unimanual or bimanual bipolar diathermy is routinely applied to sites of persistent bleeding other than the optic nerve (Fig. 13.8). The incidence of haemorrhage can be reduced by avoiding segmentation of highly vascularised membranes and ensuring that the patient's blood pressure is normal. Elevation of intraocular pressure is used to minimise bleeding during the dissection of vascularised tissue. Further elevation of intraocular pressure to a level above systolic blood pressure for 1–2 min will frequently stop persistent bleeding. Preoperative use of intravitreal anti-VEGF also reduces the risk and severity of intraoperative bleeding as discussed earlier.

Treating retinal breaks and detachments

When attempting the removal of diabetic fibrovascular membranes, the general principle is to avoid creation of retinal tears. In some cases the surgeon may therefore elect to leave some areas of traction behind as mentioned previously, particularly if this traction is present outside the macular arcades and the membranes are judged to be very adherent to the underlying retina. However, if retinal tears do occur during membrane dissection, it is

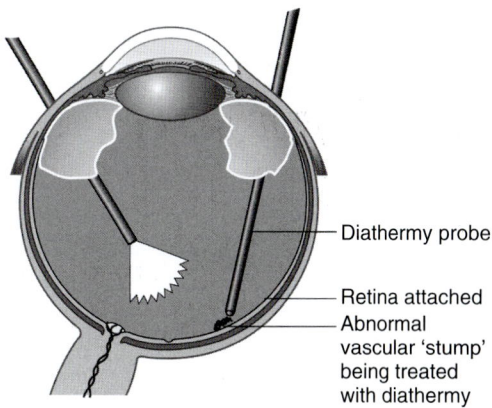

Fig. 13.8 Intraocular diathermy is employed to treat bleeding foci on the surface of the retina.

then important to continue with membrane removal to relieve any traction around the tear(s). Retinal breaks, whether iatrogenic or pre-existing before the surgery in cases of combined rhegmatogenous and tractional detachment, are treated with endolaser before the operation is completed. To achieve this, subretinal fluid is evacuated through suitable posterior breaks and fluid in the vitreous cavity is then exchanged with air to flatten the retina against the pigment epithelium, permitting laser retinopexy. If internal drainage of subretinal fluid fails to significantly re-attach the retina under air despite release of all obvious fibrovascular tissues, the surgeon should search for thin avascular membranes peripheral to the sites of neovascularisation and remove them. Staining of membranes with triamcinolone acetonide or dyes as trypan blue could be helpful in this context. Most surgeons then place additional scatter laser photocoagulation to the entire peripheral retina unless it has been treated previously.

Intraocular tamponade

Intraocular tamponade is usually not required in the absence of retinal tears. In cases where retinal tears exist, intraocular gas is usually preferred over silicone due to its superior tamponade effect and because silicone oil use in diabetic patients could trigger recurrent epiretinal membrane proliferation. Nevertheless, silicone oil might be of advantage if retinal tears are associated with significant residual traction that could not be relieved by surgery and in complex cases that involved retinectomies, or in eyes with rubeosis iridis. Other situations where silicone oil is also considered include monocular patients and those who need to fly soon after surgery.

POST-OPERATIVE COMPLICATIONS

Although vitrectomy surgery for diabetic retinal traction remains one of the challenging types of surgery for the vitreoretinal surgeon, the risk of significant post-operative complications is generally low nowadays with the use of contemporary vitrectomy instrumentation and advancements in endoillumination and retinal viewing systems.

Cataract formation is the most common complication encountered after diabetic vitrectomy surgery, and is more common in older patients with pre-existing nuclear sclerosis.

Recurrent post-operative vitreous cavity haemorrhage is also a common complication of diabetic vitrectomy surgery, and could occur in up to 50% of cases. Early bleeding usually results from leaking blood vessels after fibrovascular membranes removal or due to leaking of residual vitreous haemorrhage that was not removed during the surgery. Late bleeding usually originates from retinal or optic nerve neovascularisation and rarely from pars plana neovascularisation at the site of the vitrectomy ports (entry site neovascularisation). The latter type of neovascularisation is usually difficult to diagnose, but could sometimes be identified by ultrasound microscopy or visualised during surgery. In general, it is reasonable to observe cases with vitreous cavity haemorrhage initially as they may spontaneously resolve, and consider repeat vitrectomy/vitreous wash in those where vitreous cavity bleeding persists.

Post-operative retinal detachment is an uncommon complication after diabetic vitrectomy mainly encountered in eyes that required extensive membrane dissection and during the surgeon's learning phase. Careful dissection of epiretinal membranes could help avoid the creation of retinal tears, and examination of the peripheral retina at the end of surgery to detect retinal tears at the vitrectomy entry site is important to further decrease the risk of retinal detachment.

A further post-operative complication after diabetic vitrectomy that deserves attention is rubeosis iridis; although it is uncommonly encountered (<2%), it could result in intractable glaucoma with severe pain and significant loss of vision. The risk of developing rubeosis is high in patients with severe preoperative ischaemia, particularly if PRP laser treatment was not adequately employed, and also after complex vitrectomy surgery with retinectomy or in cases complicated with rhegmatogenous retinal detachment post-operatively. Treatment usually involves urgent intravitreal anti-VEGF as well as additional PRP laser; IOP-lowering measures and further vitrectomy surgery might be indicated in some cases.

> **Case History 13.1: Vitrectomy for severe vitreous haemorrhage and neovascularisation on the disc (NVD)**
>
> A 57-year-old man with type 2 diabetes presented with a vitreous haemorrhage in his right eye (Fig. 13.9a and b) and panretinal photocoagulation commenced.
> The vitreous haemorrhage recurred and then obscured the whole retinal view, and vision was reduced to counting fingers. A right pars plana vitrectomy was performed with delamination and PRP endolaser. Following this procedure (Fig. 13.10) his VA improved to 20/40 (LogMAR 0.34).

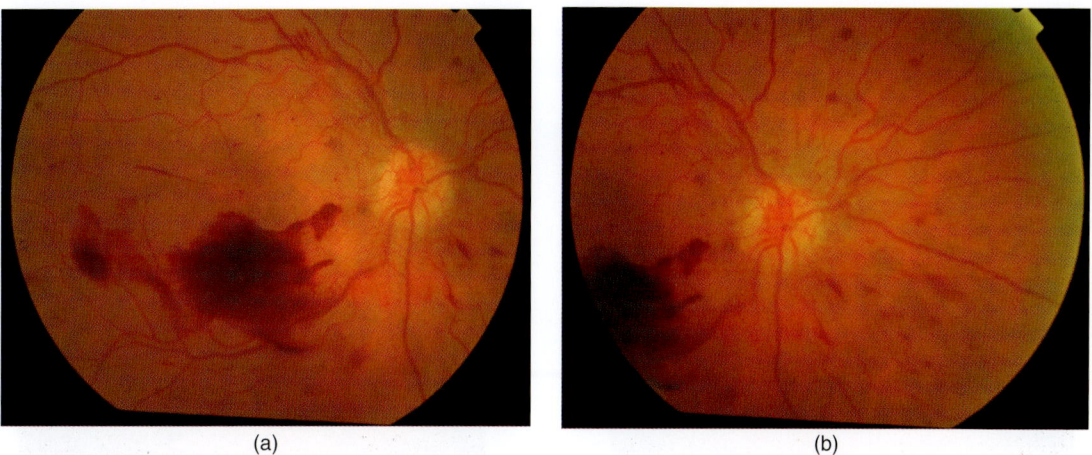

Fig. 13.9 (a, b) Vitreous haemorrhage in the right eye with neovascularisation at the right optic disc.

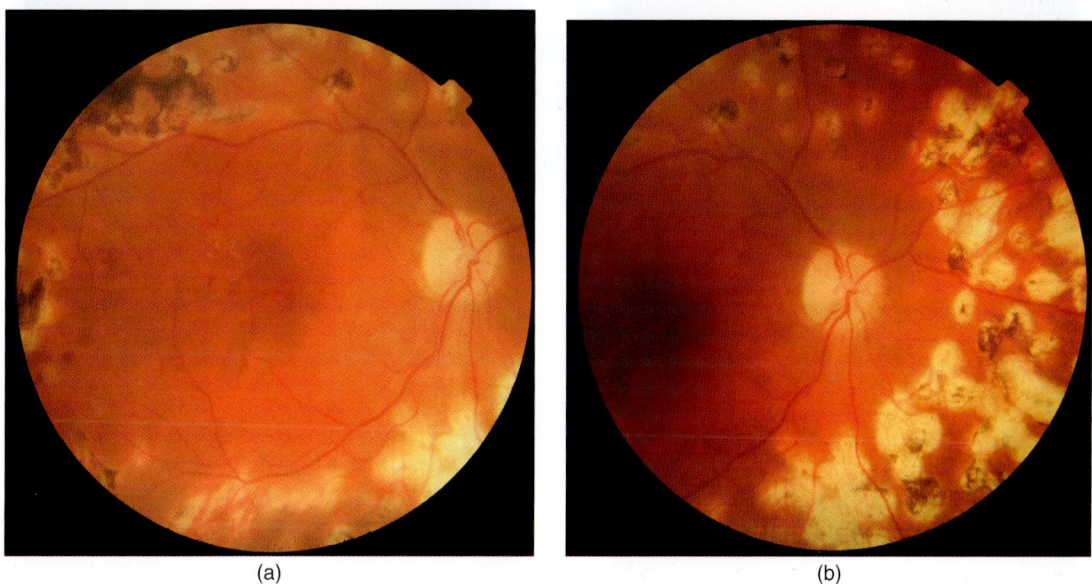

Fig. 13.10 (a, b) Retinal appearance post-vitrectomy with laser scars from the panretinal laser treatment.

Case History 13.2: **Vitrectomy for tractional retinal detachment and vitreous haemorrhage due to PDR**

A young woman with type 1 diabetes since the age of 6 years presented at the age of 27 years with a tractional retinal detachment and vitreous haemorrhage in her left eye (Fig. 13.11). Her right eye showed signs of preretinal haemorrhage. Her visual acuities were right 20/30 (LogMAR 0.1) and left hand movements only.

Her left vision improved to a level of 20/40 (LogMAR 0.3) and remained at this level when she was seen in clinic 12 years later (Fig. 13.12). Her right eye also required a vitrectomy one year after her left eye.

TREATMENT TECHNIQUES FOR DMO

Most cases of diabetic macular oedema are observed in eyes with NPDR and insignificant antero-posterior or

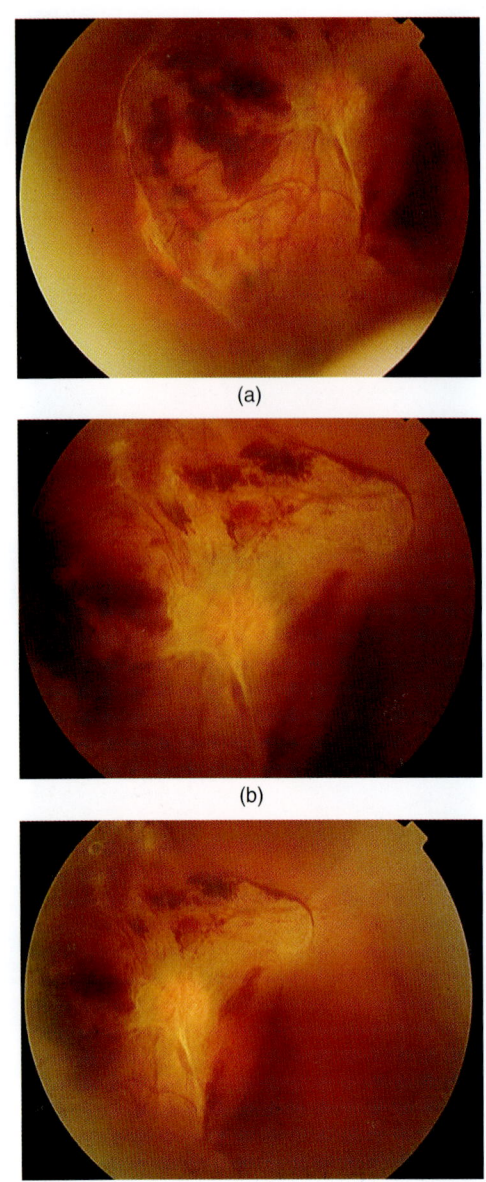

Fig. 13.11 (a–c) Signs of the tractional retinal detachment and vitreous haemorrhage in her left eye.

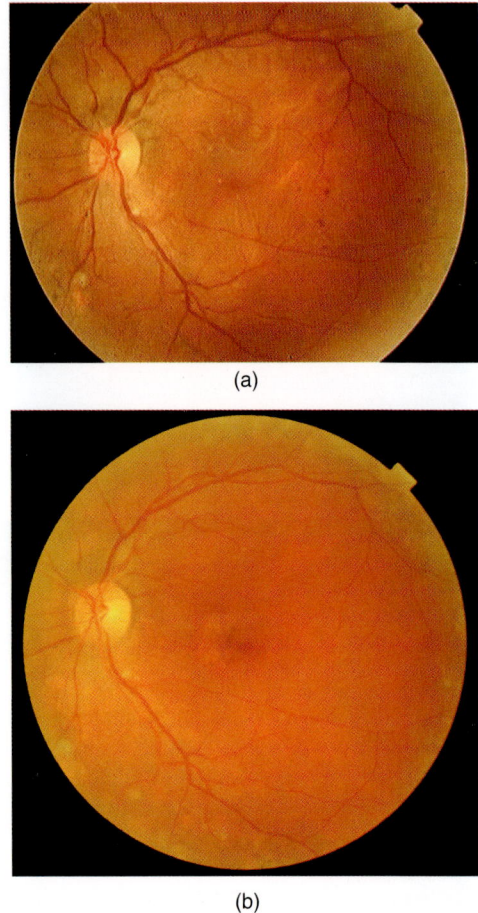

Fig. 13.12 The appearance of her left retina (a) 6 months and (b) 12 years after the vitrectomy.

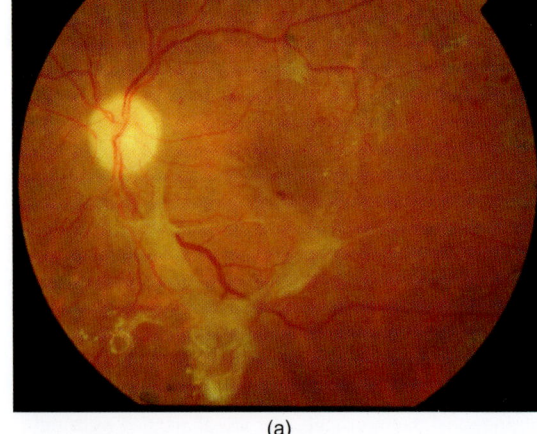

Fig. 13.13 (a) The appearance of the left retina with traction from the fibrotic neovascular complexes and (b) the OCT of the macular area demonstrating the traction.

Vitrectomy surgery in diabetic retinopathy 179

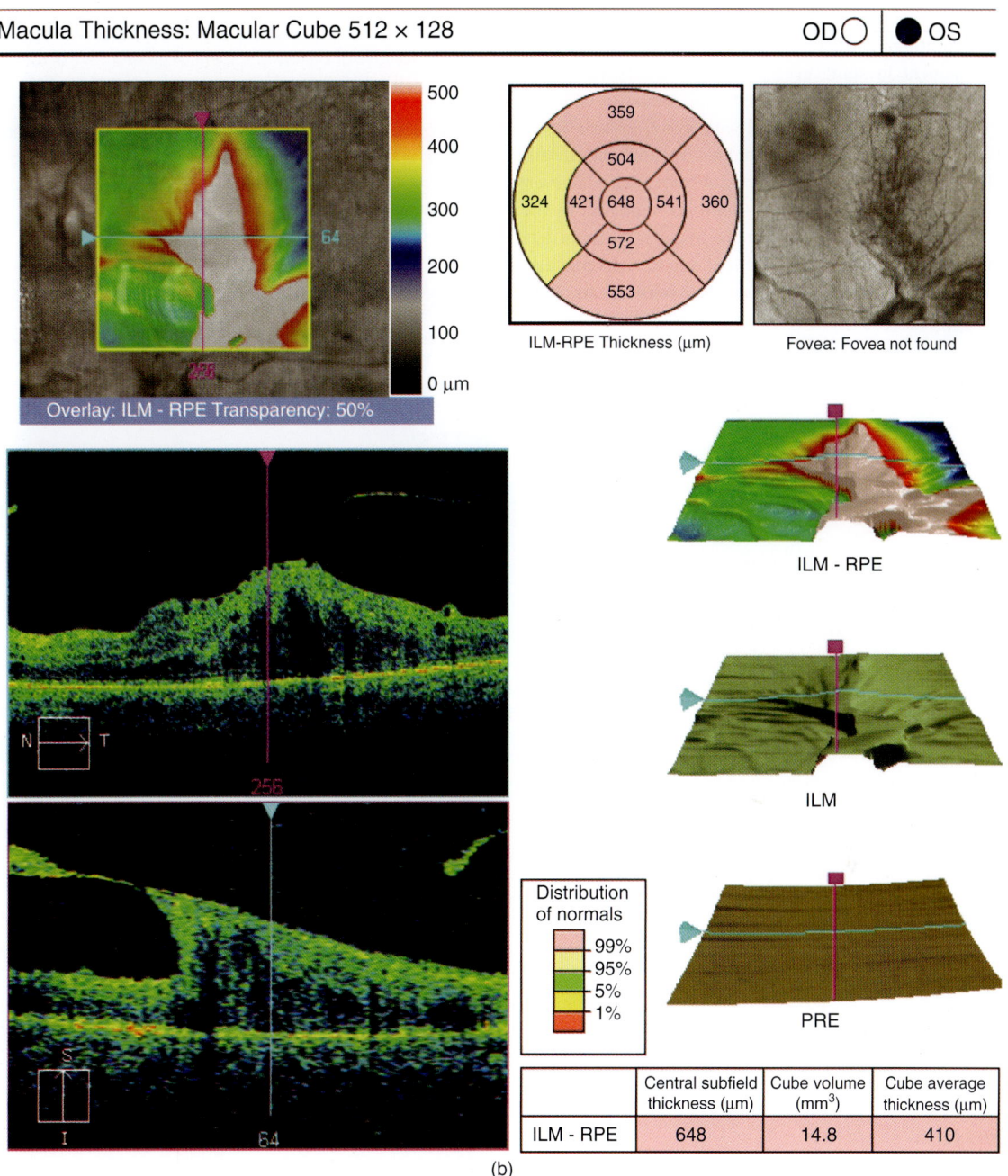

(b)

Fig. 13.13 (*Continued*)

tangential vitreous traction upon the macula. In these eyes, although vitrectomy was shown to provide possible benefit in some eyes that have failed to respond to anti-VEGF treatment in reducing macular oedema, this was not always associated with visual improvement and the role of vitrectomy in eyes without significant vitreomacular traction remains controversial. However, vitrectomy could be a useful treatment modality in the subset of diabetic patients where macular oedema has an associated tractional component due to vitreomacular traction (Fig. 13.2), taught posterior hyaloid or fibrocellular epiretinal membranes[6,7]. In all of these situations, the surgical goals include removal of the posterior cortical vitreous surface and all epimacular membranes, and elimination of vitreomacular traction forces. This is usually accomplished with vitrectomy picks, forceps and scissors, as described earlier.

Case History 13.3: Vitrectomy for macular off-tractional detachment

A 49-year-old lady presented with a shower of floaters in her right eye and was diagnosed with type 2 diabetes and proliferative diabetic retinopathy. Her visual acuity on first presentation was 20/40 (0.3 LogMAR) in each eye, using a pinhole. She commenced panretinal photocoagulation to both eyes and her diabetes was controlled on tablets. Her vision remained at this level over the next 2 years, but then her left vision deteriorated over a few months to a level of 20/200 (1.0 LogMAR). She was found to have a macular off-tractional detachment in her left macular area (Fig. 13.13).

She had a left pars plana vitrectomy, panretinal photocoagulation (endolaser, internal tamponade) SF6 gas, fibro vascular membrane delamination (Fig. 13.14). Over the next 2 years her left vision gradually improved to 20/40 (LogMAR level of 0.32).

Case History 13.4: Vitrectomy for epiretinal membrane formation with macular traction

A woman was diagnosed at the age of 55 years with type 2 diabetes, requiring a combination of tablets and insulin. Soon after diagnosis she was found to have signs of maculopathy treated with macular laser treatment, and 2 years later she required bilateral panretinal photocoagulation because of the development of proliferative diabetic retinopathy. Following this treatment her visual acuity levels were 20/40 (0.3 LogMAR) in each eye. She subsequently dropped her left visual acuity to a level of 13/200 (1.2 LogMAR) due to a combination of vitreous haemorrhage and epiretinal membrane formation with macular traction (Fig. 13.15a). Her preoperative OCT demonstrated the macular changes.

She underwent left phacoemulsification + IOL (first eye), pars plana vitrectomy, fibro vascular membrane segmentation, panretinal photocoagulation, endolaser, fibro vascular membrane delamination. Her post-operative VA improved to 0.3 LogMAR with an improvement in macular appearance (Fig. 13.15b).

PRACTICE POINTS

Both PDR and NPDR with macular oedema can be indications for a variety of surgical options, and specific stages of retinopathy represent evidence-based indications for these procedures.

Although PDR is usually managed initially with laser photocoagulation and/or anti-VEGF therapy, vitrectomy procedures are invaluable in managing severe complications of PDR, including major vitreous haemorrhage and retinal detachment.

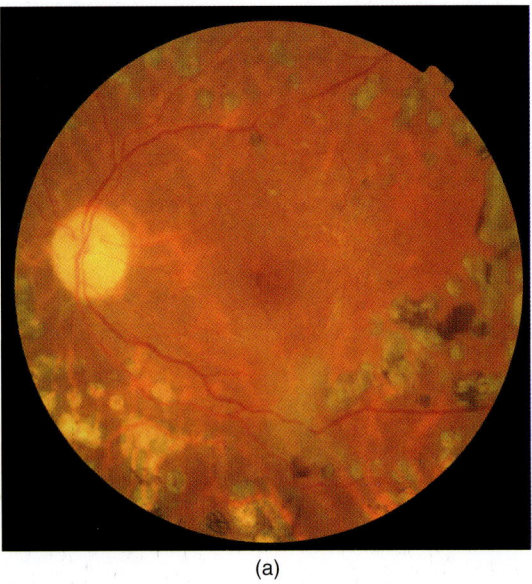

(a)

Fig. 13.14 (a, b) The appearance of the left retina and the OCT following surgery.

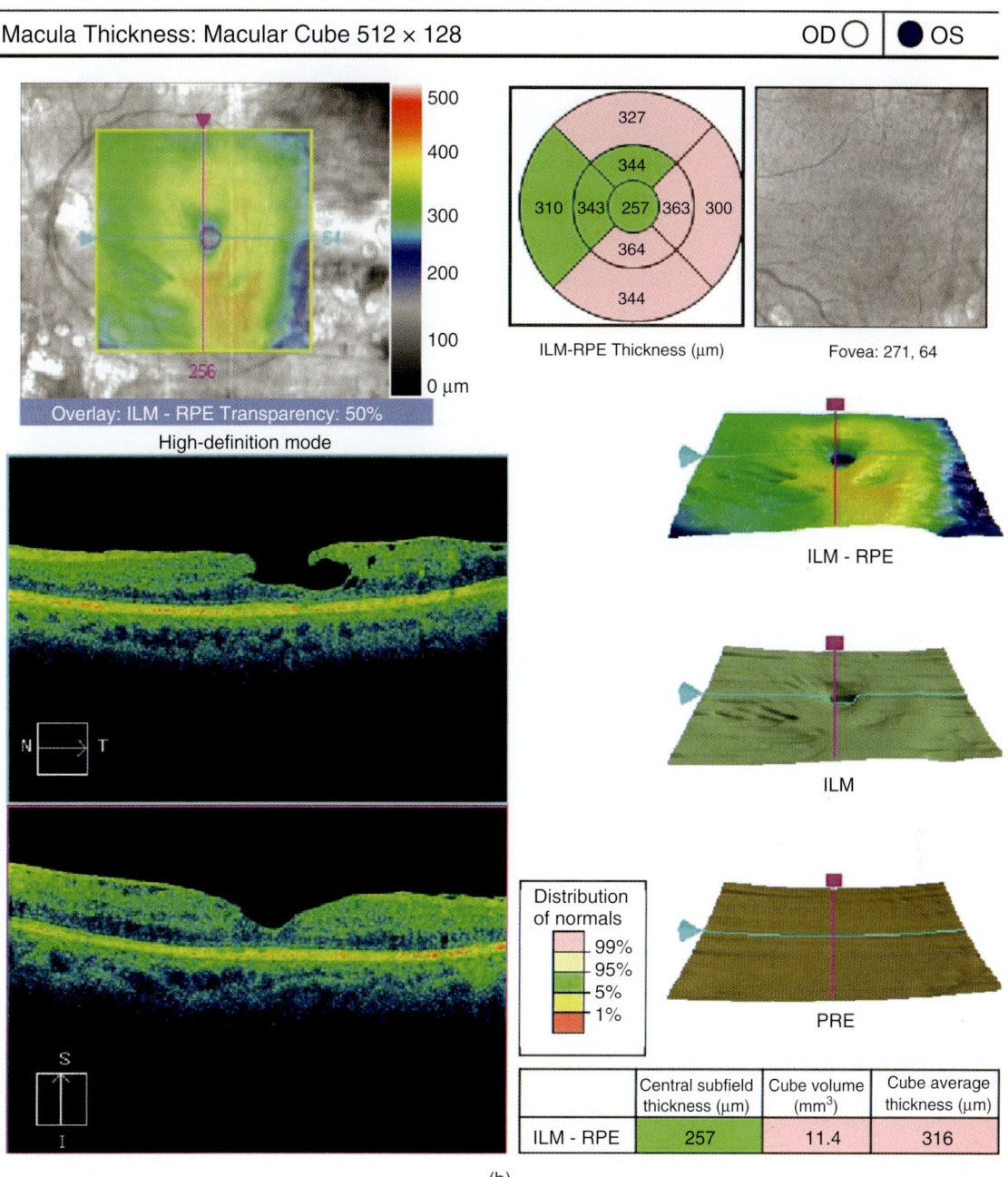

Fig. 13.14 (Continued)

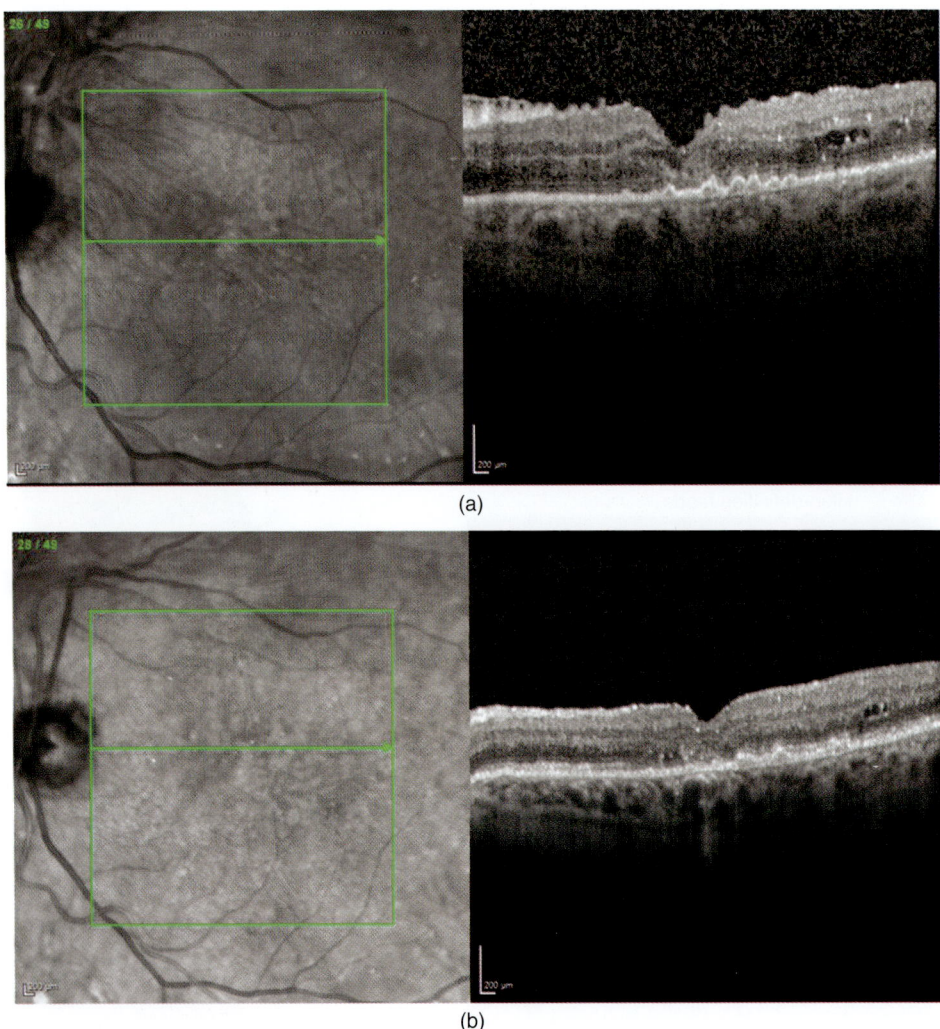

Fig. 13.15 OCT that shows the appearance of the macular area (a) with epiretinal membrane pre-surgery and (b) post-surgery.

Diabetic macular oedema is usually managed initially with anti-VEGF injections and/or laser photocoagulation, and vitrectomy is employed in selected cases in which vitreous or epimacular traction forces appear to be significant.

REFERENCE

Please visit www.wiley.com/go/scanlon/diabetic_retinopathy

14 Cataract surgery in the diabetic eye: Pre-, intra- and postoperative considerations

Abdallah A. Ellabban[1] & Ahmed Sallam[2]

[1] Suez Canal University, Egypt
[2] University of Arkansas for Medical Sciences, USA

INTRODUCTION

Cataract is a frequent occurrence in patients with diabetes mellitus (DM). The incidence of cataract in patients with diabetes ranges from 8 to 25%, with the risk of developing cataract being higher in older patients and in patients with longer duration of diabetes mellitus (DM) or poor glycaemic control. In general, around 40% percent of patients undergoing cataract surgery have DM. Compared to patients without diabetes, cataract in patients with diabetes usually develops at a younger age and progresses more rapidly[1–6].

Cataract surgery in patients with diabetes can be associated with certain intraoperative difficulties and challenges due to associated ocular co-morbidities such as poor pupillary dilatation. Diabetes is also a well-known risk factor for certain postoperative complications such as uveitis and pseudophakic macular oedema that may have impact on the rate of visual recovery and final visual outcome. Furthermore, cataract extraction could also negatively influence the rate of progression of diabetic maculopathy and may have some effect on retinopathy progression in eyes with advanced diabetic retinopathy. Taken together, these factors underscore the importance of preoperative planning of cataract surgery in patients with diabetes so that the visual outcome is not adversely affected.

Phacoemulsification is currently the standard technique for cataract surgery. This chapter reviews the management of cataract in patients with diabetes and highlights current agreements and possible controversies before, during and after cataract surgery.

PATHOGENESIS OF CATARACT DEVELOPMENT IN DIABETES

Different types of cataract can occur in patients with diabetes including nuclear, cortical, posterior subcapsular and mixed cataracts[5,7,8]. Overall, the most frequent cataract types in patients with diabetes are nuclear sclerotic and mixed cataracts. The risk of lens opacification has been linked to hyperglycaemia and higher levels of glycosylated haemoglobin at baseline[8,9]. The pathogenesis of cataract in diabetes is not fully understood, but it is thought to be due to osmotic and/or oxidative stress within the crystalline lens.

Osmotic stress pathway

The high level of glucose in the aqueous humour results in increased concentration of glucose within the lens. This leads to activation of the polyol pathway where glucose is reduced by the enzyme aldose reductase to sorbitol. The accumulation of sorbitol within the lens leads to secondary osmotic overhydration of the lens fibres and subsequent cataract development[10,11].

Oxidative stress pathway

Increased glucose levels in the aqueous humour can induce glycation of the lens proteins and therefore increase the level of free radicals and advanced glycation end-products. Since lenses of people with diabetes have an impaired antioxidant capacity, they are more susceptible to oxidative stress and cataract development[12–15].

Studies suggest that earlier cortical cataract formation is related to osmotic stress, whereas the oxidative stress pathway tends to cause later development of nuclear and mixed-type cataracts in patients with diabetes[10,11]. The classic cataract in a person with diabetes consists of snowflake-like cortical opacities. It is usually found in type 1 young diabetic patients and is thought to be due to osmotic over-hydration of the lens. With the recent advent of effective therapies for controlling hyperglycaemia, this type of cataract is rarely seen in clinical practice.

PREOPERATIVE CONSIDERATIONS

Indication for surgery

The main indication for cataract surgery in a patient with diabetes is visual rehabilitation; however, surgery may be primarily required in some patients for cataract that precludes adequate assessment or treatment of their diabetic retinopathy[16].

The advances in vitreoretinal surgical techniques have led surgeons to advocate more combined procedures[17-19]. Combined cataract and vitrectomy may be indicated in the course of diabetic retinopathy to simultaneously deal with lenticular opacity and associated vitreoretinal pathology such as vitreous haemorrhage or visually significant macular traction. In patients over the age of 55–60 years, there is a high likelihood of developing cataract after vitrectomy surgery. Some surgeons therefore routinely undertake lens extraction, even in the absence of significant cataract, at the time of vitrectomy surgery in this age group[20].

Senn et al.[21] compared the outcome of combined surgery in 26 eyes versus sequential surgery in 26 eyes. They postulated that, in selected patients, combined surgery is a safe and effective approach, and outcomes are comparable to sequential surgery. In general, the advantages of combined surgery are: only one operation is needed; earlier visual rehabilitation that is not masked by post-vitrectomy cataract formation is achieved; and a clear fundal view to allow further treatment of retinopathy at the time of the operation or later is also provided. On the other hand, the combined approach has certain disadvantages such as longer operative time, increased severity of anterior chamber inflammation and increased risk of intraocular lens (IOL) decentration, particularly in eyes where intraocular gas tamponade is used[18,21].

Control of diabetes and associated systemic co-morbidities

Patients with diabetes should have their blood sugar controlled before their surgery with the help of their primary care doctor or internist. Preoperative tight control of diabetes, reflected in a low HbA1c level, may help to reduce the risk of postoperative progression of retinopathy[22-24]. There are no published guidelines to recommend a certain cut-off limit for blood glucose level above which patients should be cancelled, but most surgeons are not comfortable operating on patients with a random blood sugar of ≥ 18–20 mmol/L (325–360 mg/dL).

Patients with diabetes often have associated co-morbidities such as hypertension, cardiac and renal diseases and some of them may be on anticoagulants. It is important to optimise the control of modifiable vascular risk factors, particularly hypertension, before the surgery. The risk of bleeding during cataract surgery is generally minimal so it is usually not essential to stop anticoagulants before the surgery. It is also worth noting that patients with diabetes, particularly those with poor control, may be susceptible to various types of systemic infections which, if untreated, may result in bacteraemia and an increased risk of postoperative endophthalmitis[25,26].

Anterior segment evaluation

As with other patients undergoing evaluation for cataract surgery, preoperative examination of the anterior segment should include level of vision, corneal status and evaluation of anterior chamber depth and cataract density. It is important to correlate the level of vision with the density of cataract in patients with diabetes, as in some patients decreased vision could also be related to an existing maculopathy. It is prudent to assess the pupillary mydriasis preoperatively. Autonomic dysfunction in patients with diabetes can lead to poor pupillary dilatation[27,28], which in turn may pose a challenge to the surgeon, rendering some aspects of surgery such as capsulorrhexis or cortical lens matter clean-up difficult and subsequently increase the risk of iris trauma or posterior capsular rupture. Finally, it is important to evaluate the iris for the presence of rubeosis iridis, as sometimes this may be subtle and could be overlooked. If present, iris neovascularisation indicates significant ischaemic retinopathy, which requires immediate aggressive treatment before surgery to decrease the risk of progression to neovascular glaucoma postoperatively[26,29].

Case History 14.1: Subtle neovascularisation of the iris (NVI) in a patient with diabetes

This 47-year-old man with type 2 diabetes was referred for cataract surgery. The pupil was mid-dilated due to mydriatic drops used at the time of his preoperative assessment. A subtle NVI was seen on the temporal border of the iris (Fig. 14.1, arrow heads). He had previously received PRP in this eye for PDR. The patient was listed for further laser photocoagulation and intravitreal bevacizumab treatment to further stabilise his retinopathy before cataract surgery. Careful examination of the pupil is of paramount importance, as such subtle NVI may be overlooked particularly when the pupil is dilated for fundus examination. The green filter may be helpful to highlight small NVI.

Posterior segment evaluation

Preoperative slit-lamp biomicroscopy examination of the macula and peripheral retina when planning cataract surgery in patients with diabetes is of paramount importance to evaluate the level and severity of any pre-existing maculopathy or retinopathy.

Because subtle macular pathology such as mild macular oedema or vitreomacular traction that could influence the visual prognosis after surgery may be overlooked during preoperative clinical examination, optical coherence tomography (OCT) is currently regarded as an indispensable tool for evaluation of macular thickness and anatomy in patients with diabetes before surgery. We recommend preoperative macular OCT scanning for all patients with diabetes; however, since this may not be feasible for all practices, it should be at least performed in eyes with pre-existing maculopathy as well as in those where the view of the macula is compromised by lens opacity or when the severity of cataract does not appear to fully explain the loss of visual acuity. It is of note that the image-averaging technology in most spectral domain OCTs can often yield quantifiable images through mild to moderate cataract. Superior resolution could also achieved with recent long-wavelength (~1050 nm) swept-source OCT that has enhanced penetration through lenses with cataract[30].

OPERATIVE CONSIDERATIONS IN CATARACT SURGERY FOR PATIENTS WITH DIABETES

Anaesthesia

Cataract surgery is usually performed under local (regional) anaesthesia without sedation. This allows the patient to take their usual medication and their regular meals, without the need to be fasting before surgery. Furthermore, as cataract surgery is usually performed under blunt-needle sub-Tenon anaesthesia or local anaesthetic drops in most centres, stopping anticoagulant therapy before surgery is often unnecessary.

Corneal epithelium and endothelium protection

The corneal epithelium is more fragile in patients with diabetes as a result of poor attachment of epithelial cells to their basement membrane, and it could be easily sloughed at the time of surgery due to minor accidental trauma such as forceful corneal irrigation[31-33]. While it is important to protect the corneal epithelium during surgery, this is of concern mainly in complex cataract cases that are expected to be lengthy.

Diabetes is also a risk factor for corneal endothelial dysfunction, which may affect both the number and function of endothelial cells[34]. This puts patients with diabetes at a higher risk of developing postoperative corneal oedema that may also take longer time to recover compared to other patients. It is therefore important to reduce endothelial trauma during surgery when operating on cataracts in patients with diabetes. This is of particular importance when operating on dense cataracts or eyes that

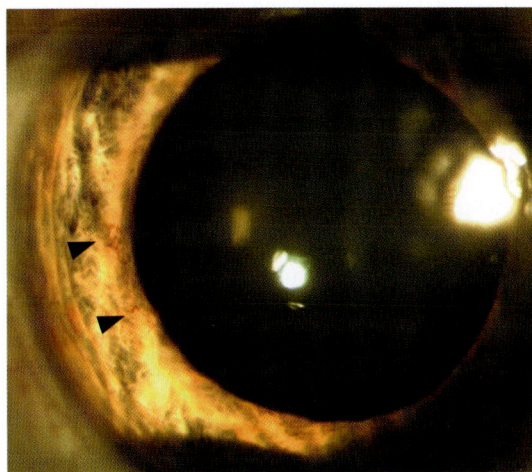

Fig. 14.1 Neovascularisation of the iris.

have co-existing corneal endothelial disease such as Fuch's endothelial dystrophy. In these cases, we use a dispersive ophthalmic viscosurgical device (OVD) to protect the corneal endothelium from the outset of the surgery.

Anterior capsulorrhexis

Anterior capsule contraction or capsulophimosis is more common in patients with diabetes as compared to patients without diabetes[35,36] and, when severe, could interfere with postoperative fundus visualisation. To decrease its occurrence, a large anterior capsulorrhexis is advised, provided that it still covers the edge of the IOL optic by 0.5–1.0 mm to maximize IOL centration and also lessen the risk of posterior capsular opacification, since IOL edge-capsule contact helps to prevent migration of lens epithelial cells.

> **Case History 14.2:** Anterior capsular contracture following cataract surgery in a patient with diabetes
>
> A 70-year-old female with type 2 DM underwent combined lens extraction and vitrectomy for vitreomacular traction and cataract. At the time of surgery, the surgeon elected to perform a small capsulorrhexis in order to decrease the risk of postoperative IOL decentration that occurs occasionally after combined surgery. This has resulted in significant anterior capsular contraction (Fig. 14.2). Anterior capsular contracture does not usually affect the patient's visual acuity or visual field unless very severe, but the main concern is that it may interfere with further visualization and treatment of the peripheral retina.

Pupil management

We routinely use adrenaline (0.5 mL of 1:1000 added to 500 mL of balanced salt solution) in the irrigating solution to assist and maintain pupillary dilatation in all our cataract surgery, including those for people with diabetes[37,38]. In general, eyes with a pupil diameter of 6 mm or more can be operated without any additional measures to dilate the pupil. In those with smaller pupil, we favour mechanical methods for enlarging the pupil using devices such as iris hooks (Fig. 14.3) or a 6.25 mm Malyugin ring (Fig. 14.4).

Phacodynamics

Maintaining the stability of the anterior chamber during surgery is an essential concept for successful

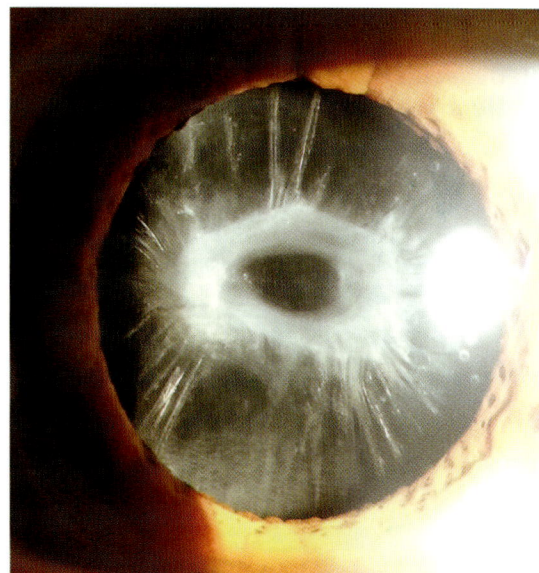

Fig. 14.2 Contraction of the anterior capsule.

phacoemulsification and is particularly important in eyes of patients with diabetes. Anterior chamber fluctuation is thought, at least theoretically, to result in disruption of the blood-aqueous barrier and consequently an increased risk of postoperative inflammation and cystoid macular oedema. Movement of the iris-lens diaphragm can also result in pupillary constriction as surgery progresses, and surgically induced miosis is more frequent in patients with diabetes[39,40].

Posterior capsule rupture

The reported rates of posterior capsular rupture are often higher in patients with diabetes compared to patients without diabetes[41]. While there is no evidence that diabetes is an independent risk factor for posterior capsular rupture, DM may indirectly influence the rate of posterior capsular rupture due to associated poor pupillary dilation or excessive iris-lens diagram movements in eyes that had previous pars plana vitrectomy[42,43]. Posterior capsular rupture in an eye of a person with diabetes can negatively influence the visual outcome after surgery because of exaggerated postoperative inflammation, progression of retinopathy and maculopathy as well as an increased risk of developing iris rubeosis[44].

Type of intraocular lens implant

It recommended to use IOLs with a larger optical diameter (6.0–7.0 mm) in eyes of patients with diabetes so that the

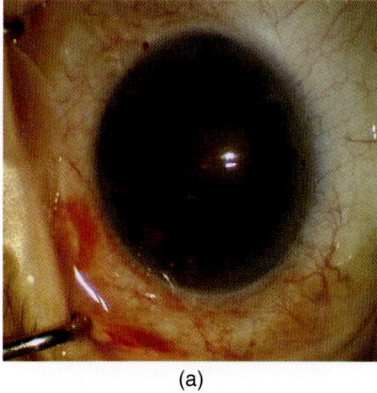 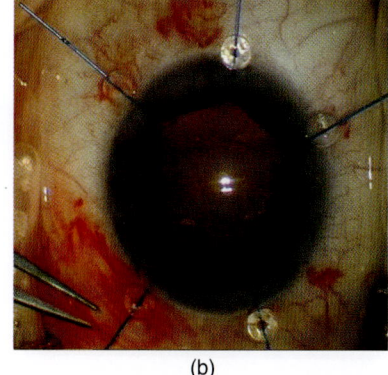

(a)   (b)

Fig. 14.3 Pupillary dilatation by flexible iris retractors (or hooks): (a) before dilation and (b) after dilation by iris hooks. The retractors are used to mechanically stretch and stabilise the pupil during surgery. Usually 4–5 hooks are used for pupillary dilation, according to surgeon preference.

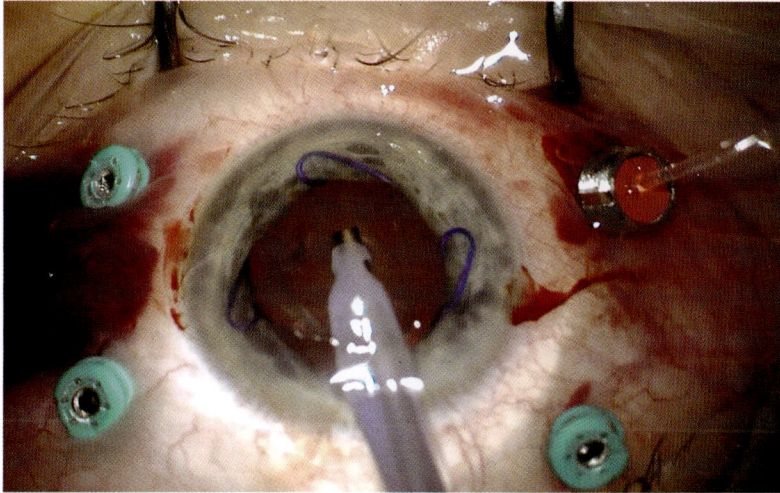

Fig. 14.4 Pupillary dilatation during surgery using a 6.25 mm Malyugin ring at the time of combined cataract and vitrectomy surgery. This ring has two sizes (6.25 and 7 mm) and is injected into the anterior chamber via a special device through the main cataract incision. We prefer the 6.25 mm size as we find it easier to insert, it provides good pupillary dilation and is less traumatic to the iris tissue.

edge of the lens optic is less likely to impede visualisation of the retinal peripheral during peripheral laser treatment or if par plana vitrectomy surgery is indicated later[45].

The standard 'in the bag' IOL implantation is the recommended site of implantation to maintain the barrier between the anterior and posterior segment. Hydrophobic acrylic IOLs are preferred over silicone lenses in patients with diabetes. The deposition of precipitates on the anterior surface of silicone lenses is much more common than with other lenses. Additionally, patients with diabetes may require vitrectomy in the future; if YAG capsulotomy laser was performed before vitrectomy surgery, silicone lenses may hinder visualisation during vitrectomy surgery when the eye is filled with air. Furthermore, if silicone oil is used as a tamponade during vitrectomy, silicone oil droplets could firmly adhere to the IOL causing reduced visualisation of the fundus postoperatively[46,47].

Anterior chamber and iris-supported implants are generally not recommended in patients with diabetes, and better avoided whenever possible as they are associated with greater risk of anterior segment inflammation.

Multifocal IOLs are also not recommended in patients with diabetes with pre-existing retinopathy since light dispersion along the visual axis can cause visual disability which may render future laser treatment or macular surgery difficult.

> **Case History 14.3: Silicone oil droplets on the back surface of silicone IOL**
>
> This 68-year-old man had previous cataract surgery with a foldable silicone IOL implanted on the bag. One year later, he developed a macula-off rhegmatogenous retinal detachment that was treated by vitrectomy and gas endotamponade. Unfortunately, he went on to develop recurrent detachment which required silicon oil tamponade. After silicon oil removal, there were multiple oil droplets adherent to the back of the IOL limiting his visual acuity to less than 6/60 with significant visual blurring (Fig. 14.5). Finally, his IOL was exchanged with an anterior-chamber IOL, after which his vision improved to 6/36 and his blurring of vision significantly improved.

Post-vitrectomy surgery cataract

Cataract is one of the most common complications after vitrectomy surgery in patients with diabetes. Approximately 50% of phakic eyes develop cataract within 3 years and 75% will subsequently have cataract surgery in the first 10 years after vitrectomy in patients with diabetes[48,49]. Loss of vitreous support following vitrectomy could result in exaggerated movements of the iris-lens diaphragm during cataract surgery. In addition, extreme deepening of the anterior chamber during phacoemulsification could sometimes occur due to intraoperative reverse pupillary block between the iris diaphragm and anterior lens capsule. This may lead to difficult or prolonged surgery with increased risk of intraoperative complications[50,51]. An established reverse pupillary block can be broken by separating the iris from the anterior capsule rim with the second instrument[52]. In our hands this manoeuvre is very effective; this often needs to be repeated during the course of surgery however as the pupillary bock will recur each time the surgeon initiates the infusion anteriorly.

In our view, cataract surgery in patients with diabetes is best undertaken by an experienced cataract surgeon who has the capacity to handle complex cases and can employ compensatory measures to manage intraoperative difficulties and challenges such as a small pupil or exaggerated iris movements. Even mild complications such as iris trauma, let alone posterior capsular rupture or vitreous loss, can negatively influence the visual prognosis of a diabetic eye[39,41].

POSTOPERATIVE CONSIDERATIONS

Patients with diabetes are known to have a higher risk of developing certain postoperative complications compared to those without diabetes. These include anterior segment inflammation[53], pigment dispersion with precipitates on the IOL surface[53], pseudophakic cystoid macular oedema and postoperative endophthalmitis[53-55]. Cataract extraction could also negatively influence the rate of progression of diabetic maculopathy[56].

Anterior segment inflammation

The degree of anterior chamber inflammation in the early postoperative period can be more pronounced in patients with diabetes and, in some cases, may be complicated by posterior synaechiae or fibrinous exudation[53,57]. Diabetes is associated with the breakdown of the blood-aqueous barrier that is further exacerbated by cataract surgery[58-60]. Takamura et al.[61] evaluated anterior segment inflammation and found significantly more aqueous flare intensity in the early postoperative period in patients with diabetes

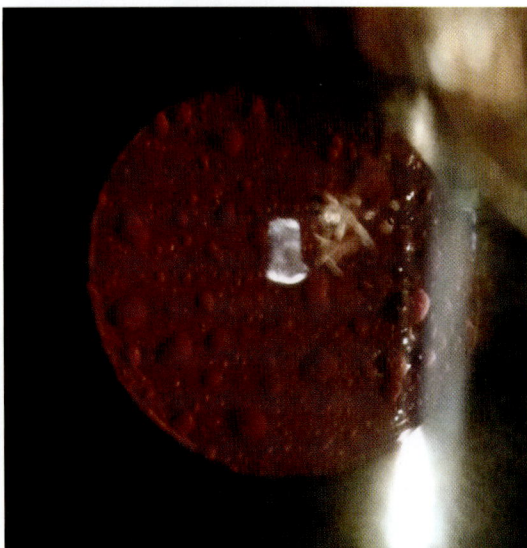

Fig. 14.5 Silicon oil droplets on the posterior surface of the posterior chamber intraocular lens.

than in those without diabetes. In another quantitative study using an aqueous flare meter, Oshika et al.[60] found higher flare levels in eyes with diabetic retinopathy than those without retinopathy, and their results also demonstrated that the intensity of aqueous flare rose proportionately with increasing severity of diabetic retinopathy.

Iris neovascularisation

In the past era of large incision intracapsular and extracapsular surgery, cataract extraction in eyes with severe NPDR or PDR was associated with a high likelihood of development of iris rubeosis and neovascular glaucoma postoperatively[62,63]. While these complications are still seen after modern phacoemulsification surgery their frequency has substantially decreased, particularly as clinicians are now more aggressive in treating proliferative retinopathy before surgery. As mentioned earlier, it is important to look for iris rubeosis when evaluating patients with diabetes before surgery, particularly in eyes with signs of retinal ischaemia (e.g. severe NPDR).

Progression of diabetic retinopathy

There is evidence to inform of a causal relationship between the progression of DR and large-incision cataract extraction surgery[64–66]. However, modern cataract surgery is associated with significantly less disturbance of the blood ocular barriers; whether contemporary phacoemulsification techniques accelerate DR progression remains unclear. Some studies compared the rate of progression of DR between eyes when monocular phacoemulsification was performed[67–69]. Romero-Aroca at al.[68] prospectively compared the progression of DR and DMO between 132 eyes after monocular cataract surgery versus their contralateral eyes as control. They found uneventful cataract surgery was not associated with DR or maculopathy progression. Similar results were also found by Squirrell et al.[69] and Krepler et al.[67] in two other independent but smaller studies. Conversely, Hong et al.[70] showed in a retrospective study that undergoing phacoemulsification doubles the rate of DR progression 12 months after surgery.

In the absence of uncontrolled active PDR, it is unlikely that uneventful phacoemulsification surgery poses significant risk to the progression of DR or negatively influence the natural course of the disease[67–69]. Modern phacoemulsification surgery is associated with significantly less disturbance of the blood ocular barriers as compared to large-incision cataract surgery. It is also possible that the reduced risk of DR progression after modern cataract surgery is related to the recent advances in medical treatment of DM with tighter control of hyperglycaemia, more optimum preoperative control of PDR with laser treatment and the widespread use of intravitreal anti-VEGF for treatment of diabetic maculopathy.

Macular oedema following cataract surgery

The presence of macular oedema following cataract surgery in a patient with diabetes can either be predominantly due to diabetes, that is, diabetic macular oedema, or in relation to cataract surgery, that is, pseudophakic macular oedema.

Table 14.1 lists the differentiating features between diabetic and pseudophakic macular oedema and outlines their main lines of treatment. Of all the features, the timing of onset of visual symptoms is usually the most indicative of the nature of the macular oedema, followed by their OCT features. Diabetic macular oedema (DMO) is usually present before the surgery although in some cases it might only be diagnosed after the operation, having been overlooked preoperatively because of the cataract. Pseudophakic macular oedema (PMO) usually occurs in the early postoperative period around 4–6 weeks, but not immediately post-surgery. Diabetes, even in the absence of retinopathy, is associated with an increased risk of pseudophakic macular oedema, which is typically cystoid in nature.

Differentiation between these two types of macular oedema is helpful since their management strategy is different; for example, while intravitreal anti-VEGF is currently the first line of DMO treatment, the present literature does not provide robust evidence to support the use of anti-VEGF treatment for PMO[71–73]. In some cases, macular oedema following cataract surgery in patients with diabetes can have overlapping features of both types, which makes the distinction difficult. In these situations, we usually commence treatment with a combination of topical steroids/NSAID and move on to intravitreal anti-VEGF treatment if the macular oedema fails to significantly improve in 6 weeks.

There is variation in the results of studies reporting on incidence of macular oedema after cataract surgery in patients with diabetes. Whereas some previous reports have shown no difference in progression of maculopathy after phacoemulsification surgery[67–69], data

Table 14.1 Types of post-cataract-surgery macular oedema in patients with diabetes.

	Diabetic macular oedema	Pseudophakic macular oedema
Onset	May be present preoperatively, or in the early postoperative period	Usually occurs 4–6 weeks after surgery but not immediately following surgery
Macular biomicroscopy	Lesions associated with diabetic macular oedema including microaneurysms, retinal haemorrhage and hard exudates are usually present in addition to the macular oedema	Mainly cystoid changes without prominent lesions associated with diabetic macular oedema
Fluorescein angiogram	Leakage takes different patterns; may be focal or diffuse, within any part of the macula; no disc leakage unless neovascularization exists	Perifoveal leakage with petalloid appearance and sometimes with disc leakage.
Optical coherence tomography	Cystoid changes can occur anywhere in the macular region; evidence of microstructural features of diabetic retinopathy changes such as microaneurysms, hyper-reflective foci and hard exudates	Cystoid changes, mainly in the foveal and parafoveal regions
Course	Unlikely to resolve spontaneously and need further treatment	May resolve spontaneously, especially if retinopathy is mild, but occasionally may take a chronic or recurrent course
Main lines of treatment	Intravitreal pharmacotherapy with anti-VEGF	Topical steroids and NSAIDS; periocular steroids; intravitreal steroids

from contemporary OCT-based studies demonstrate an increased risk of significant macular thickening post-cataract-surgery in patients with diabetes compared to those without[56,74]. Several factors could account for such differences in results between studies, including whether the diagnosis was confirmed by clinical examination alone or with OCT or fluorescein angiography, variation in study definition of postoperative macular oedema and whether a distinction was made between postoperative DMO progression and PMO.

In an OCT-based prospective study, Kim et al.[56] reported an incidence rate of 22% for DMO exacerbation (defined as ≥30% increase in OCT centre-point thickness from baseline) 1 month after cataract surgery. The degree of postoperative macular thickness appears to be influenced by the grade of preoperative diabetic retinopathy, with significant differences in macular thickness found between eyes with no DR or mild retinopathy compared to eyes with moderate or severe retinopathy. Furthermore, it was also shown that in eyes with no centre-involved DMO before the surgery, the risk of developing new-onset central macular thickening after surgery is higher in eyes that had treatment for DMO in the past or exhibited non-centre-involved DMO preoperatively[74].

Case History 14.4: Tomographic appearance of diabetic macular oedema

A 53-year-old male patient had type 2 DM of 23 years duration, controlled by insulin and tablets. Infra-red fundus image (Fig. 14.6, left side) shows non-proliferative diabetic retinopathy fundus changes (multiple dot-blot haemorrhage, microaneurysms and hard exudates). The OCT (Fig. 14.6, right side) shows multiple cystoid spaces in the foveal and parafoveal region with different reflectivity within the cystoid spaces. There are multiple large hyperreflective spots denoting hard exudates (red arrow). He was treated with a combination of macular laser to the oedema on the temporal side of the macula outside the foveal avascular zone and intravitreal ranibizumab. The ranibizumab was given as a loading dose of five injections at monthly intervals, which cleared the oedema, followed by treatment as required depending on the recurrence of oedema.

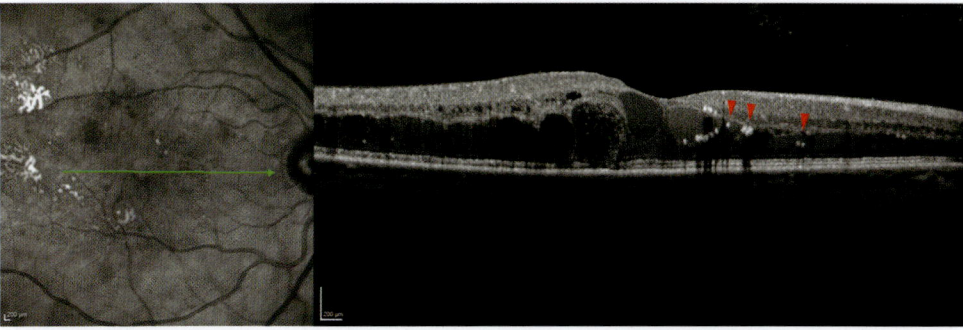

Fig. 14.6 Diabetic macular oedema.

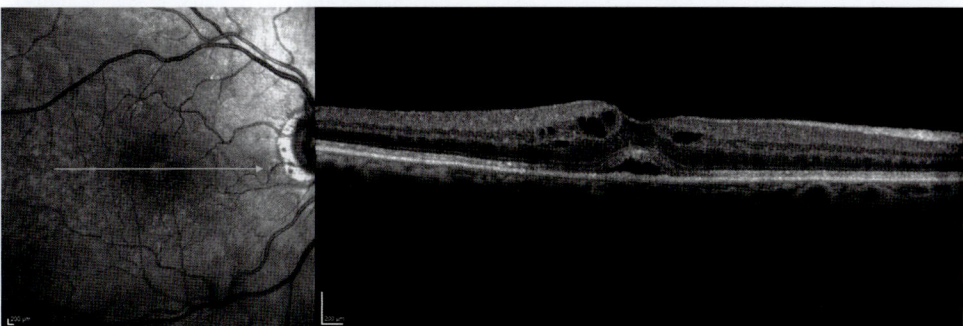

Fig. 14.7 Cystoid macular oedema following cataract surgery.

Case History 14.5: Tomographic appearance of pseudophakic macular oedema following cataract surgery

This 65-year-old type-2 patient with diabetes noticed marked improvement in vision immediately after cataract surgery. However, three weeks later he started to notice blurring of his vision and VA dropped to 6/12 (Fig. 14.7, left). Infrared fundus image appears unremarkable (Fig. 14.7, left). An OCT scan (Fig. 14.7, right) through the fovea shows multiple cystoid spaces mainly involving the foveal centre and small serous detachment. All cystoid spaces appear hyporeflective and clear. There are no features associated with diabetic macular oedema seen on the OCT scan. The patient received a course of topical NSAIDs and topical corticosteroid drops for a month. Macular oedema completely resolved after 1 month with improvement of vision to 6/6.

Endophthalmitis

Endophthalmitis is a devastating complication after cataract surgery. Reported rates of endophthalmitis following cataract has dramatically declined in the past two decades with estimated prevalence in recent major cohorts of 0.014–0.029[75,76]. Precise information regarding the relative risk of endophthalmitis following cataract surgery in a population with diabetes is still lacking, but several reports have shown that DM is one of the possible systemic risk factors for endophthalmitis[76–80]. Patients with diabetes are known to have altered systemic immunity and are susceptible to different types of infections including endogenous endophthalmitis and endophthalmitis following ocular surgery[77–79]. Phillips and Tasman[79] reviewed records of 162 consecutive patients of endophthalmitis after ocular surgery and found that 21% of these had diabetes mellitus. Moreover, the visual outcome after endophthalmitis in eyes of people with diabetes has been shown to be worse than in eyes of those without diabetes[81,82].

ADJUNCTIVE PRE- AND INTRAOPERATIVE PHARMACOTHERAPY

Several pharmacotherapeutic agents are currently used as adjuncts before or at the time of cataract surgery in patients with diabetes to prevent or minimise the risk of postoperative complications, particularly PMO or DMO progression.

Topical non-steroidal anti-inflammatory drugs (NSAIDs)

Topical non-steroidal anti-inflammatory drugs (NSAIDs) are nowadays used prophylactically in patients with diabetes undergoing cataract surgery to reduce the risk of surgically associated ocular inflammation and PMO[72,83,84]. NSAIDs achieve their effect on inflammation through suppression of cyclooxygenase enzyme that is responsible for the production of prostaglandin and thromboxane. Several NSAIDs are available for topical use including ketorolac, diclofenac, bromfenac and nepafenac. The latter is a prodrug that is activated inside the eye and was shown to have superior ocular penetration and bioavailability.

The role of topical NSAIDs as a prophylactic treatment against postoperative CMO in patients with diabetes was examined in several studies[84–87]. In a multicentre, randomised, double-masked, controlled study that included 236 patients with NPDR without macular thickening, patients received either topical nepafenac or placebo three times daily beginning 1 day prior to surgery through day 90, in addition to a 2 week course of topical corticosteroids postoperatively. In the nepafenac group, only 2.4% developed macular oedema (defined as a >30% increase in central subfield macular thickness from baseline) versus 8.7% in the placebo group ($P<0.029$) at 1 month and the difference was even wider at the 2 month and 3 month time points.

In another study by Endo et al.[86], 62 eyes with moderate NPDR or less and central retinal thickness of <250 μm were prospectively randomised to either bromfenac ($n=31$) or corticosteroid drops ($n=31$). For all patients, bromfenac drops were at least comparable to steroids and were even superior at 4 week ($P<0.0001$) and 6 week ($P<0.0001$) time point in patients who had features of NPDR before surgery. This study also assessed anterior chamber flare, and in patients with NPDR flare values were found to be significantly lower in the bromfenac group at 4 weeks ($P=0.0009$) and 6 weeks ($P=0.005$).

Nepafenac is currently our NSAID drug of choice for prophylaxis against macular oedema in patients with diabetes without diabetic macular oedema undergoing cataract surgery, and has been approved in the European Union for this indication since 2012. It is advised to instil one drop every 15 min for 1 hour before cataract surgery and to continue for at least 4 weeks after surgery[83].

Posterior sub-Tenon triamcinolone acetonide injection

Sub-Tenon triamcinolone injection (40 mg) at the end of cataract surgery was shown to have an equivalent therapeutic effect to a course of topical prednisolone in controlling postoperative inflammation with less effect on IOP[88].

Kim et al.[89] compared the effect of single sub-Tenon triamcinolone acetonide at the end of cataract surgery in eyes with no or mild/moderate NPDR with almost similar stage of retinopathy in both eyes undergoing sequential cataract surgery. At 1 month, the triamcinolone-treated eyes showed improved visual recovery and reduced incidence of macular oedema by OCT compared to fellow eyes (control), but there was no difference between both groups in macular thickness, vision or DR progression at 6 months.

In our practice, we use sub-Tenon triamcinolone (in addition to routine topical corticosteroid drops) at the end of the surgery in eyes with anticipated risk of pronounced postoperative inflammation due to intraoperative iris manipulation or prolonged surgery. Its short duration makes it unsuitable alone for preventing postoperative macular thickening[89].

Intravitreal anti-vascular endothelial growth factor

The efficacy of intravitreal anti-VEGF therapy in improving the vision has revolutionised the treatment of DMO as demonstrated in pivotal studies[90–94], with the role of macular laser being currently diminished. In eyes with co-existing DMO and cataract, the presence of lens opacity also renders treatment with macular laser difficult and makes the use of intravitreal pharmacotherapy at the time of surgery more feasible.

Over the past few years, several prospective, randomised studies have also advocated the use of anti-VEGF at the time of cataract surgery to minimise the risk of postoperative cystoid macular oedema and/or worsening of pre-existing diabetic maculopathy[35,95–98]. In aggregates, these studies demonstrated that anti-VEGF might be associated with a short-term benefit (6 months or less) in reducing postoperative macular thickness when used in combination with cataract surgery; however, the improved anatomical outcomes observed with the use of anti-VEGF did not always translate into better visual acuity outcomes (Table 14.2). In addition to its effect on macular thickness, anti-VEGF was also

Table 14.2 Summary of studies evaluating intravitreal anti-VEGF use for prevention or treatment of diabetic macular oedema at the time of cataract surgery.

Study ($P \leq 0.05$)	Diabetic retinopathy grading	Number of eyes (treatment/control)	Adjunct intravitreal drug (dose)	Follow-up (months)	Mean BCVA changes in ETDRS letters (treatment/control)	Mean CRT changes in microns (treatment/control)
Takamura et al. (2009)[35]	NPDR and DMO	(21/21)	Bevacizumab 1.25 mg	3	+26/+16 $P=0.034$	−25/+28 $P=0.0217$
Lanzagorta-Aresti et al. (2009)[98]	NPDR and DMO	(13/13)	Bevacizumab 1.25 mg	6	+5/−5 $P=0.008$	0/+77 $P=0.001$
Chae et al. (2014)[95]	NPDR without DMO	(37/39)	Ranibizumab 0.5 mg	6	+16/+10 $P=0.046$	+16/+46* $P=0.22$
Fard et al. (2011)[97]	NPDR without DMO	(31/30)	Bevacizumab 1.25 mg	6	+26 /+24 $P=0.1$	0/+23 $P=0.3$
Salehi et al. (2012)[96]	DR of any grade, with or without DMO	(27/30)	Bevacizumab 1.25 mg	6	+20/+24 $P=0.50$	+3/+41 $P=0.54$

DR: diabetic retinopathy; NPDR: non-proliferative diabetic retinopathy; DMO: diabetic macular oedema; BCVA: baseline best-corrected visual acuity; CRT: central retinal thickness; IVR: intravitreal ranibizumab; IVB: intravitreal bevacizumab.
*Central subfield thickness is the macular thickness metric used.

shown to reduce the short-term progression of diabetic retinopathy in patients undergoing cataract surgery. In a prospective study of 68 eyes with diabetic retinopathy and cataract randomised to standard phacoemulsification with intraocular lens implantation alone ($n=33$, control group) or to receive 1.25 mg intravitreal bevacizumab at the end of surgery ($n=35$, intervention group), progression of DR at 6 months occurred in 45.5% in the control group and 11.4% in the intervention group ($P=0.002$)[99].

Rarely, cataract surgery alone or combined with vitrectomy may be indicated in patients with active proliferative retinopathy and dense cataracts precluding preoperative laser treatment. In these cases, although not supported by data from controlled studies, preoperative use of anti-VEGF treatment has been shown to be efficacious in causing a rapid but short-term regression of the iris neovascularisation and stabilisation of the diabetic retinopathy[100,101]. Anti-VEGF treatment can also be repeated at the end of the surgery followed by prompt or deferred PRP laser treatment.

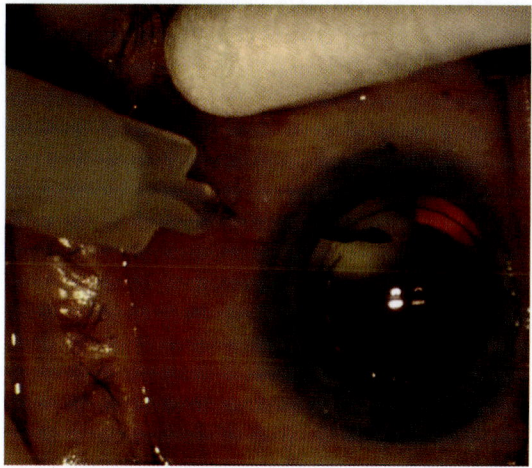

Fig. 14.8 Intravitreal triamcinolone acetonide injection in a patient with co-existing diabetic macular oedema and cataract. The injection (4 mg in 0.1 mL) is performed through the pars plana near the end of the cataract surgery before removing the ophthalmic viscosurgical device from the eye.

Intravitreal injection of triamcinolone acetonide

Intravitreal corticosteroids are another modality to treat DMO when associated with significant cataract. Intravitreal triamcinolone (Fig. 14.8) was one of the first steroid preparations to be used for intravitreal injection and, while more frequently used in the past for treatment of DMO, the advent of VEGF-blocking therapy and recent corticosteroids implants has dramatically reduced its use.

Intravitreal triamcinolone acetonide (4 mg/0.1 mL) was studied in several reports alone, combined with laser or at the time of cataract surgery for treatment of DMO[102–104]. In a prospective randomised controlled study by Ahmadabadi et al.[102] 41 eyes with DMO were randomly assigned to a treatment group that received an intravitreal triamcinolone at the end of phacoemulsification, or a control group which had only routine phacoemulsification surgery. Although there was no statistically significant difference between the two groups in the mean corrected distance visual acuity at any follow-up examination ($P>0.05$), the mean change in central retinal thickness measurement was significantly lower in the treatment group than in the control group at all follow-up visits ($P<0.05$) with less risk of developing CMO. As expected with the use of intravitreal triamcinolone, IOP rise was encountered in a significant number of eyes (15%) in the treatment group.

Intravitreal dexamethasone implant

Dexamethasone intravitreal implant (Ozurdex, Allergan, Inc., Irvine, CA) is a biodegradable 0.7 mg dexamethasone implant that gradually dissolves into the vitreous cavity. The implant was evaluated in several reports to treat DMO either alone or with other modalities (Fig. 14.9)[32,105–108]. The implant is injected through a 22-gauge injector and achieves a measurable effect for about 3–4 months. The main concerns with the dexamethasone implant use in pseudophakic eyes is IOP elevation, although this is less frequent compared to either intravitreal triamcinolone acetonide or fluocinolone acetonide implant[109,110].

In a small prospective study, 9 eyes received dexamethasone implant at the time of surgery and a similar number of eyes were only treated with cataract surgery. A significant difference in visual acuity levels and CRT was observed between the 2 groups at 6, 12 and 24 month time points with a visual acuity gain of 18 letters achieved by week 12 in the treatment group (0.22 letters in the control group)[110]. IOP rise was not observed in the dexamethasone implant treated eyes; however, the small number of patients in this study and its short duration render it unsuitable for judging safety of a dexamethasone implant during cataract surgery. Corticosteroid-induced IOP rise has been reported in nearly one-third of patients when a dexamethasone implant was used for diabetic macular

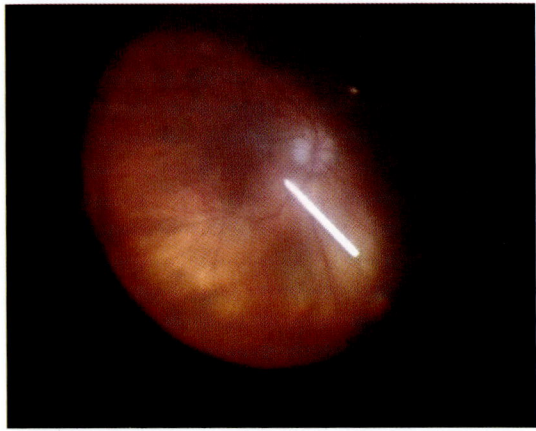

Fig. 14.9 Operative photograph of intravitreal cavity dexamethasone implant administered after combined cataract surgery and pars plana vitrectomy surgery. Note the posterior location of implant, which is usually the case in vitrectomised eyes.

oedema in a recent trial with a large dataset and long follow-up[111].

Intravitreal fluocinolone acetonide implant

Fluocinolone acetonide implant (Iluvien) is a 190 μg fluocinolone acetonide sustained-release drug-delivery system. Due to a very high risk of cataract, this implant is used for chronic DMO in pseudophakic eyes that are refractory to other therapeutic modalities[112]. The implant is inserted via a 25-gauge device and can be combined with cataract surgery. For further details on the outcomes and safety of fluocinolone acetonide implant in DMO, please refer to Chapter 6.

ADJUNCTIVE PANRETINAL PHOTOCOAGULATION LASER

Eyes with proliferative diabetic retinopathy need prompt laser treatment before the time of cataract surgery. Operating in eyes with active proliferative retinopathy increases the risk of developing severe postoperative inflammation, progression of retinopathy and development of rubeosis iridis[62,63]. In some cases with dense cataract, it may not be possible to perform/complete

PRP treatment before surgery. In this context, laser could be applied directly after removing the cataract while the patient is still on the operating table using the laser indirect ophthalmoscope or in the early postoperative period. Suto et al.[113] compared the outcomes of patients with diabetic retinopathy and cataract who had PRP first and cataract surgery second (1–3 months after surgery) in 1 eye (n=29 eyes) and cataract surgery followed by PRP (3 months after surgery) in the fellow eye (n=29 eyes). They found that the order in which PRP and cataract surgery were performed had no effect on postoperative retinopathy. However, this study only included eyes with severe NPDR or early PDR.

Recent multicolour laser photocoagulators have the facility to use different wavelengths. The longer wavelengths in the yellow (577 nm) and red (647 nm) spectrum are more effective in delivering laser treatment through mild to moderate cataracts as compared to traditionally used green (532 nm) laser[114].

VISUAL OUTCOME AFTER CATARACT SURGERY IN PATIENTS WITH DIABETES

There has been a change towards performing cataract surgery at an earlier stage in patients with diabetes[67,115,116] compared to the 1980–1990 era, where ophthalmologists recommended delaying surgery because of the expected poor visual outcome in patients with diabetes[63,65,117].

In 1995, Dowler et al.[118] carried out a meta-analysis of 10 studies published between 1983 and 1993 on the visual outcome of cataract surgery in patients with diabetes. They found the mean proportions of eyes achieving a postoperative visual acuity ≥ 6/12 to be: 80% non-proliferative retinopathy with no maculopathy eyes; 57% in quiescent proliferative retinopathy with no maculopathy; 41% in non-proliferative retinopathy with maculopathy; 11% in stable proliferative retinopathy with maculopathy; and none in the eyes with active proliferative retinopathy. In contrast, using data from 1999 to 2008 a Danish registry study on the outcome of cataract surgery in 285 diabetic patients with different levels of retinopathy demonstrated overall improvement in vision postoperatively, regardless of the level of retinopathy[116]. Furthermore, in 2011 Eriksson et al.[115] found that the final visual outcome in eyes with mild to moderate retinopathy without previous DMO is as good as in normal eyes.

The current trend in improvement of cataract surgery results over the past 30 years is likely to be related to the adoption of less traumatic small-incision cataract surgery techniques as well as the witnessed changes in diabetes management over the past years including tighter control of hyperglycaemia, better treatment of retinopathy and recent advances in the pharmacotherapy for DMO.

Visual outcome following cataract surgery in patients with diabetes may vary between patients; while some patients improve to near-normal levels, others may have poor vision postoperatively. In general, worse outcomes are expected in old age or those with poor glycaemic control and longstanding DM. Additionally, eyes with a higher level of retinopathy, diabetic macular oedema, significant macular ischaemia and those that suffered intraoperative complications are also more likely to have worse visual outcome[116,118,119].

CONCLUSIONS

The advances in treatment of diabetic retinopathy, widespread implementation of retinopathy screening programs, modern surgical and laser techniques and recent intravitreal pharmacotherapies have markedly improved the outcome of cataract surgery in patients with diabetes. Careful pre-, intra- and postoperative planning of surgery and optimisation of retinopathy and maculopathy control can impart significant protective effect in preventing unfavourable outcomes after diabetic cataract surgery.

PRACTICE POINTS

To maintain a good postoperative view of the macula and peripheral retina, we recommend wide anterior capsulorrhexis, an acrylic large-diameter IOL implanted in the capsular bag as well as meticulous clearance of lens cortex during cataract surgery.

Since uveitis and posterior synechiae are more common in eyes with diabetes, we tend to increase the frequency of topical steroids in these eyes and we may also use short-term mydriatic drops as well as sub-Tenon triamcinolone acetonide if there was iris manipulation at the time of surgery.

Postoperative macular thickening after cataract surgery in patients with diabetes could be due to progression of DMO or PMO or both.

For patients with cataract and no DMO, we use topical NSAID drops for prophylaxis against postoperative macular thickening. For eyes where DMO co-exists with cataract, we prefer to start treatment and stabilise the maculopathy before undertaking cataract surgery, but treatment may be commenced at the time of cataract surgery in eyes with dense cataract precluding macular assessment. As for most eyes with DMO, intravitreal anti-VEGF is our main line of treatment and intravitreal corticosteroids implants are considered as a second line of treatment in patients who have demonstrated previous resistance to anti-VEGF therapy.

We treat patients with PDR before cataract surgery. For those with advanced cataract precluding PRP treatment, we usually perform laser at the end of the cataract surgery while the patient is still on the operating table, using the laser indirect ophthalmoscope. In eyes with florid retinopathy, we may also use intravitreal anti-VEGF at the time of surgery to 'buy time' until the effect of laser starts in order to lessen the risk of postoperative iris rubeosis.

When cataract surgery is combined with additional procedures such as intravitreal injection or laser indirect ophthalmoscopy, we prefer to undertake these procedures near the end of cataract surgery after placing the IOL implant, but before removing the OVD from the anterior chamber to prevent collapse of the globe at the time of the injection or when applying pressure on the sclera with laser.

REFERENCE

Please visit www.wiley.com/go/scanlon/diabetic_retinopathy

15 Pregnancy and the diabetic eye

Peter H. Scanlon

Harris Manchester College, University of Oxford; Medical Ophthalmology, University of Gloucestershire, UK

RISK FACTORS FOR PROGRESSION OF DIABETIC RETINOPATHY DURING PREGNANCY

Progression of diabetic retinopathy may occur during pregnancy. The worsening of retinopathy during pregnancy can be quite significant and may require photocoagulation during pregnancy, more frequently in those patients with pre-existing diabetic retinopathy. The known risk factors for progression of diabetic retinopathy in pregnancy are summarised in the following sections.

Pregnancy independently associated with DR progression

Two studies found pregnancy to be independently associated with progression of diabetic retinopathy. A prospective study was undertaken within the Wisconsin Epidemiological Study of Diabetic Retinopathy in 1990[1] to determine the effect of pregnancy on diabetic retinopathy. Insulin-taking diabetic women were enrolled; one group comprised 171 pregnant women and the other group comprised 298 women who were not pregnant. Women were evaluated on referral and again during the postpartum period. A total of 133 pregnant women and 241 non-pregnant women attended and had gradable photographs at both visits. The severity of diabetic retinopathy was based on grading of fundus photographs of seven standard photographic fields. The glycosylated haemoglobin, duration of diabetes, current age, diastolic blood pressure, number of past pregnancies and current pregnancy status were evaluated as risk factors for progression of diabetic retinopathy. After adjusting for glycosylated haemoglobin, current pregnancy was significantly associated with progression ($P<0.005$, adjusted odds ratio 2.3).

In the Diabetes Control and Complications Trial[2] (DCCT) in 2000, a multicentre controlled clinical trial that compared intensive treatment with conventional diabetes therapy, 180 women who had 270 pregnancies and 500 women who did not become pregnant during an average of 6.5 years of follow-up were studied. Women assigned to the conventional treatment group were changed to intensive therapy if they were planning pregnancy or as soon as possible after conception. Fundus photography was performed every 6 months. Compared with non-pregnant women, pregnant women had a 1.63-fold greater risk of any worsening of retinopathy from before to during pregnancy ($P<0.05$) in the intensive treatment group; the risk was 2.48-fold greater for pregnant v. not pregnant women in the conventional group ($P<0.001$). Although individual patients had transient worsening of retinopathy during pregnancy, which persisted for as long as 12 months post-pregnancy, at the end of the DCCT mean levels of retinopathy in subjects who had become pregnant were similar to those in subjects who had not become pregnant within each treatment group. It was therefore concluded that because pregnancy in type 1 diabetes induces a transient increase in the risk of retinopathy, increased ophthalmologic surveillance is needed during pregnancy and the first year postpartum. The long-term risk of progression of early retinopathy does not however appear to be increased by pregnancy in this study.

A further study described the progression of diabetic retinopathy in pregnancy in type 2 diabetes. Rasmussen et al.[3] studied 80 of 110 (73%) consecutively referred pregnant women with type 2 diabetes. Progression of diabetic retinopathy was observed in 11 (14%) women. Progression was mainly mild, but one woman with poor glycaemic control and uncontrolled hypertension progressed from mild retinopathy to sight-threatening retinopathy with proliferations, clinically significant macular oedema and impaired vision in both eyes. Progression of diabetic retinopathy was associated with a longer duration of diabetes ($P=0.03$) and insulin treatment before pregnancy ($P=0.004$).

A Practical Manual of Diabetic Retinopathy Management, Second Edition.
Edited by Peter Scanlon, Ahmed Sallam, and Peter van Wijngaarden.
© 2017 John Wiley & Sons Ltd. Published 2017 by John Wiley & Sons Ltd.
Companion Website: www.wiley.com/go/scanlon/diabetic_retinopathy

Baseline severity of retinopathy

Baseline severity of retinopathy is a risk factor for progression of retinopathy during pregnancy. In the Diabetes in Early Pregnancy Study[4], 155 diabetic women were followed from the periconceptional period to 1 month postpartum. In the 140 patients who did not have proliferative retinopathy at baseline, progression of retinopathy was seen in 10.3% of patients with no retinopathy, 21.1% with microaneurysms only, 18.8% with mild non-proliferative retinopathy and 54.8% with moderate-to-severe non-proliferative retinopathy at baseline. Proliferative retinopathy developed in 6.3% with mild and 29% with moderate-to-severe baseline retinopathy.

These findings are supported by three further studies. Phelps et al.[5] monitored 35 women with insulin-dependent diabetes mellitus for changes in diabetic retinopathy in 38 pregnancies. Three of 13 patients with no retinopathy at baseline developed retinopathy during pregnancy. Thirteen of 20 with background retinopathy at baseline showed progression of retinopathy during pregnancy. Two of 20 developed proliferative retinopathy. All five patients with proliferative retinopathy at baseline deteriorated during pregnancy.

Rosenn et al.[6] followed 154 women with type 1 diabetes through pregnancy and found progression of diabetic retinopathy in 18/78 (23%) with no retinopathy, 28/68 (41%) with background retinopathy and 5/8 (63%) with proliferative retinopathy at baseline.

Arun and Taylor[7] studied 59 women with type 1 diabetes who had retinal photographs before pregnancy and yearly for 5 years post-pregnancy. At baseline, 43 (72.9%) women were free of retinopathy, 15 had non-proliferative retinopathy and one woman had previously had laser therapy. During pregnancy four women required laser therapy. Over the next 5 years none required laser therapy, although retinopathy worsened in 14 women. Ten-year follow-up data were available on 22 women, one of whom required laser therapy 8 years after pregnancy. Baseline retinopathy status was the only independent risk factor which predicted progression of retinopathy. The article concluded that, although worsening of retinopathy occurs in some women with diabetes in pregnancy, pregnancy is not associated with postpartum worsening of retinopathy.

Poor metabolic control at conception

Poor metabolic control at conception is a risk factor for progression of diabetic retinopathy in pregnancy. In the Diabetes in Early Pregnancy Study[4], the risk for progression of diabetic retinopathy was increased by initial glycosylated haemoglobin elevations as low as 6 SD above the control mean. This increased risk may be due to suboptimal control itself or to the rapid improvement in metabolic control that occurred in early pregnancy.

Rapid improvement of glycaemic control

Rapid improvement of glycaemic control may be a contributing factor in worsening of retinopathy as shown in four studies[2,4–6]. The effect of rapid improvement in glycaemic control is impossible to separate from the effect of elevated glycosylated haemoglobin levels at conception and the associated increased proportion of retinopathy (both mild and severe) that occurs in this group of patients. The progression of retinopathy following commencement of intensive treatment has also been observed in non-pregnant adults with diabetes[8]. The established benefits of excellent diabetic control during pregnancy clearly outweigh the relatively minor effects noted in the fundi of the majority of patients who do not have significant pre-existing retinopathy.

Poor metabolic control during pregnancy and early postpartum

Poor metabolic control during pregnancy or the early postpartum period is a risk factor for progression as shown in four studies[1,2,6,9]. Tight glycaemic control is recommended to avoid progression of retinopathy. Attention should be given to the period after delivery, when the tight regulation may be more difficult to achieve.

Duration of diabetes

Duration of diabetes is a risk factor for progression of retinopathy during pregnancy as shown in three studies[6,10,11]. The effect of duration of diabetes on progression of retinopathy during pregnancy is difficult to separate from the effect of the severity of retinopathy at conception, as the two are correlated. For example, the Diabetes in Early Pregnancy Study[4] found that the baseline retinopathy level was a significant risk factor for progression ($P= 0.025$) but duration of diabetes was not ($P=0.10$).

Chronic hypertension and pregnancy-induced hypertension

Chronic hypertension and pregnancy-induced hypertension are risk factors for progression of retinopathy during pregnancy. Rosenn et al.[6] followed 154 women with type 1 diabetes through pregnancy and found progression of diabetic retinopathy in 29/11 (25%) with no hypertensive disorder, 11/22 (50%) with pregnancy-induced hypertension and 11/18 (61%) with chronic hypertension with or without superimposed pregnancy-induced hypertension.

Vestgaard et al.[12] conducted a prospective study of 102 (87%) out of 117 consecutive pregnant women with type 1 diabetes for median 16 years (range 1–36) and HbA1c 6.7% (4.9–10.8) in early pregnancy. Diabetic retinopathy was present at inclusion in at least one eye in 64 (63%) women and proliferative retinopathy and macular oedema were present in 9 and 16 women, respectively. Progression of retinopathy occurred in 28 (27%) women. Sight-threatening progression occurred in six women; in three, visual acuity deteriorated and four required laser treatment. Sight-threatening progression was associated with the presence of high blood pressure ($P=0.016$) in early pregnancy.

Pre-eclampsia or pregnancy-induced hypertension as a possible risk factor for progression of diabetic retinopathy later in life. A study by Gordin et al.[13] re-examined 203 women with type 1 diabetes who were followed during pregnancy within the Finnish Diabetic Nephropathy Study. A total of 158 women were included from 203 pregnant women with diabetes, after excluding 45 women with pre-pregnancy hypertension and those who had had laser treatment or whose retinopathy was graded as proliferative before or during pregnancy. As a surrogate marker for SDR, retinal laser photocoagulation was used. Women with pre-eclampsia (26% v. 6%; $P=0.003$) or pregnancy-induced hypertension (24% v. 6%; $P=0.008$) more often had incident SDR during follow-up compared to those with normotensive pregnancy. The article concluded that women with type 1 diabetes and a hypertensive pregnancy have an increased risk of severe diabetic retinopathy later in life.

BEFORE AND DURING PREGNANCY

Laser treatment

Dibble et al.[10] studied 55 insulin-dependent diabetic patients throughout pregnancy with serial retinal examinations by ophthalmoscopy and photographs. During gestation 3 of 19 patients (16%) with minimal or background retinopathy and 6 of 7 patients (86%) with untreated proliferative retinopathy experienced deterioration of their eye disease. In 4 patients with proliferative retinopathy, progression of retinal disease was arrested with photocoagulation during pregnancy. Only 1 of 6 who had received laser treatment prior to pregnancy experienced progression of her retinopathy.

Recommendations for retinal assessment

The following are recommendations by the National Institute for Clinical Excellence in the UK (NICE guidelines in pregnancy[14]).

1. Annual screening for diabetic retinopathy is recommended in the preconception period.
2. It is recommended that screening in the preconception period should include annual mydriatic digital photography to provide a hard copy for comparison purposes. In the UK, two 45-degree fields are taken (one macular-centred and one disc-centred).
3. Women with type 1 and type 2 diabetes should be offered mydriatic retinal assessment at the first antenatal clinic visit and again at 28 weeks gestation. Digital photography is recommended at these visits to provide a hard copy for comparison purposes.
4. If any diabetic retinopathy is present at booking, an additional screen should be performed at 16–20 weeks.
5. If diabetic retinopathy is found to be present in early pregnancy, careful ophthalmological supervision is required depending on the level of retinopathy both during pregnancy and for at least 6 months postpartum.

A recent study by Hampshire et al.[15] of 180 pregnant women with diabetes confirmed that the above guidelines provide a safe pathway with 93 patients (50%) remaining free of diabetic retinopathy throughout pregnancy. Eighteen (10%) presented with sight-threatening retinopathy at their first antenatal screen and were referred to the hospital eye service. Fifty patients (27%) were shown to have relatively stable retinopathy throughout pregnancy, with only two patients (1%) deteriorating and requiring referral to hospital eye service. Twenty-three (12%) failed to complete the screening protocol after their first screen.

Case History 15.1: Proliferative diabetic retinopathy in pregnancy

A young woman of 16 years was screened and referred to the Hospital Eye Service due to the presence of exudates in both macular areas (Fig. 15.1a and b).

Despite the exudates in the macular areas there was only minimal oedema and so no treatment was given. The following year increasing oedema was forming in the right macular area (Fig. 15.1c and d) and so focal laser therapy

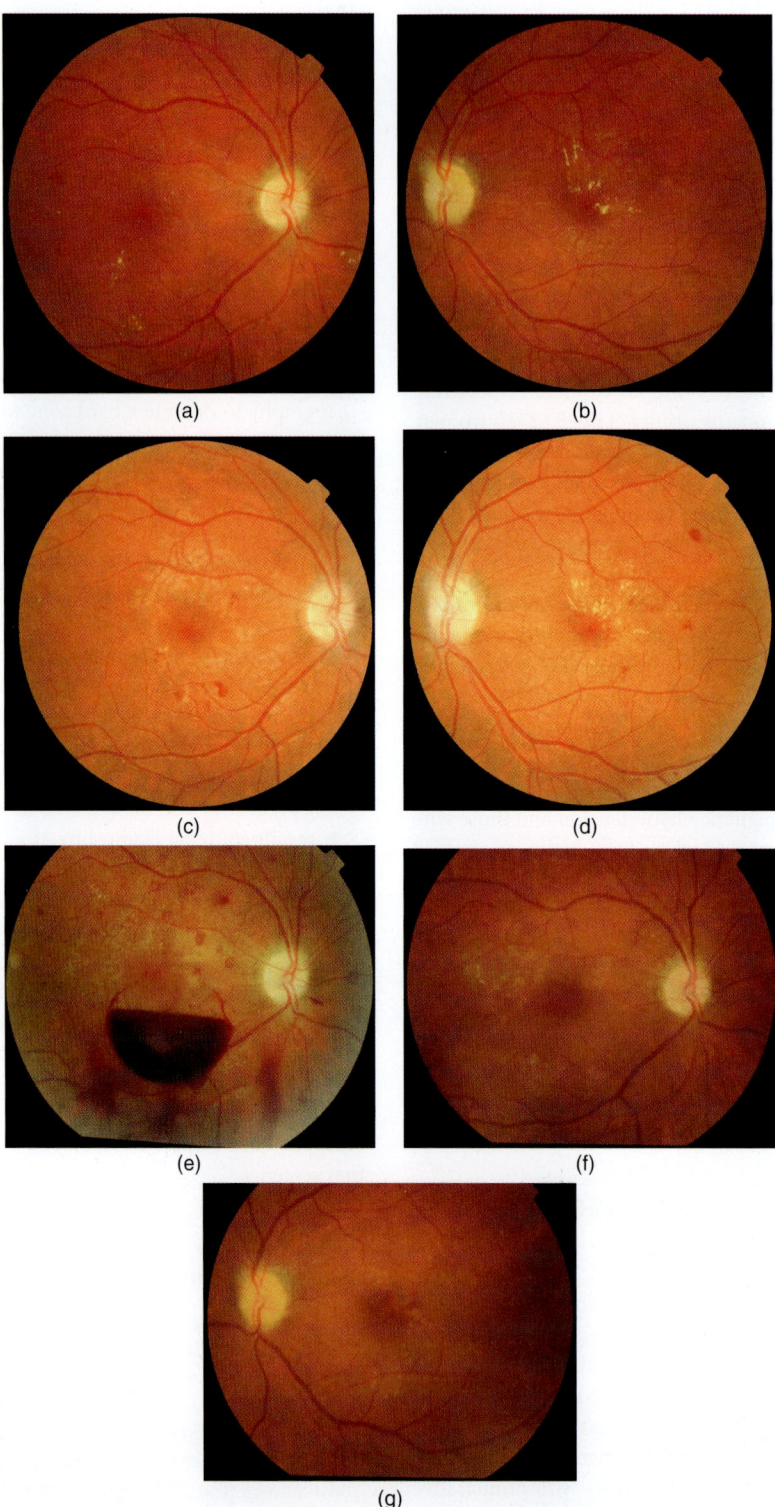

Fig. 15.1 Colour (a) right and (b) left macula at presentation. Colour (c) right and (d) left macula 1 year after presentation. (e) Colour right macula 2 years after presentation at about 34 weeks gestation. Colour (f) right and (g) left macula 8 years after presentation.

was undertaken: 23 burns, 100 micron size, 150 mW, 0.05 s, Pascal focal laser with the Area Centralis lens.

Eighteen months after the initial presentation, she commenced her first pregnancy and there was a progression of retinopathy during pregnancy with new vessels forming at the right disc at a gestation of about 24 weeks. Laser treatment of 1507 burns of 200 micron spot size, 225–275 mW, 0.03 s, Superquad lens, Pascal scatter laser was given over two sessions. At about 34 weeks gestation, a preretinal haemorrhage formed in the right macular area (Fig. 15.1e).

A further 1590 burns, 200 micron spot size, 225–275 mW, 0.03 s, Superquad lens, Pascal scatter laser was given over two sessions. The left eye showed signs of severe non-proliferative DR with maculopathy and required macular laser treatment of 10 burns, 100 micron size, 125 mW, 0.05 s, Pascal focal laser with the Area Centralis lens was given.

A health boy was born at 38 weeks gestation. In the postpartum period, a non-clearing vitreous haemorrhage formed at approximately 4 months postpartum and a right pars plana vitrectomy with panretinal endolaser, retinopexy, cryotherapy and internal tamponade with C2F6 gas was undertaken.

Two months later there were signs of proliferative diabetic retinopathy (NVE) and some further macular oedema developing in the left eye which required panretinal and macular laser treatment of 1750 burns, 250–275 mW, 0.03 s, 200 micron size Superquad lens, Pascal scatter laser over two sessions. Treatment of 17 burns 100 micron size, 100 mW, 0.05 s, Pascal focal laser with the Area Centralis lens was given at the first of these sessions.

Over the next 5 years the eyes have remained stable (Fig. 15.1f and g) with a vision of right 0.02, left 0.16 LogMAR and she managed to maintain good control of her diabetes with HbA1c levels of 33, 45, 42, 48, 48, 47, 48, 61 and 58 mmol/mol.

Case History 15.2: Proliferative diabetic retinopathy in pregnancy

A woman of 33 years was routinely referred to hospital by the diabetic eye screening service who photographed her eyes at 17/40 weeks of pregnancy. She was found to have proliferative diabetic retinopathy in both eyes. A red-free photograph of each macular area is shown in Figure 15.2a and b. Panretinal photocoagulation was commenced to each eye: 1409 burns of 200 micron spot size, 250–300 mW, 0.02 s, Superquad lens, Pascal scatter laser over two sessions.

A health boy was born at 38 weeks gestation. A further 2229 burns of scatter laser treatment was given over the next 6 months in the postpartum period. Due to personal circumstances she did not attend further follow-up appointments, but attended screening 20 months after the birth of her son (3 years and 6 months) after her initial presentation (Fig. 15.2c–f). She was given further panretinal photocoagulation to both eyes. Her right eye received a further 5037 burns over 3 sessions over 3 months (Fig. 15.2g) and her left received a further 5586 over 4 sessions over 4 months (Fig. 15.2h). The right eye then developed a non-clearing vitreous haemorrhage. At 4 years and 4 months after the original presentation, a right pars plana vitrectomy, endolaser, fibrovascular membrane delamination, internal limiting membrane peel and internal tamponade with SF6 gas was undertaken. Two weeks postoperatively she is seeing 0.3 LogMAR (6/12) in her right eye and has been listed for a similar procedure to her left eye.

Over this period of time her diabetes has been poorly controlled until the last 12 months with Hba1c levels of 104, 107, 102, 103, 103, 102, 99, 113, 110, 110, 111, 100, 49, 90, 59 and 69 mmol/mol.

Case History 15.3: Diabetic retinopathy in pregnancy

A 29-year-old woman with type 1 diabetes for 21 years was seen in the eye clinic with mild non-proliferative diabetic retinopathy (Fig. 15.3a–d). Her BP was 138/74 and HbA1c 8.8.

The following year she was seen in the eye clinic at 11/40 weeks pregnant. The fundi did not appear to have changed and no photographs were taken. At 25/40 pregnant the photographs in Figure 15.3e–h were taken. Figure 15.3i and j show the photographs at 29/40 pregnant, while Figure 15.3k–n were taken at the 34/40 pregnant stage.

The retinal appearance gradually settled during the postpartum period. At 1 year postpartum, no treatment having been given, the photographs in Figure 15.3o–r were taken. Her visual acuity remained good at 6/6 (20/20), right and left, throughout this time.

POSTPARTUM REGRESSION

Postpartum regression of diabetic retinopathy does occur in a proportion of patients. In the study by Rosenn et al.[6] of 154 women with type 1 diabetes followed through pregnancy, 51 women had progression of retinopathy

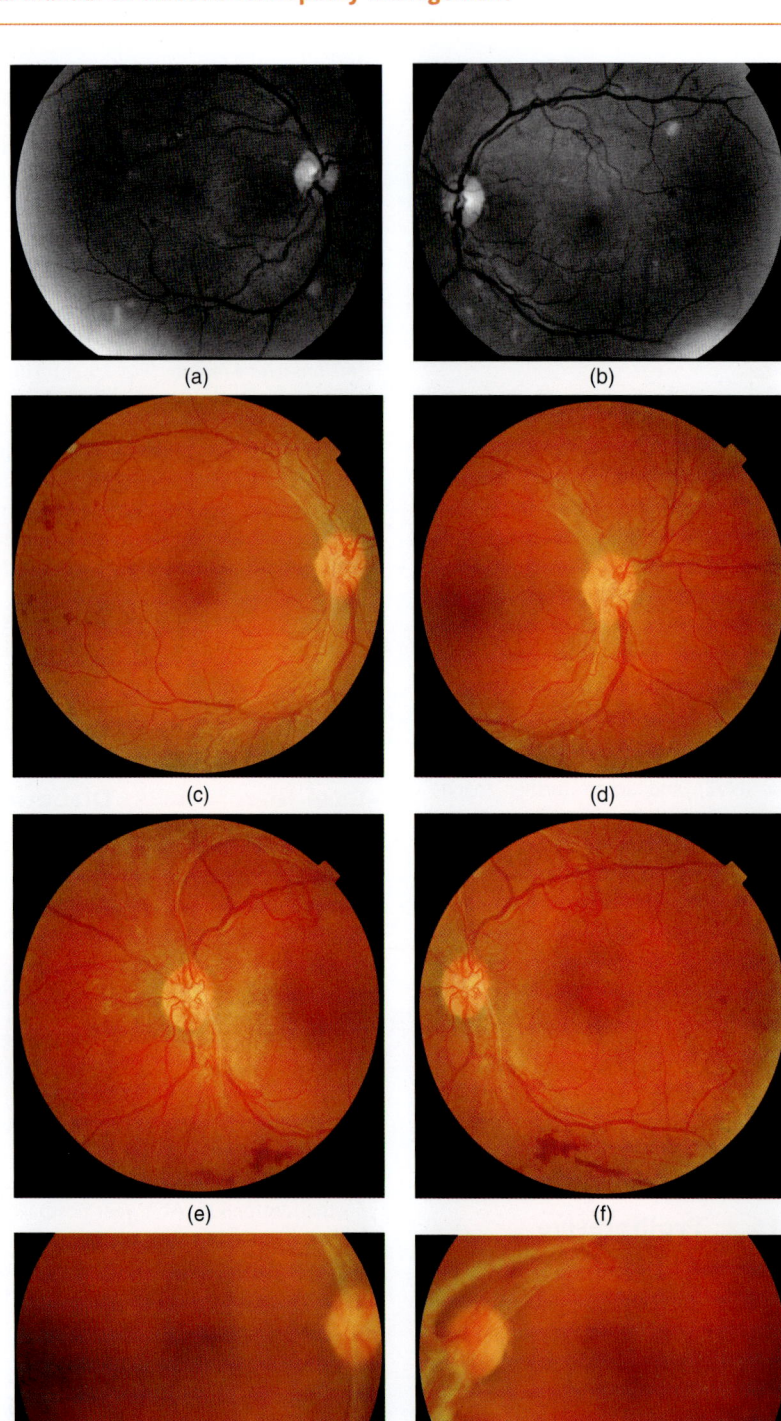

Fig. 15.2 Red-free (a) right and (b) left macula at presentation. Colour (c) right macula, (d) right disc, (e) left disc and (f) left macula 3 years and 6 months after initial presentation. Colour (g) right and (h) left macula 3 years and 10 months after initial presentation.

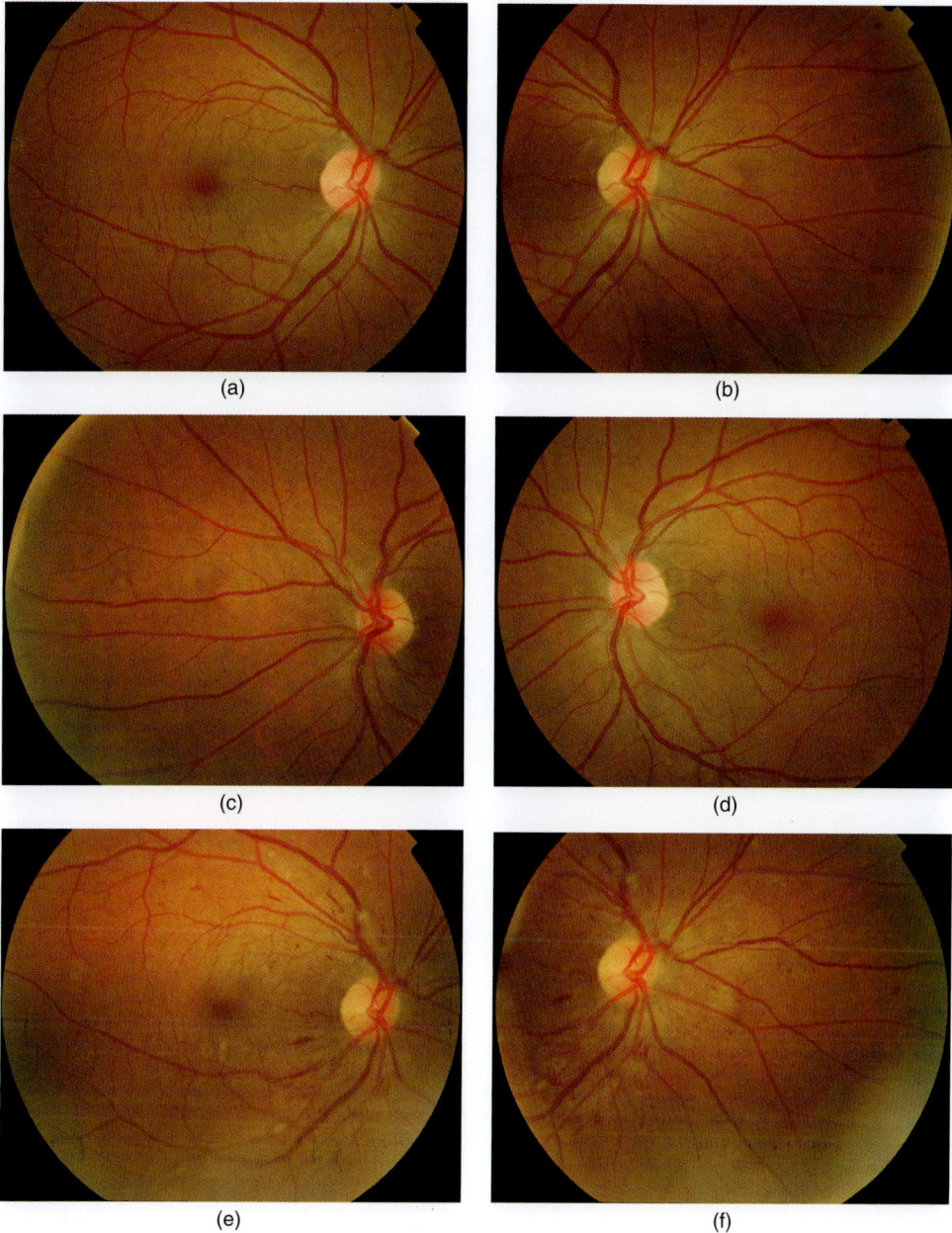

Fig. 15.3 Right (a) macula and (b) nasal colour, and left (c) nasal and (d) macula colour at presentation. Right (e) macula and (f) nasal colour, and left (g) nasal and (h) macula colour at 25/40 pregnant. (i) Right and (j) left macula colour at 29/40 pregnant. Right (k) macula and (l) nasal colour, and left (m) nasal and (n) macula colour at 34/40 pregnant. Right (o) macula and (p) nasal colour, and left (q) nasal and (r) macula colour at 1 year postpartum.

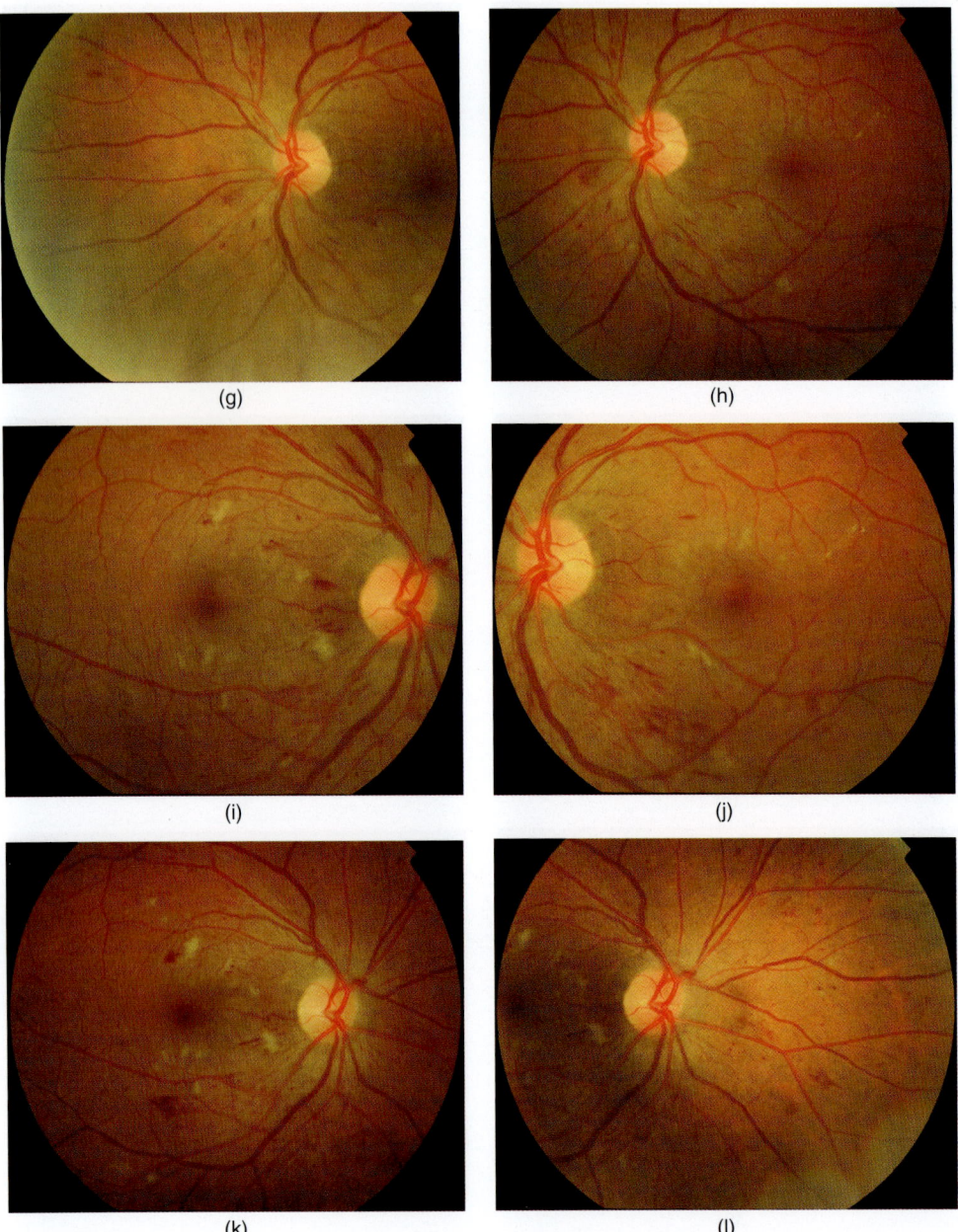

Fig. 15.3 (*Continued*)

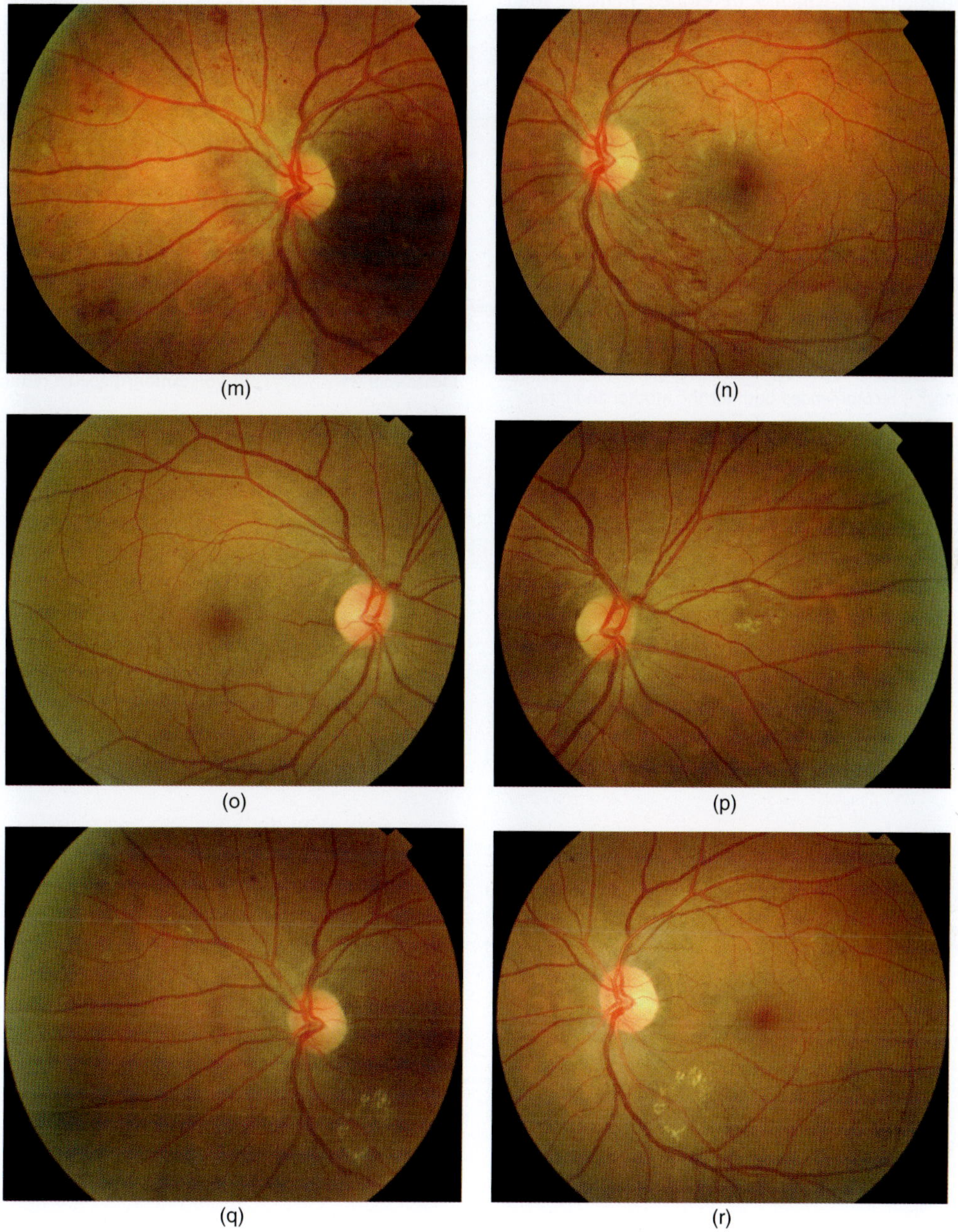

(m) (n)
(o) (p)
(q) (r)

Fig. 15.3 (*Continued*)

during pregnancy of which 7 developed PDR. A total of 13 women experienced postpartum regression. None of the women who developed PDR during pregnancy experienced postpartum regression.

PRACTICE POINTS

Recommendations for patients are as follows.
1. Women with type 1 diabetes should be encouraged to plan pregnancies early in life[9].
2. Improving metabolic control before conception[4] is recommended both for the mother and infant.
3. Improving metabolic control during pregnancy[1,2,6,9] is recommended both for the mother and infant.
4. Control of hypertension both before conception and during pregnancy[6] is recommended both for the mother and infant.
5. Photocoagulation before conception and during pregnancy[10] is recommended. If a patient is found to have significant retinopathy before conception, it is recommended that pregnancy is delayed where possible until appropriate laser treatment has been applied and good metabolic control has been achieved for a 9-month period to overcome any effects of the early worsening phenomenon[8]. Photocoagulation before pregnancy may protect against rapidly progressive proliferative retinopathy. Aggressive treatment of proliferative retinopathy developing in pregnancy may prevent further progression of the disease.

REFERENCE

Please visit www.wiley.com/go/scanlon/diabetic_retinopathy

16 Low vision and blindness from diabetic retinopathy

Peter H. Scanlon

Harris Manchester College, University of Oxford; Medical Ophthalmology, University of Gloucestershire, UK

DEFINITION OF BLINDNESS

Legal blindness (Fig. 16.1) is defined in the USA as best corrected visual acuity in the better eye worse than or equal to 20/200 or a visual field extent of less than 20 degrees in diameter. Vision impairment is defined as having a best corrected visual acuity of 20/40 or worse vision in the better-seeing eye. Legal blindness is defined by the World Health Organization in the same way as for the USA, that is, a best corrected visual acuity in the better eye worse than or equal to 20/200.

The definition of blindness and partial sight in the UK is:
- blind (severely sight impaired): acuity below 3/60; or acuity better than 3/60 but below 6/60 with a very restricted visual field; and
- partial sight (sight impaired): from 3/60 to 6/60 with a full field; up to 6/24 with moderate restriction of visual field (e.g. glaucoma); or 6/18 or better with a gross field defect (e.g. hemianopia) or a marked constriction of the field (e.g. retinitis pigmentosa).

In 2005 the Certificate of Visual Impairment is the new form used in the UK (replacing the BD8) to register people as severely sight impaired (blind) or sight impaired (partially sighted). The definitions remain as above.

IN THE USA

Vision Problems in the US is a publication produced jointly by Prevent Blindness America (a volunteer eye health organisation) and the National Eye Institute. The 2002 publication reported that legal blindness affects more than one million Americans age 40 and older and affects blacks more frequently than whites. Hispanics have higher rates of visual impairment than other races, but not blindness. The overall national rate of blindness in the total US population age 40 and older is 2.85%, varying between 1.3% in Alaska and 3.74% in North Dakota. The 2002 report estimated the numbers of people in the US with mild or worse diabetic retinopathy are 5,353,233, of whom 74% were white, 10% black, 10% Hispanic and 6% other ethnicity. This compares to the 2000 US Census total US population aged 40 years of 119,386,252, of whom 78% were white, 10% black, 7% Hispanic and 5% other ethnic backgrounds.

Diabetic retinopathy is a leading cause of adult blindness in the US reported by Fong et al.[1] in 2004 to result in blindness for over 10,000 people with diabetes per year. Moss et al.[2] reported the 10-year incidence of blindness in the Wisconsin Epidemiological study of Diabetic Retinopathy to be 1.8%, 4.0% and 4.8% in the younger-onset, older-onset-taking-insulin and older-onset-not-taking-insulin groups, respectively. Respective 10-year rates of visual impairment were 9.4%, 37.2% and 23.9%. The Diabetes 2000 program of the American Academy of Ophthalmology (AAO) was established to disseminate the recommendations of various nationwide controlled studies[3-6] that demonstrate that effective therapy exists for diabetic retinopathy and also the Preferred Practice Patterns (PPP) for diabetic retinopathy in an effort to improve the overall quality of care for patients with diabetes and those specifically at risk for diabetic retinopathy. A review of clinicians'[7] practice patterns over time suggests that practitioners are becoming increasingly aware of Diabetes 2000 and adopting the guidelines outlined within the PPP.

The report used data from the 1996–2002 Medical Expenditure Panel Survey aged 40 and older. The majority (70,711) of the 77,511 participants over the seven years reported no visual impairment; 6288 reported visual impairment; and 512 reported being blind. Of the 70,711

A Practical Manual of Diabetic Retinopathy Management, Second Edition.
Edited by Peter Scanlon, Ahmed Sallam, and Peter van Wijngaarden.
© 2017 John Wiley & Sons Ltd. Published 2017 by John Wiley & Sons Ltd.
Companion Website: www.wiley.com/go/scanlon/diabetic_retinopathy

reporting no visual impairment, 9% were diagnosed with diabetes. Of the 6288 reporting visual impairment, 18% were diagnosed with diabetes. Of the 512 reporting blindness, 22% were diagnosed with diabetes.

Black and Asian populations in the USA have a greater risk of developing diabetic eye disease compared to the white population[8]. Zhang et al.[9] reported that the estimated prevalence of diabetic retinopathy and vision-threatening diabetic retinopathy was 28.5% (95% confidence interval or CI, 24.9–32.5%) and 4.4% (95% CI, 3.5–5.7%) among US adults with diabetes.

IN EUROPE

In 1990, the St Vincent Declaration[10] recognised diabetes and diabetic retinopathy to be a major and growing European health problem, a problem at all ages and in all countries. The first of the five-year targets that were unanimously agreed by Government Health Departments and patient's organisations from all European countries was to reduce new blindness due to diabetes by one-third or more. In 2002, Kocur and Resnikoff[11] reported that in people of working age in Europe diabetic retinopathy

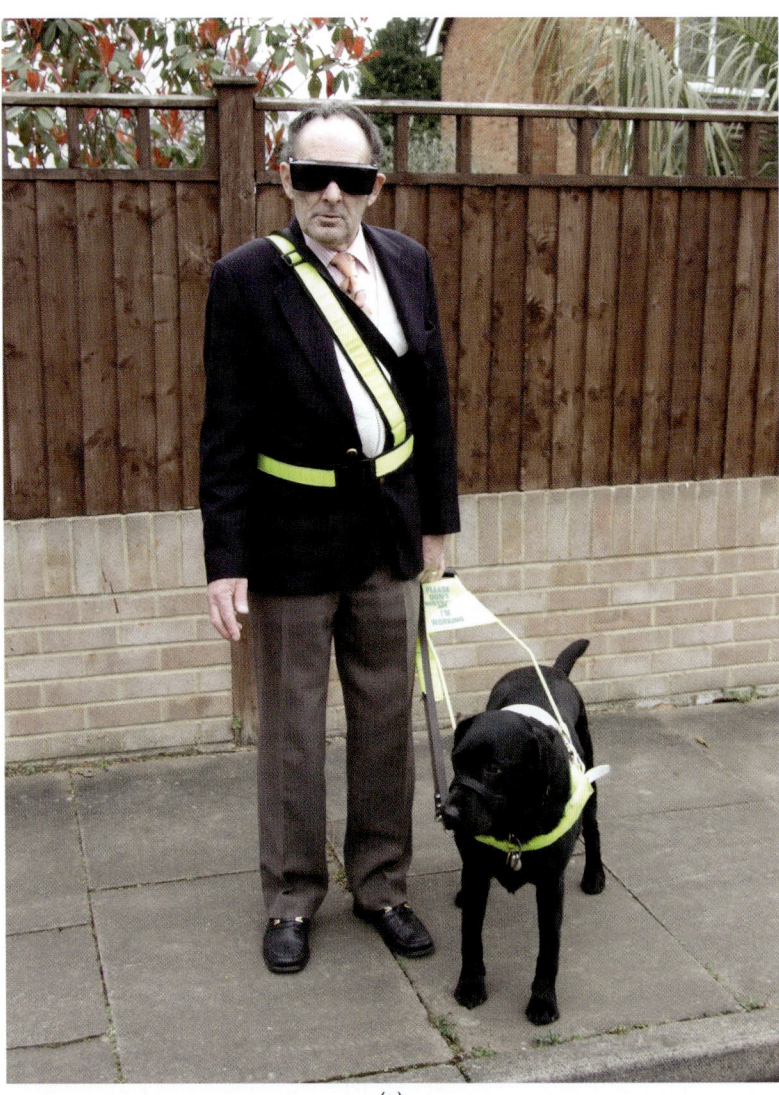

(a)

Fig. 16.1 (a, b) A blind patient using his guide dog.

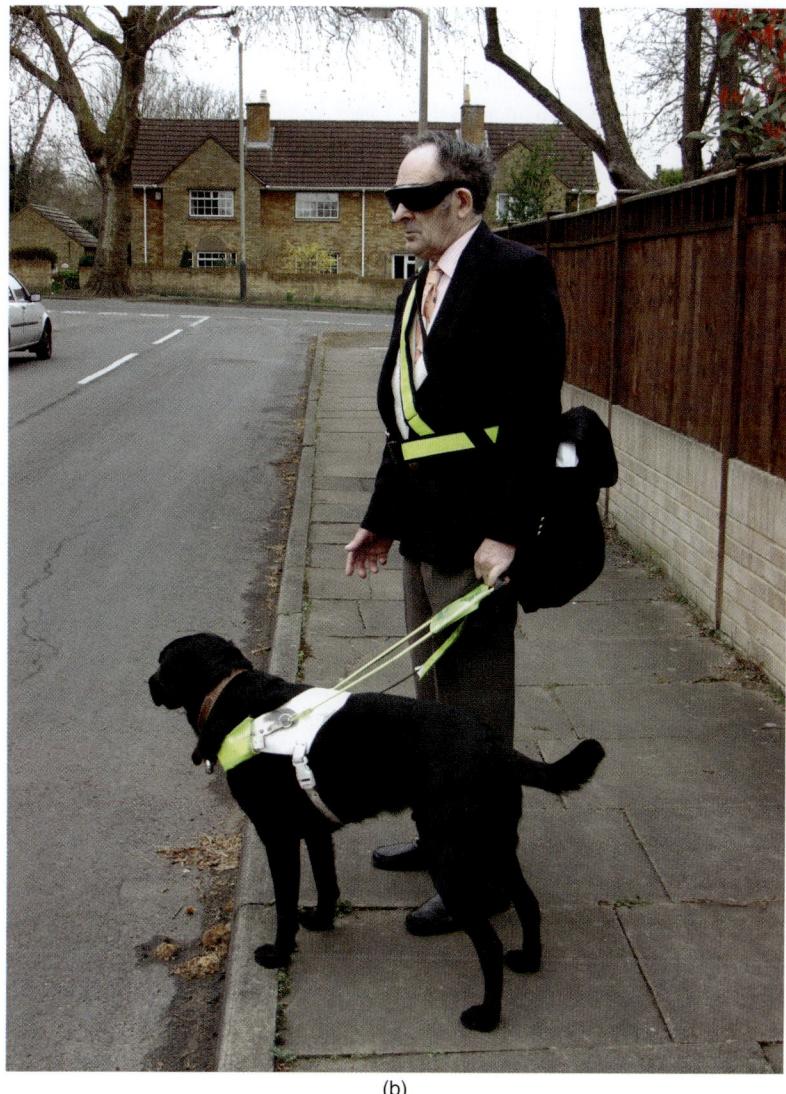

(b)

Fig. 16.1 (Continued)

is the most frequently reported causes of serious visual loss.

In Liverpool on the 17 and 18 November 2005 a conference took place to review progress in the prevention of visual impairment due to diabetic retinopathy since the writing in 1989 and publication in 1990 of the St Vincent Declaration. Formal invitations were sent to all known diabetes and ophthalmology organisations in 43 countries in Europe, and official national representatives of 29 European countries attended. Each country was asked to submit a poster which reviewed their current position. In posters from Denmark, England, Finland, Iceland, Northern Ireland, Norway, Scotland, Sweden and Wales the reported prevalence of diabetes varied between 2.9 and 4.7%. However, in Turkey the reported prevalence of diabetes was 7.2% and in the Czech Republic 7%.

Over the past 15 years most countries appear to have made genuine progress in an effort to reduce blindness due to diabetic retinopathy. However there were certain key issues that affected some European countries more than others: lack of data; inadequate resources; lack of awareness and education; and lack of co-ordination and communication within the individual health system.

In 1995, Evans[12] reported on the causes of blindness and partial sight in England and Wales from an analysis of all registration forms for the year April 1990 to March 1991. Among people of working age (ages 16–64), diabetes was the most important cause of blindness (13.8%) with 11.9% due to diabetic retinopathy.

In 2006, Bunce and Wormald[13] repeated this analysis of all registration forms for the year April 1999 to March 2000. Overall, the age-specific incidence of all three leading causes (age-related macular degeneration, glaucoma and diabetic retinopathy) has increased since 1990–1991. Changes in diabetic retinopathy are the most marked, particularly in the over 65s where figures have more than doubled. In the figures from 1999–2000, diabetic retinopathy was again reported as the most common cause of severe visual impairment (combining blind and partial sight registrations) in the working age group.

A total of 813 people were registered blind and 1414 people registered partially sighted due to diabetic retinopathy in the year April 1999–March 2000, making a total registered with visual impairment of 2227. A publication[14] from a clinic in Birmingham UK suggested that only 55% or eligible people are registered because of the voluntary nature of the registration and the individual variations in interpretation by ophthalmologists. It might therefore be assumed that the actual number of people who should have been registered as blind or partially sighted in England in the year April 1999–March 2000 should have been 4049 people. Of concern in the Bunce and Wormald[13] paper was that the numbers in the age group 16–64 had increased from 1.26 in 1990–1991 to 2.05 per 100,000 population in 1999–2000, in the age group 65–74 had increased from 7.28 to 15.06, in the age group 75–84 had increased from 8.27 to 17.08, and in the age group 85 and over had increased from 3.92 to 11.02. This may be partly explained by increased ascertainment and people with diabetes living longer.

Black and Asian populations in the UK also have a greater risk of developing diabetic eye disease compared to the white population[15].

The most progress in reduction of blindness has been made in Iceland where the prevalence of legal blindness from diabetic retinopathy dropped from 4.0% to 0.5% over 15 years, beginning in 1980. The prevalence of diabetes is relatively low in Iceland (2.9%) and the country has a very strong centralised medical system regarding all aspects of diabetes control and screening. However, the example that Iceland has shown is that optimal management is very effective in preventing and/or reducing severe complication of diabetes.

Other reports of successful reductions of blindness have come from Poland[16] and Sweden[17] and more recently in England and Wales[18]. This recent study[18] has shown that, for the first time in at least five decades, diabetic retinopathy/maculopathy is no longer the leading cause of certifiable blindness among working-age adults in England and Wales, having been overtaken by inherited retinal disorders. This may relate in part to introduction of nationwide diabetic retinopathy screening programmes and improved glycaemic control.

IN THE REST OF THE WORLD

The World Health Organization definition of blindness is the same as that of legal blindness in the US, that is, a best corrected visual acuity in the better eye worse than or equal to 20/200. In 2001, Cunningham[19] reported that 45 million people worldwide fulfil the World Health Organisation's criterion for blindness. More than 90% of all blind and visually disabled people live in the developing world, where common causes of bilateral vision loss include cataract, glaucoma, trachoma, vitamin A deficiency and onchocerciasis. Additional causes of bilateral vision loss, which together comprise nearly one-quarter of all blindness and which affect people in both developed and developing nations, include diabetic retinopathy and macular degeneration.

Zheng et al.[20] reported that, globally, the number of people with DR will grow from 126.6 million in 2010 to 191.0 million by 2030, and estimated that the number with vision-threatening diabetic retinopathy (VTDR) will increase from 37.3 million to 56.3 million in that time.

COSTS OF BLINDNESS DUE TO DIABETIC RETINOPATHY

In 2003, Meads and Hyde[21] reported the costs of blindness and equated the published estimates of the annual cost of blindness in diabetic retinopathy to December 2002 rates. The 1983 estimate of Foulds et al.[22] was inflated to £7433 in 2002 costs (converts to US$ 14,654). Dasbach et al.'s 1991 estimate[23] was inflated to £5391 in 2002 costs (converts to US$ 10,628). Wright et al.'s 2000 estimate[24] was inflated to £7452 (£4070–11,250) in 2002 costs (converts to US$ 14,690 US dollars with a range of US$ 8023–22,183).

He suggested that much of the uncertainty in any sensitivity analysis of the cost of blindness in older people is associated with the cost of residential care, because the excess admission to care homes caused by poor vision was impossible to quantify at that time. In the publication *The Economic Impact of Vision Problems* produced by Prevent Blindness America in 2007, it reported that visual impairment, compared to no visual impairment, is associated with over $1000 of excess annual medical expenses and a little more than a day of informal care days. Compared to no visual impairment, blindness is associated with over $2000 of excess annual medical expenditures per year and more than five extra days of informal care from someone outside the household. Excess medical expenses are tied mainly to home healthcare expenditures, particularly from private providers. The authors also published a paper[25] that reported the annual total financial burden of major adult visual disorders in the US is $35.4 billion and that the annual governmental budgetary impact is $13.7 billion.

A recent report[26] on the economic effects of blindness for the Royal National Institute for the Blind in the UK estimated that partial sight and blindness in the adult population places a large economic cost on the UK, totalling £22 billion in 2008. Direct healthcare system costs amount to £2.14 billion and indirect costs amount to £4.34 billion. The report estimated that there were 1.8 million people with partial sight and blindness in the UK and 62,000 (3.5%) had partial sight and blindness due to diabetic retinopathy. Of an estimated total of 218,000 blind people, approximately 19,000 (8.7%) were blind due to diabetic retinopathy. The report estimated that from 2010 to 2050 the share of partial sight and blindness from diabetic retinopathy would decrease from 3.4% to 2.3% (a 46% increase in absolute numbers, however, to 93,000 people).

COSTS OF TREATMENT FOR DIABETIC RETINOPATHY

Brown et al.[27] reported results from a retrospective literature review that demonstrated that ophthalmologic interventions for diabetic retinopathy and other eye diseases are cost-effective because of the substantial value that ophthalmologic interventions confer to patients for the resources expended. In another publication[28] it was reported that laser surgical procedures, such as for diabetic retinopathy, appear to be especially cost-effective as a group.

The cost of diabetic retinopathy treatment was estimated[26] assuming four laser treatments per year and a follow-up ophthalmologist visit, amounting to £1151 per eye in 2008 values (NHS, 2004). However, when diabetic retinopathy is present with symptomatic disease in one eye, the other eye is also likely to have retinopathy and the additional laser treatment required in the second eye could amount to a further cost of £830–1107. Taking the average of the additional laser treatment, the estimated cost of treating diabetic retinopathy in both eyes was £2120 per person (in 2008 prices).

The costs of treating diabetic macular oedema have increased in the last few years with the introduction of VEGF inhibitors. A recent review[29] by the London Medicines Evaluation Network estimated the number of required intravitreal injections based on the VISTA and VIVID trials and the NICE TA for ranibizumab as approximately eight intravitreal injections in the first year and two in the second year. The cost of the vial for intravitreal injection was reported at varying over £742–816 and hence the cost for eight intravitreal injections in the first year would be £5937–6928. In addition there would be outpatient costs as well as the cost of a monitoring visit and a fluorescein angiogram (if undertaken), estimated at £194, £139 and £117, respectively.

REDUCED VISION AND QUALITY OF LIFE

There is a substantial prevalence of vision-related quality of life impairment in both the UK[30] and USA. Major complications relating to diabetes are generally associated with worse health-related quality of life[31] and with lower utility scores, although Brown et al.[32] found that visual loss seems to cause a similar diminution in self-assessed quality of life in those who do and do not have serious associated systemic co-morbidities. A review of evidence[33] evaluating the effect of diabetic retinopathy and diabetic macular oedema on health-related quality of life found several articles that demonstrated both a qualitative and a quantitative reduction in health-related quality of life in persons with diabetic retinopathy.

A study in which the author of this chapter was involved reported symptoms and quality-of-life impacts in patients having laser treatment for sight-threatening diabetic retinopathy showed that fewer of the multi-treatment patients were free of symptoms at their post-treatment follow-up interviews (13% compared to 26% of first treatment patients), which cascaded into a variety of life impacts. Concurrent progression of both the underlying diabetes and the eye disease adds other progressive complications and life impacts into the picture. First-time-treatment patients reported both relief in visual disturbances and a general decrease in level of anxiety associated with the worry about what the treatment would be like. Multi-treatment patients seemed to have considerably less pain and anxiety about the treatment, but their anxiety and worry appears to grow in relation to their increasing visual disturbances and daily life limitations. Their worry or fear tended to be more focused on the progression of their condition.

A recent study[34] has demonstrated that quality-of-life scores are most closely associated with a weighted VA measure of 0.75 in the better and 0.25 in the worse eye.

LOW-VISION REHABILITATION

Despite major advances in treatment and early detection of diabetic eye disease, the aging demographic and increased incidence of diabetes is resulting in greater numbers of diabetic visually impaired people in the population.

Low-vision aids (LVAs) have been shown[35,36] to be useful in aiding important near and distance daily living tasks, and in contributing to increased quality of life in those using them.

Low-vision clinics in the UK have been traditionally hospital based with low-vision aids (LVAs) supplied on permanent loan to patients. This service has historically been patchy[37], and following national consultation[38] in the UK and the formation of local Low-Vision Services committees, a number of clinics have evolved[38,39] to suit local needs and are increasingly multidisciplinary with the involvement of rehabilitation, mobility and voluntary services, among others.

Low-vision assessments (LVAs) typically encompass detailed task and lifestyle analysis, measurement of functional vision, the selection of an appropriate LVA and development of modified approach to attempt the task, and the provision of information to access additional support.

Identifying a need or task is often attempted on a problem-solving basis, and correctly defining a suitable activity is known to affect the successful use of LVAs. Chosen or preferred tasks are patient specific and may be divided into spot or rapid tasks (e.g. looking at a cooker dial or shop price) or prolonged (e.g. reading a book or newspaper). A greater level of magnification is normally required for the latter[40]. They are significantly influenced by lifestyle. An elderly diabetic patient living alone may raise issues about viewing medication and reading their mail and correspondence, while a younger person of working age may be more concerned with work-related visual problems.

Information about a patient's visual function is used in conjunction with this to select an initial aid to attempt a given task. Useful measures of visual function for all low-vision assessments include: best corrected visual acuity (preferably logMAR[41]); near acuity; and basic visual field assessment. Peak contrast sensitivity function (such as Peli-Robson) has been shown to be a useful tool for selecting a preferred eye for viewing[42] and assessment of reading speed may be valuable[43].

There are many hundreds of low-vision aids commercially available[44], in different designs and magnification availability. They can be divided into different categories. Hand magnifiers are relatively inexpensive, portable, easy to use and widely accepted. If the patient has a hand tremor or has difficulty in maintaining a good grip, then stand magnifiers (often with internal illumination) can be more useful. To obtain the largest field of view for a given magnification and to maintain a 'hands-free' approach, for example when reading a book, an aid such as a high reading add or spectacle microscope might be tried initially. If the longest possible working distance is required, a near telescope (usually Galilean) would be the first LVA of choice; these are normally spectacle-mounted. If a distance task is identified, then a distance telescope (either Galilean or astronomical with a righting device) can be tried. These are usually hand-held devices and magnification of up to 8× can be commonly utilised if the user has a reasonable steady hand. More modern telescopic devices have been developed with an auto-focus facility for distance and near, although the considerable cost has limited their supply from most clinics.

CCTV reading aids electronically magnify print onto a TV screen and have enabled many more people to be able to read print. Simpler devices that plug into the user's own TV have become available for a couple of hundred pounds, as opposed to several thousand for the most sophisticated models. Portable pocket video devices have become increasingly popular for spot tasks.

The development of enlargement software for computers (which can often be used in conjunction with speech synthesis) has enabled many visually impaired people to embrace modern technology and has revolutionised the way they can access information; there are a number of commercially available products.

Finally, there are many non-optical ways of tackling visual difficulties ranging from optimum task lighting, correct use of contrast in cooking, a template for signing a name or cheque, a device that buzzes when a cup is filled, talking scales and watches, bumper stickers for cooker dials to symbol canes to aid crossing roads. Examples of this last group are available from Social Services as part of the community care provision, and many low-vision clinics have direct access to these services.

Low-vision clinics are often able to supply written information about sight loss and the availability of local services such as clubs and support groups, for example newly registered groups as well as computer access and large-print text. They can provide a gateway to additional support and information from other agencies such as the RNIB Sightline Directory, which is a directory of low-vision services available for blind and partially sighted people in the UK[45], the Disability Employment Advisers (DEAs) in most local job centres and the Access to Work programme, which provides advice and equipment to visually impaired people in the work place.

Low-vision aids have been shown to be beneficial in the rehabilitation of those who have lost acuity because of diabetic retinopathy changes and those who have temporary sight reduction in sight. LVAs have been shown[46] to be more successful in patients with visual difficulties related to diabetic retinopathy than those with age-related macular degeneration. This was thought to be related to a more useable central field and lack of a dense central scotoma in most cases.

Successful usage of correctly selective LVA is relatively high and considered cost-effective[47], and many people are able to continue to live independently and carry out their everyday tasks if the right help has been made available[48,49].

CAUSES OF LOSS OF VISION IN DIABETES AND DIABETIC RETINOPATHY

Visual loss occurs due to involvement of the macula in the following circumstances: (1) advanced proliferative DR with traction on the macular area; (2) ischaemic maculopathy; (3) chronic macular oedema; or (4) can occur in intracerebral visual pathway interruptions.

Case History 16.1: Blindness due to advanced proliferative DR with traction on the left macular area

A young woman presented at the age of 35 years with advanced retinopathy in both eyes with a visual level of right perception of light only and left hand movements only. There was extensive fibroproliferative disease in both eyes with a tractional detachment of her left macular area caused by contraction of fibro-proliferative vessels, and the visual acuity in her left eye did not improve despite successful vitrectomy surgery. Her right eye had a long-standing combined tractional/rhegmatogenous retinal detachment (Fig. 16.2) with a vision of NPL (no perception of light), and was considered too advanced for surgery. She has been registered as Severely Sight Impaired.

Case History 16.2: Blindness associated with macular ischaemia

A 32-year-old man who has had type 1 diabetes since the age of 11 years presented with reduced vision in both eyes at a level of right 1.22 (4/60) and left 1.30 (3/60).

Colour photographs (Fig. 16.3a and b) and a fluorescein angiogram (Fig. 16.3c and d) were taken, and show a combination of severe ischaemia involving both macular areas and new vessels elsewhere.

He was treated with bilateral panretinal photocoagulation and later required vitrectomy surgery in both eyes for non-clearing vitreous haemorrhages. His vision never recovered, and his vision remains at a level of right 1.22 (4/60) and left 1.30 (3/60) and he has been registered as Severely Sight Impaired.

Case History 16.3: Blindness due to chronic diabetic macular oedema prior to VEGF inhibitor treatments

This 83-year-old woman (BMI 32) with type 2 diabetes, diagnosed at the age of 62 years, commenced initially on tablets and is now controlled on insulin. She presented to the Ophthalmology Department at the age of 72 years with extensive haemorrhages and oedema in her right macular area and a reduced VA to a level of right 6/36 (20/180). The left VA was satisfactory at 6/9 (20/30). At the time her BP was elevated at 180/110 and, although she had been treated with insulin since the age of 64 years, her blood sugars had been consistently high at her diabetic clinic appointments running between 10.9 and 20.7. Her BP had also been poorly controlled, with readings recorded of 200/95, 200/85 and 180/110.

At 72 years, laser treatment was given to the extensive thickening in the right macular area with right 95 burns, 100 micron size, 170–240 mW, Area Centralis lens, argon laser. The right vision improved a little to 6/24 (20/80) and the retinal thickening reduced, but no further visual improvement occurred. At 73 years, blurring then started to develop in the left eye (Fig. 16.4a, b).

Extensive oedema was present in both macular areas and the VAs were right 6/60 (20/200) and left 6/18 (20/60). Treatment was given to the right macular area of right 160 burns, 100 micron size, 150 mW, Area Centralis lens, argon laser. Treatment was given to the left macular area of left 70 burns, 100 micron size, 130–150 mW, Area Centralis lens, argon laser.

Unfortunately the vision did not improve and the vision in her left eye subsequently deteriorated over the next 18 months to a level of 3/60, despite one further laser treatment to her left eye of left 85 burns, 100 micron size, 180 mW, Area Centralis lens, argon laser. Registration on the partial register of Visual Impairment was made. At 73 years, pan retinal photocoagulation was commenced to the right eye because of the increasing signs of peripheral retinal ischaemia. Treatment was given of right 2022 burns, 500 micron size, 260–300 mW, Karickhoff 4 mirror lens, argon laser over 3 sessions separated by 1 week. Photographs taken at the age of 76 years are presented in Figure 16.4c–f.

At 77 years, her VA had fallen to right counting fingers and left 1/60 (3/200) due to severe ischaemic maculopathy. There were also signs of increasing ischaemia in her left retina. Panretinal photocoagulation was therefore commenced to the left eye. Treatment was given of right 2275 burns, 200 micron size, 250–300 mW, Quadraspheric lens, argon laser over 2 sessions separated by 1 week. Registration on the full register of Visual Impairment was made.

HbA1c results that have been recorded in the last 10 years have been 9.9, 9.5, 11.4, 11.4, 10.6, 11.0, 8.5, 10.0, 10.6, 12.9, 8.6 and 10.8. BP results that have been recorded in the last 10 years have been 170/90, 150/82, 176/60, 181/88, 164/100, 155/85, 140/70, 165/95, 130/70, 118/68, 150/82, 138/70, 153/71 and 212/93. The combination of difficulties with glycaemic control, blood pressure control and the development of ischaemic maculopathy that has been difficult to treat with conventional argon laser treatment have lead to this loss of vision.

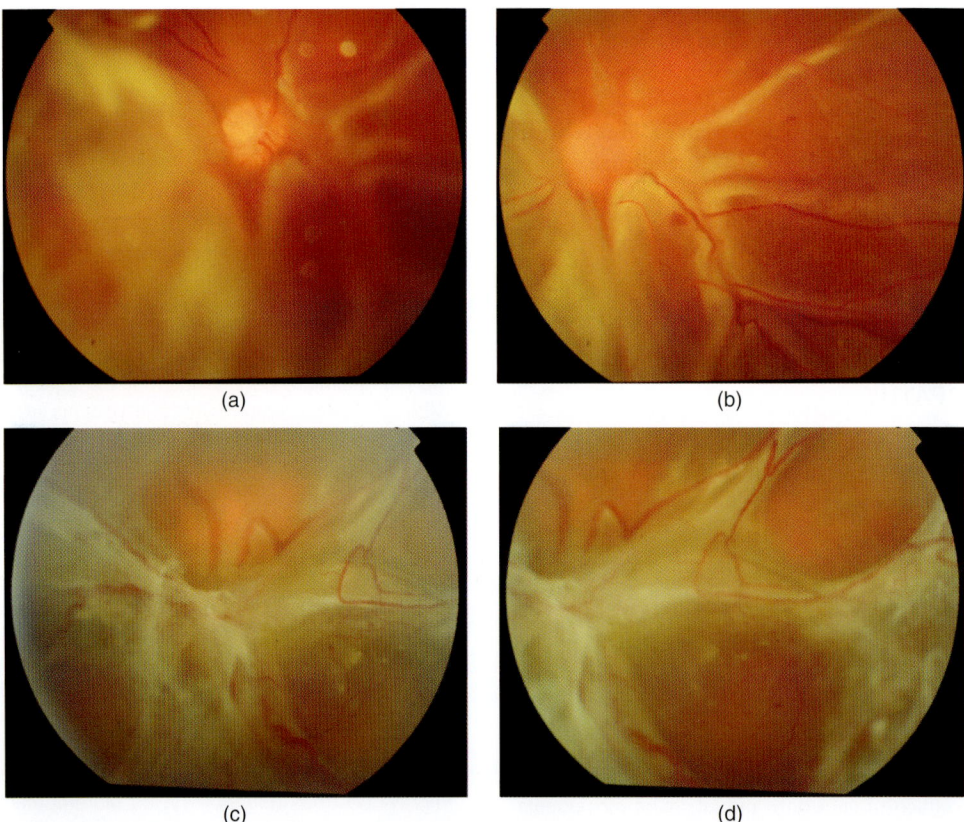

Fig. 16.2 Right (a) macula and (b) disc colour. Left (c) disc and (d) macula colour. (e) OCT left macular area.

Low vision and blindness from diabetic retinopathy 215

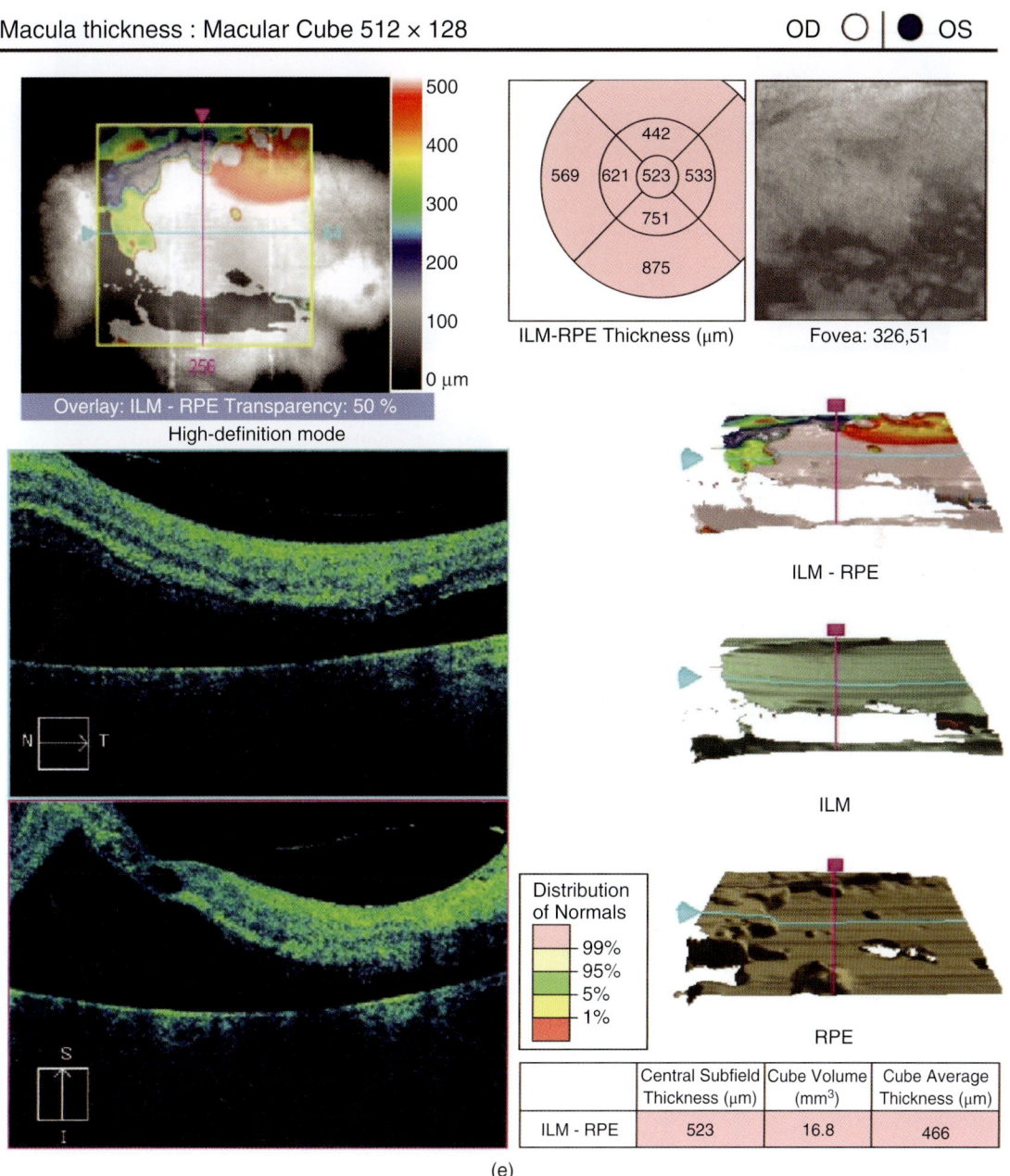

(e)

Fig. 16.2 (*Continued*)

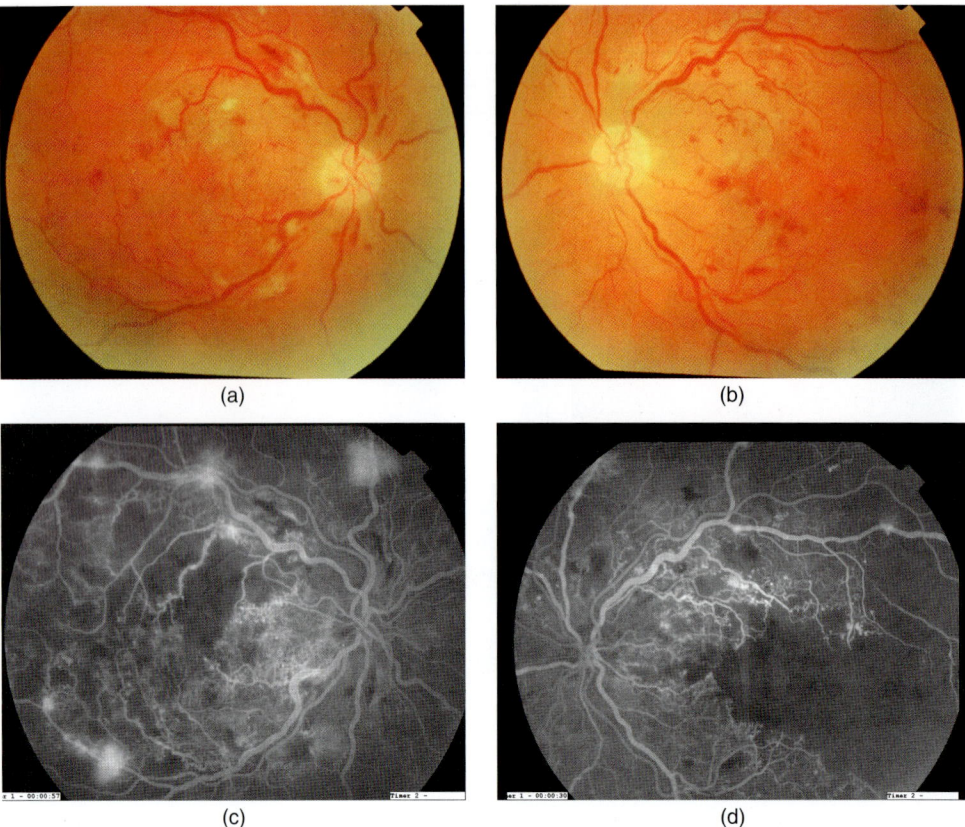

Fig. 16.3 (a) Right and (b) left macula colour at presentation. Fluorescein (c) right macula 1 min 57 s and (d) left macula 1 min 30 s after injection.

Case History 16.4: Cortical blindness following a cardiac arrest in a patient treated for proliferative diabetic retinopathy

This 64-year-old man presented with a vitreous haemorrhage in his left eye. He had a past history of panretinal photocoagulation and macular laser treatment to both eyes and his visual acuity was right 6/24, left hand movements. The haemorrhage in his left eye gradually cleared and he was found to have active neovascularisation in both eyes and a chronically oedematous right central foveal area. Over the next 2 years he required infilling laser treatment to both eyes. However, he developed a further non-clearing vitreous haemorrhage in his left eye at the age of 66 years with visual acuities of right 6/24 left HM and was listed for a left vitrectomy and endolaser. His left vision improved to 6/7.5 in his left eye following this procedure and he retained a level of vision of right 6/24, left 6/7.5 over the next few years (Fig. 16.5a–d), although he required a left cataract extraction 1 year after the vitrectomy procedure. At the time his blood glucose control had improved from a HbA1c value of 11.2 to 8.6 and he commenced insulin treatment at the age of 69 years. At the age of 72, he had an asystolic arrest due to prerenal failure and hyperkalaemia. This resulted in loss of vision to a level of right 3/60, left 5/60 with significant field loss (Fig. 16.5e, f) and he was registered Severely Sight Impaired. He continues to live an active life getting out on a regular basis with National Blind Associations and using modern computer software to read his e-mails to him.

Low vision and blindness from diabetic retinopathy 217

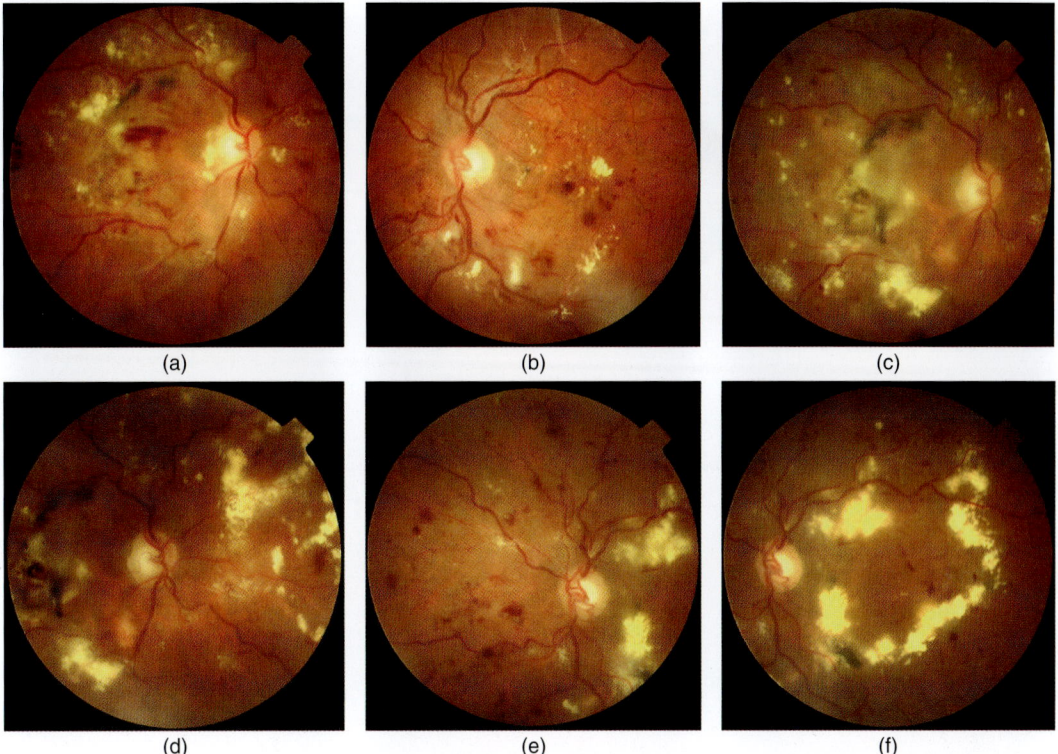

Fig. 16.4 (a) Right and (b) left macula colour. Right (c) macula and (d) nasal colour. Left (e) nasal and (f) macula colour.

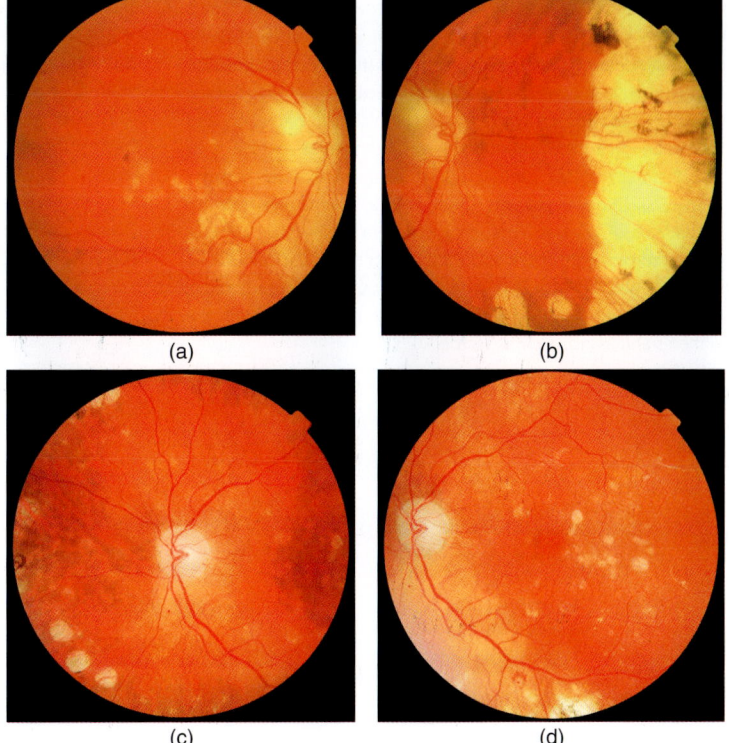

Fig. 16.5 Right (a) macula and (b) nasal colour. Left (c) nasal and (d) macula colour. (e) Right and (f) left eye visual field after recovering from cardiac arrest.

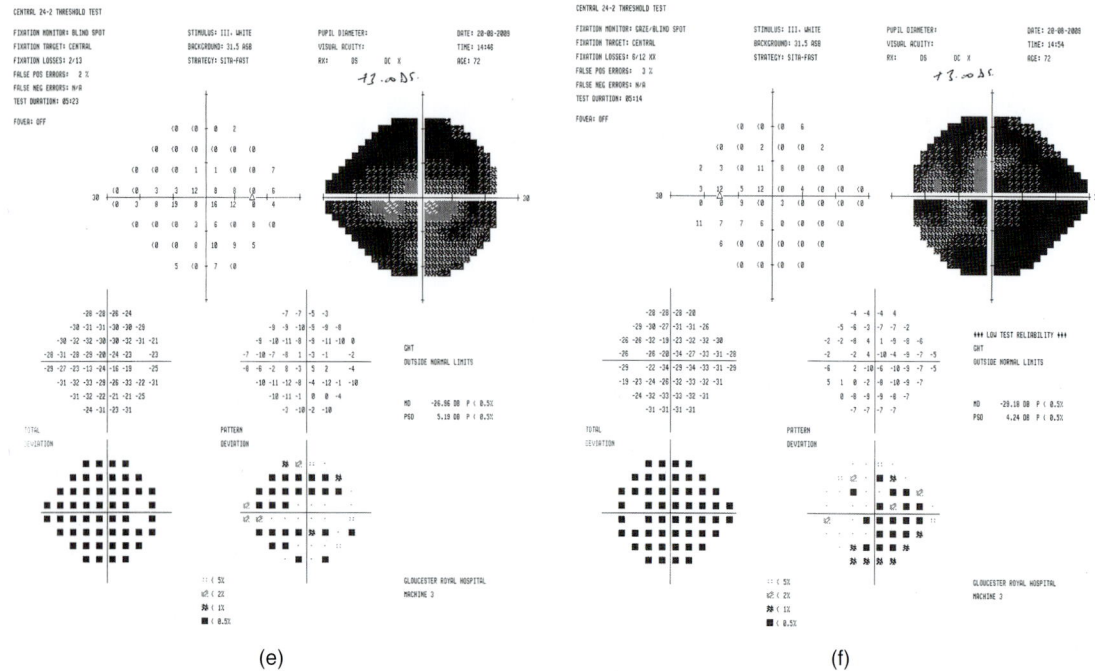

(e)   (f)

Fig. 16.5 (*Continued*)

PRACTICE POINTS

In the Wisconsin study[50], proliferative retinopathy occurred in 67% in persons with type 1 diabetes for 35 or more years. One would therefore expect that two-thirds of people with type 1 diabetes would need laser treatment for proliferative diabetic retinopathy during their lifetime, although the rate of progression to proliferative DR has reduced in more recent generations. Klein et al.[51,52] reported on the 25-year cumulative progression and regression of diabetic retinopathy and cumulative incidence of macular oedema (ME) and clinically significant macular oedema (CSME) in type 1 patients. The 25-year cumulative rate of progression of DR was 83%, progression to proliferative DR was 42%, improvement of DR was 18% and the 25-year cumulative incidence was 29% for DME and 17% for CSME. These findings may reflect an improvement in medical management of the diabetes and associated risk factors.

In patients with type 2 diabetes, the rate of proliferative diabetic retinopathy is not as high but it is estimated that 1 in 3 patients with type 2 diabetes will develop sight-threatening diabetic retinopathy, requiring laser during their lifetime.

The prevalence of blindness is influenced by duration of diabetes, blood glucose and pressure control, and by the presence or absence of screening and preventive laser treatment.

Achieving a high compliance as achieved in Iceland[53] and in England and Wales[18] can lower the risk of blindness to very low levels.

REFERENCE

Please visit www.wiley.com/go/scanlon/diabetic_retinopathy

17 Future advances in the management of diabetic retinopathy

Peter van Wijngaarden

Consultant Ophthalmologist, Centre for Eye Research Australia, Royal Victorian Eye and Ear Hospital, Australia
Ophthalmology, Department of Surgery, University of Melbourne, Australia

While great progress has been made in our ability to diagnose and treat diabetic retinopathy, the enormous burden of vision loss from diabetes indicates that further progress is urgently required. Key future advances in the management of diabetic retinopathy will likely centre on the following:

- the use of personalised risk stratification derived from genetic, biochemical and clinical biomarker profiling to inform screening intervals, preventive strategies and tailored therapeutics;
- more timely, convenient and cost-effective detection of retinopathy through population-wide screening and the implementation of streamlined health service pathways to facilitate appropriate medical and surgical intervention;
- retino-protective therapies to prevent or delay retinopathy progression;
- enhanced anti-angiogenic and anti-inflammatory therapies to better manage proliferative retinopathy and macular oedema, as well as improved methods of drug delivery;
- regenerative therapies to repair or replace damaged retinal vessels and perhaps even retinal neurons.

Initiatives to improve the management of diabetic retinopathy must go hand-in-hand with improved comprehensive care of people with diabetes. Effectively addressing key modifiable risk factors for the complications of diabetes (e.g. suboptimal glycaemic control, hypertension, dyslipidaemia and smoking) rests not only on appropriate prescribing practices, but also on personalised evidence-based programs that are grounded in the science of health behaviour change. Emerging evidence suggests that improvements in glycaemic control are rarely achieved with clinical counselling alone[1]. Health system changes to ensure co-ordination of care and seamless data sharing between people with diabetes and healthcare providers is important. In addition, societal reforms to promote healthy eating and physical activity may also help to stem the tide of T2DM[2]. Underpinning each of these advances is the need for governments to commit to policy reform and appropriately funded health programs; tackling the world's most rapidly growing chronic health problem demands no less.

PREDICTING RISK OF DIABETIC RETINOPATHY AND ITS PROGRESSION

There is growing interest in the potential for individualised prediction of risk for the complications of diabetes. Accurate risk prediction would allow tailored screening and the identification of key pathogenic pathways at play in a given individual[3,4]. This will inevitably lead to personalised medicine through tailored medical therapy, environmental risk factor modification and eventually genetic treatment strategies. Validated biomarker profiles will also serve as useful surrogate end-points for clinical trials in diabetic retinopathy, facilitating more timely translation of drug discovery research into clinical practice. Clinical translation is currently hampered by a reliance on conventional clinical markers of retinopathy progression that typically change slowly. Furthermore, accurate stratification of study participants according to risk of progression is of great importance to the conduct of clinical trials of novel therapies for diabetic retinopathy.

A Practical Manual of Diabetic Retinopathy Management, Second Edition.
Edited by Peter Scanlon, Ahmed Sallam, and Peter van Wijngaarden.
© 2017 John Wiley & Sons Ltd. Published 2017 by John Wiley & Sons Ltd.
Companion Website: www.wiley.com/go/scanlon/diabetic_retinopathy

Genetic risk profiling and the role of epigenetics

The genetics of diabetic retinopathy are complex and little understood at present, and this currently poses a barrier to personalised genetic risk profiling. It is clear that diabetic retinopathy is a multifactorial, heterogeneous disorder and progress in the field of gene discovery has been hampered by relatively small sample sizes, and sample heterogeneity associated with a lack of phenotypic standardisation within and between studies[5]. Accurate phenotyping of retinopathy status and clinical risk factors is an important prerequisite to progress in this field that is likely to be aided significantly by the wide-scale adoption of digital health records and archiving of serial digital retinal photos. As has been the case in fruitful genetic studies of diabetic nephropathy, the establishment of large multicentre genetic consortia, utilising standardised approaches to phenotyping and study protocols is key[5–7]. Equally, the judicious application of state-of-the-art genetic technologies, including next-generation sequencing and exome sequencing, is likely to be important in unravelling the complex genetic determinants of retinopathy risk.

It has long been known that gene–environment interactions, manifest as epigenetic changes, have a major bearing on the risk of diabetic retinopathy. Interest has focused on unravelling the epigenetic basis of metabolic memory (Box 17.1) as therapeutic modulation of metabolic memory may profoundly alter risks of developing the complications of diabetes, including retinopathy. Furthermore, understanding the enduring effects of early glycaemic control is also likely to be important in the design of clinical trials of new therapeutic agents, as the recruitment of subjects who are inherently predisposed to progression despite improvements in metabolic parameters is likely to confound trial outcomes. It is speculated that metabolic memory may be a factor contributing to the low success of translating of therapeutics with strong pre-clinical results to favourable performance in clinical trials[8]. While epigenetic mechanisms in diabetes are not completely characterised, evidence suggests that hyperglycaemia induces histone modifications, alterations in DNA methylation and the expression of non-coding RNAs, which may have enduring effects on the expression of genes implicated in the complications of diabetes, including retinopathy[9,10].

The identification of the epigenetic basis of metabolic memory as well as other epigenetic changes that contribute to the pathogenesis of diabetic retinopathy may open new therapeutic pathways. For example, the progression of diabetic retinopathy has been associated with the acetylation of histones in retina and the use of minocycline, a non-specific acetylation inhibitor, has been shown to reduce early signs of retinopathy in diabetic rodents[11]. Moreover, expression of inflammatory mediators by retinal Müller cells during culture in high-glucose medium was reduced by histone acetyltransferase inhibitors and by activators of histone deacetylases[11]. Histone methylation is also considered to play a central role in the complications of diabetes[12]. Other *in vitro* work has identified an epigenetic basis for glucose-induced upregulation of the pro-inflammatory transcription factor NF-κB with increased expression of vascular adhesion molecules (VCAM-1) and chemokines (MCP-1) that are known to play roles in the pathogenesis of diabetic retinopathy[13].

Epigenetic changes in diabetes have also been linked with reactive oxygen species (ROS) and advanced glycation end-products[12,13]. Accordingly, antioxidants may have a role in preventing epigenetic changes that occur in diabetes[14]. The underwhelming responses seen in clinical trials of non-specific antioxidants in diabetes point to the need for selective targeting of key ROS producers and the bolstering of appropriate antioxidant defences[15]. Numerous studies have identified associations between altered microRNA (miRNA) expression and diabetic complications, including retinopathy[16–18]. miRNAs are small, non-coding RNAs that modify gene expression by binding complementary mRNA sequences and triggering mRNA degradation – through cleavage or destabilisation – or reduced translational efficiency. miRNA profiles may serve as biomarkers of retinopathy risk and may be of value for therapeutic purposes: selective expression or inhibition of miRNAs known to regulate key genes in the pathogenesis of diabetic retinopathy may be powerful tools in delaying or preventing retinopathy[8]. Advances in miRNA expression profiling mean that this will soon become a standard biomarker in population studies of diabetic retinopathy, and may well have utility for individual risk prediction[19].

Box 17.1: Metabolic memory

Metabolic memory refers to a phenomenon whereby the level of glycaemic control during a critical period, typically soon after the onset of diabetes, sets a rheostat for the risk of developing complications of the disease that appears to be relatively independent of the intensity of glycaemic control once this rheostat has been set[20]. Follow-up studies of several large clinical trials, including the Diabetes Control and Complications Trial (DCCT) and the UK Prospective Diabetes Study (UKPDS), provide compelling evidence of this effect[21–23]. The Epidemiology of Diabetes, Interventions and Complications (EDIC) study followed DCCT trial participants with T1DM to assess the effects of prior DCCT randomisation to intensive versus conventional control on the development of complications. Despite rapid convergence of glycaemic control and maintenance of similar levels over the ensuing 20 years, the cumulative incidence of retinopathy continued to diverge for at least the first 10 years of study, with an overall hazard reduction of 56% in subjects randomised to intensive control in the DCCT, relative to those in the conventional control group[21,22]. Similarly, of subjects with T2DM followed for 10 years after cessation of the UKPDS, subjects randomised to the intensive glycaemic control group maintained a lower risk of microvascular complications (composite measure) than those randomised to conventional control, despite the early loss of glycaemic differences between the groups[23].

Blood and ocular fluid biomarkers

In addition to miRNA profiling, numerous studies have identified alterations in a range of peripheral blood and ocular fluid biomarkers. Serum markers of inflammation and vascular endothelial cell dysfunction including retinol-binding protein 4, advanced glycation end-products, laminin, homocysteine and vascular cell adhesion molecules have been associated with diabetic retinopathy in a number of studies[24]. High-sensitivity c-reactive protein has been associated with risk of diabetic macular oedema in an analysis of biomarkers in stored samples from participants in the Diabetes Complications and Control Trial (DCCT), consistent with the known role of inflammation in the pathogenesis of this complication[25]. Interestingly, no associations were found between macular oedema and serum levels of vascular cell adhesion molecules (VCAM-1) and a pro-inflammatory cytokine (TNF-alpha) in the DCCT study[25]. Another study of high-sensitivity c-reactive protein found a positive association between levels of the factor and risk of proliferative diabetic retinopathy in subjects with T1DM; however, this association was non-significant in multivariate analysis[26]. Similarly, lipid and lipoprotein levels have been associated with retinopathy risk in a number of cross-sectional and longitudinal studies, but as yet no marker or combination of markers has sufficient predictive value at the level of individual subjects[8,27–29].

Endothelial progenitor cells comprise a low-frequency population of circulating bone-marrow-derived cells that home to sites of vascular injury and contribute to vascular repair[30]. Emerging evidence suggests that EPC numbers are reduced in diabetes, due in part to the effects of peripheral neuropathy on bone marrow. EPC function is also thought to be reduced in diabetes. Accordingly, reductions in EPC numbers and functional impairments have been proposed as potential biomarkers portending risk of poor outcomes for diabetic macular oedema and proliferative retinopathy[30]. Further characterisation of EPC number and function in diabetes and correlation of these parameters with retinopathy is required to assess the value of these cells as biomarkers of retinopathy.

Ocular fluid biomarkers may have some advantages over peripheral blood biomarkers in that they may more closely reflect changes occurring in the retinal microenvironment. Several small studies have identified associations between diabetic retinopathy and changes in tear protein composition (proteome), in the glycosylation of tear proteins and in tear inflammatory markers (TNF-α)[31–33]. Similarly, a number of small case-control studies have variously identified increases in aqueous humour levels of pro-inflammatory cytokines, markers of Müller cell activation and pro-angiogenic factors (angiopoietin-like 4, VEGF and placental growth factor) and downregulation of angiogenesis inhibitors (semaphorin 3E) in subjects with diabetic retinopathy relative to non-diabetic controls. Small sample sizes make it difficult to assess the potential of tear and aqueous humour biomarkers in diabetic retinopathy.

Numerous studies have examined vitreous biomarkers of diabetic retinopathy. A systematic review of these studies identified 12 biomarkers of proliferative diabetic retinopathy, including increased levels of pro-angiogenic factors (VEGF, erythropoietin, platelet-derived growth factor-BB), inflammatory mediators (interleukins 6 and 8; monocyte chemoattractant protein-1; transforming growth factor beta) as well as endothelin-1 and nitric oxide[34]. Vitreous levels of hepatocyte growth factor and the endogenous anti-angiogenic agent, pigment epithelium-derived factor, were reduced. It is postulated that the vitreous sampling for biomarker profiling at the time of intravitreal injection, as is commonly done to administer anti-VEGF or corticosteroid therapies, or at vitrectomy, could be used to identify the key pathogenic pathways that are active in a given individual and use this knowledge to personalise therapy[34].

There are presently no widely validated blood or ocular fluid diabetic retinopathy biomarkers beyond HbA1c. Barriers to the utility of peripheral blood biomarkers stem from the fact that they are subject to regulation by multiple factors and that, in many cases, peripheral levels of biomarkers implicated in the pathogenesis of diabetic retinopathy do not reflect local levels in the retina. While ocular fluids may more closely recapitulate the retinal microenvironment, the sampling of aqueous and vitreous humour is invasive and impractical for early disease that does not otherwise warrant invasive ocular procedures. The prospective validation of biomarkers is complicated by the long time necessary to observe retinopathy progression in clinical studies. In addition, many biomarkers that have proven useful at a population level have limited utility at the individual level[24]. The biomarker field is evolving rapidly and novel markers, such as exosomes (small vesicular structures released by cells and which carry cargo including nucleic acids and proteins, which recapitulate the intracellular environment of the cell of origin), are likely to emerge in diabetic retinopathy in coming years[35]. Despite existing barriers, it is likely that panels of validated biomarkers will be developed for retinopathy risk prediction, and these panels will most likely include a spectrum of marker types and utilise high-throughput technologies. Moreover, comprehensive risk profiling will likely include advanced clinical imaging and genetic testing as well as environmental risk factor modelling. As complex as this may seem, such approaches to diabetic retinopathy risk modelling are likely to be adopted in the not-too-distant future.

Retinal biomarkers

Developments in imaging technologies are allowing much more precise clinical phenotyping of diabetic retinopathy than ever before. Semi-automated retinal image analysis systems are currently capable of measuring retinal vascular calibres as well as a wide range of higher-order vascular parameters, such as fractal dimension (a measure of the complexity of a branching network), tortuosity and branch angle[36]. Moreover, functional imaging techniques, including flicker light-induced retinal vasodilation, provide measures of neurovascular coupling, and reductions in arteriolar and venular dilation appear to be correlated with the severity of diabetic retinopathy[37,38]. While significant associations have been identified with a range of these vascular parameters at a population level, including retinal arteriolar narrowing and venular dilation, no parameter has yet proven to be of value for retinopathy risk stratification for individual subjects[36]. Changes in retinal microaneurysm counts and distribution have also been proposed as biomarkers of risk of retinopathy progression in diabetes[24,39,40], and clinical studies using computer-assisted microanuerysm tracking have identified associations between high microaneurysm turnover and diabetic macular oedema, as well as its response to anti-VEGF treatment[41,42]. The broader utility of this measure of diabetic retinopathy risk is still to be established. Other work has identified abnormal multifocal electroretinogram (mfERG) recordings, namely prolonged implicit time, as a marker of diabetic retinal neuronal degeneration that may be predictive of retinopathy severity[24,43,44]. One of the objectives of a multicentre clinical study of neuroprotective agents in diabetic retinopathy (EUROCONDOR) is the validation of mfERG as a predictive marker of retinopathy severity[45].

As previously discussed (Chapter 5 on Imaging Techniques), the advent of ultra-widefield retinal fluorescein angiography has allowed more complete appreciation of the extent of peripheral retinal non-perfusion in patients than was previously possible with conventional angiography[46]. Given the clearly established associations between retinal non-perfusion and hypoxia-induced angiogenesis, it is likely that more complete evaluation of the extent of retinal non-perfusion afforded by ultra-widefield angiography will have value in predicting risk of proliferative retinopathy[46,47]. Associations between peripheral non-perfusion and diabetic macular oedema appear to be more complex than was previously thought[47]. While it is apparent that ultra-widefield angiography is likely to have an important role in the management of diabetic retinopathy, large clinical studies are required to establish exactly what that role will be.

A number of new and emerging retinal imaging techniques allow quantification of retinal blood flow and retinal oxygen tension, potentially providing additional prognostic value for diabetic retinopathy. Scanning laser Doppler flowmetry and the newer Doppler OCT enable a qualitative and quantitative analysis of retinal blood flow[48,49]. In addition, multispectral and hyperspectral imaging technologies are being applied to clinical retinal oximetry (Figs 17.1, 17.2). Hyperspectral imaging is a technique that was developed for remote sensing that has been widely applied in satellite imaging and a host of industrial applications. In hyperspectral retinal imaging, the absorption and scatter of light at each point in the retina is measured across a wide range of illuminating wavelengths extending beyond the visible spectrum[50]. Multispectral imaging utilises a narrower range of illuminating wavelengths[51]. A spectral signature that is indicative of tissue composition is therefore measured for each retinal point. *In vivo* retinal oximetry is possible with this technique as oxygenated and deoxygenated haemoglobin have

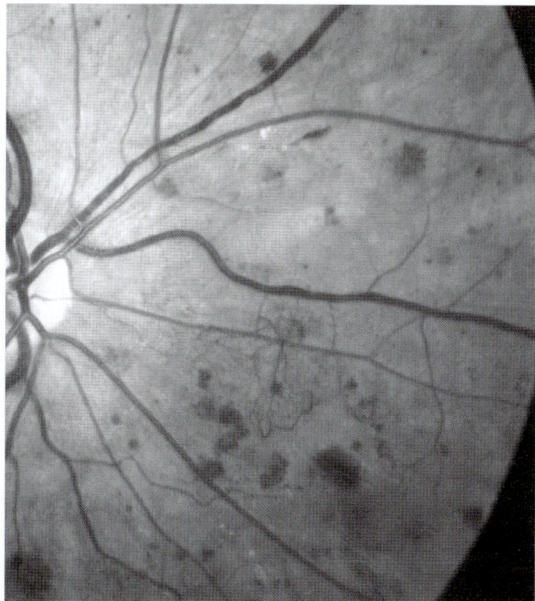

Fig. 17.1 Red-free image of NVE in nasal retina.

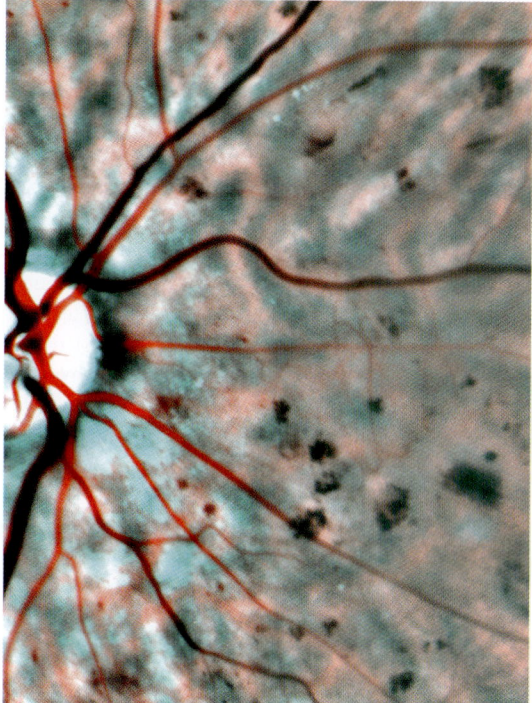

Fig. 17.2 Hyperspectral image showing high venular blood oxygenation in areas of the retina where new vessels have grown.

distinctive spectral signatures, meaning that is it possible to acquire highly accurate, spatially resolved oximetry data[52,53]. It is likely that retinal blood flow and oximetry measurements will become standard imaging techniques with roles in the stratification of risk of retinopathy progression. Further studies are needed to define the place of these imaging methods in clinical practice.

TIMELY DETECTION OF DIABETIC RETINOPATHY

The advent of non-mydriatic retinal photography and the falling price of cameras mean that retinal photography is increasingly attractive for diabetic retinopathy screening. Cost reductions will likely translate to increased uptake of screening as the positioning of cameras at locations of greater convenience for people with diabetes increases screening uptake. Mobile phones have growing roles in medical diagnostics[54–56]. Advances in smartphone camera technology are such that some mobile imaging platforms already appear to have sufficient capability for diabetic retinopathy screening[57,58]. In one study, mydriatic four-field smartphone photography had high sensitivity and specificity both for the detection of any retinopathy (92.7% and 98.4%) as well as sight-threatening retinopathy (87.9% and 94.9%), with high levels of agreement with conventional seven-field photography (kappa 0.9)[57]. A study of another smartphone retinal photography system demonstrated a high level of agreement with slit-lamp biomicroscopy for diabetic retinopathy grading (kappa 0.78) and high sensitivity and specificity for the detection of macular oedema (81% and 98%, respectively) relative to biomicroscopy. Smartphone retinal photography systems and other low-cost portable retinal cameras are likely to have major impacts on diabetic retinopathy screening in low-resource and remote areas.

Further improvements in lens and illumination systems may mean that smartphone users may one day image their own retinas and wirelessly upload them for remote assessment. Such advances would make it possible for individuals to closely monitor the progression of their own retinopathy. The analysis of data from large numbers of retinal image series could facilitate the identification of clinical biomarkers of risk of progression[24].

Remote grading is increasingly used in retinopathy screening to facilitate high-throughput retinal photography and ensure quality-controlled grading.

A variety of automated retinal image analysis systems are already available and others are in development[59–61]. State-of-the-art systems have demonstrated high sensitivity and moderate specificity for the classification of retinopathy severity[59]. Further advances in image analytics and the application of increasingly sophisticated artificial intelligence systems are likely to see computer-assisted grading become the norm for diabetic retinopathy screening. Automated retinal image analysis systems may offer advantages of cost-effectiveness, quality assurance and high throughput. This technology could have tremendous utility when coupled with next-generation smartphone retinal photography. Integration of user-operated retinal screening with electronic health records would facilitate timely follow-up for treatable retinopathy and could automatically flag progressive disease to members of the healthcare team, going some way towards closing the loop between the screening episode and definitive clinical care.

TREATMENT OPTIONS

Personalised treatments are likely to play a central role in the future management of diabetic retinopathy. It is increasingly apparent that diabetic retinopathy is a complex disease with multiple interacting mechanisms, some of which predominate in some individuals and not in others. Moreover, it is likely that these mechanisms vary considerable over the course of the disease, such that therapeutic interventions may need to be tailored accordingly. Genetic studies and biomarker profiles are likely to be important in identifying the optimal therapies for a given individual at a given time. Advances in biomarker profiling and the development of many new therapies mean that truly personalised treatment for diabetic retinopathy is foreseeable. While a detailed account of all of the new agents under development is beyond the scope of this text, key illustrative examples are provided to highlight what the future of diabetic retinopathy therapy may entail.

Anti-angiogenic therapies

The tremendous success of the anti-VEGF agents in the management of diabetic macular oedema and proliferative retinopathy has fuelled great interest from the pharmaceutical industry in generating even more effective, longer-lasting agents. The development of many of these drugs has run in parallel with their development for choroidal neovascularisation in age-related macular degeneration and in tumour angiogenesis, as the final common pathway of neovascularisation and vascular hyperpermeability in these disparate diseases share much in common. While VEGF plays a central role in diabetic retinal neovascularisation and vascular hyperpermeability, it is one of many angiogenic factors upregulated in the disease. Indeed, in health retinal angiogenesis is kept in check by a balance in the expression of endogenous pro-angiogenic and anti-angiogenic agents. The fact that a significant proportion of people with diabetic macular oedema are incompletely responsive to anti-VEGF therapy suggests that factors other than VEGF predominate in these individuals[62]. Future anti-angiogenic therapies for diabetic retinopathy are likely to be personally tailored and will typically target more than one factor. Inhibitors of pro-angiogenic factors, their receptors and signalling cascades will likely be administered in combination with drugs that augment the expression or action of endogenous anti-angiogenic agents. A case in point is the bispecific monoclonal antibody against angiopoietin-2 and VEGF that is currently undergoing clinical evaluation in cancer[63]. Bispecific antibodies are engineered such that each of the two antigen-binding domains has specificity for a different target antigen, in this case the pro-angiogenic factors VEGF and angiopoietin-2[64].

The burdensome requirement for intravitreal injections of anti-VEGF agents, as often as monthly for extended periods, has driven innovation in the development of long-acting therapies. Examples include a long-acting, single-chain antibody fragment with specificity for VEGF (RTH258) that is currently in phase III clinical trials for choroidal neovascularisation with a 3-month maintenance dosing interval[65]. Another longer-acting anti-VEGF agent at a similar stage in clinical trials for AMD and diabetic macular oedema is the darpin, abicipar pegol[66]. Clinical trials of gene therapies targeting VEGF via the expression of the soluble receptor sFLT-1 in AMD, via intravitreal (AAV2-sFLT01) or subretinal injection (AVA-101) are also well underway[67,68]. Another trial of subretinal injection of a lentiviral vector expressing the endogenous anti-angiogenic factors endostatin and angiostatin (RetinoStat) is underway in patients with AMD[69]. The translation of these gene therapy approaches to the management of diabetic retinopathy seems unlikely in the immediate future, as the potential harms of long-term VEGF suppression in relatively young patients may obviate the advantages of less frequent administration[70].

A range of topically administered small-molecule angiogenesis inhibitors are also undergoing clinical trials.

These include: squalamine lactate, an inhibitor of multiple angiogenic factors including VEGF, that is in clinical trials for proliferative diabetic retinopathy and diabetic macular oedema[71]; regorafenib, a multiple receptor tyrosine kinase inhibitor that inhibits the downstream signalling of VEGF receptor 2 and Tie2 (angiopoieitin-2 receptor) that is in clinical trials for AMD[72]; and PAN-90806, a small-molecule, selective VEGF receptor antagonist, that is in clinical trials for proliferative diabetic retinopathy[73].

The desire to avoid frequently repeated intravitreal injections has also driven technological innovation in the field of drug delivery. A range of novel anti-angiogenic drug-delivery methods, ranging from biodegradable thermoresponsive polymers to nanoparticle carriers and encapsulated cell technology implants containing retinal pigment epithelial cells that express soluble VEGF receptor for prolonged periods[74–76] are also under investigation.

Targeting key pathogenic pathways

New therapies for diabetic retinopathy that target the molecular pathways implicated in the pathogenesis of the disease are likely to be widely available in future[77]. Targets include both pathogenic processes (retinal inflammation, oxidative stress) and signalling molecules (advanced glycation end-products, vascular cell adhesion molecules and extracellular matrix molecules)[8,78,79]. Attempts at clinical translation of many such agents have failed in the past after promising pre-clinical studies. For example, systemic administration of infliximab, a monoclonal antibody with specificity for tumour necrosis factor-α, appeared to be effective in a small study of subjects with refractory diabetic macular oedema; however, a subsequent pilot study of intravitreal infliximab was associated with high rates of intraocular inflammation (uveitis)[80,81]. Similarly, the receptor tyrosine kinase inhibitor, ruboxistaurin, and an advanced glycation end-product inhibitor, aminoguanidine, failed at clinical trial stage due a lack of efficacy and adverse effects, respectively[82,83]. Advances in our understanding of the intricacies of diabetic retinopathy pathogenesis will inform a more nuanced approach to these novel therapeutic targets. As a case in point, the identification of key isoforms of the ROS-generating enzyme NADPH oxidase in diabetic nephropathy and retinopathy and the efficacy of a small-molecule, selective inhibitor of these isoforms (GKT137831) in a pre-clinical retinopathy model reinvigorates interest in antioxidant therapies[84]. Clinical studies of this drug in diabetic nephropathy are underway[85].

Retinal neuroprotection

Increasing awareness of retinal neuronal injury in diabetes and the interplay between neurons, glia and blood vessels (the 'neurovascular unit') has focused attention on neuroprotective therapies. Somatostatin has been identified as a potential neuroprotectant; it is down-regulated in diabetes and exogenous administration of the factor is neuroprotective in a pre-clinical rodent model of retinopathy[86]. Somatostatin is thought to minimise glutamate-induced excitotoxicity and neuronal apoptosis[78]. Brimonidine, an α2-adrenergic agonist, has long been recognised as having neuroprotective properties, possibly mediated through the regulation of retinal ganglion cell apoptosis[87]. A multicentre clinical trial of topical somatostatin and brimonidine in diabetic retinal neuroprotection is underway. Similarly metformin, a commonly used oral hypoglycaemic agent used in T2DM, is increasingly recognised as neuroprotective and vasoprotective[88]. These and other neuroprotective factors[78] may be used therapeutically by people with diabetic retinopathy in future.

Laser treatment

Laser photocoagulation has long been the mainstay of diabetic retinopathy treatment. While improved medical management of diabetes and diabetic retinopathy are already supplanting laser photocoagulation for diabetic macular oedema, it is likely that peripheral scatter laser photocoagulation will continue to be the treatment of choice for proliferative retinopathy until such time as regenerative therapies can restore retinal perfusion, or until chronic anti-angiogenic therapies are demonstrated to be superior to laser treatment. Navigated laser systems that incorporate gaze tracking and image registration to allow superimposition of the angiogram onto the live retinal image, as well as treatment preplanning, offer greater convenience and precision[89]. Studies suggest that this improved precision is associated with better control of diabetic macular oedema and a lower requirement for re-treatment and anti-VEGF therapy[90,91]. Large multicentre studies are necessary to validate these findings.

Recently developed sub-threshold micropulse laser systems may offer greater relative selectivity to the retinal pigment epithelium than conventional laser, reportedly with similar therapeutic efficacy for macular laser[92]. Larger studies of micropulse laser treatment are needed to draw robust conclusions on this and on its role in peripheral scatter photocoagulation[93]. Moreover, further insights into the mechanisms of laser treatments are warranted. Interestingly, the application of a small number of low-energy nanosecond laser spots to the peripheral macula of subjects with drusen has been associated with a remodelling response that led to drusen clearance and a reduction in Bruch's membrane thickness[94]. While these findings are not directly applicable to diabetic retinopathy, it could be envisaged that the use of laser therapy to promote extracellular matrix remodelling may have therapeutic utility in diabetic retinopathy.

Regenerative therapies

Endothelial progenitor cells are endogenous stem-like cells that ordinarily serve roles in vascular repair, including in the retina[30,95]. Several research groups have proposed harnessing the reparative capacity of these cells in diabetic retinopathy[30]. Work is underway to identify the most appropriate cell type for retinal vascular repair and some suggest that endothelial colony-forming cells, otherwise known as outgrowth endothelial cells, may have the ideal attributes. Potential approaches to retinal vascular regeneration could involve the isolation of EPCs from peripheral blood using conventional cell-sorting technologies (flow cytometry or immunomagnetic bead selection) for *ex vivo* expansion in culture prior to cell characterisation and administration, either to the donor (autologous transplantation) or to a new host (allogeneic transplantation). While intravitreal administration may be possible, the potential for multisystem vascular repair makes systemic administration an attractive option[30]. Measures to enhance EPC homing to the retinal vasculature may also be necessary for optimal repair. In addition, optimisation of systemic metabolic control at the time of engraftment and in the early post-graft period are likely to be needed to maximise the likelihood of successful therapy. Co-administration of pericyte progenitor cells may also be important – pericytes are lost from blood vessels in the early stages of diabetic retinopathy and the association of endothelial cells with pericytes is a key step in the stabilisation of nascent blood vessels[30,96,97]. An alternative approach may be to stimulate EPC niches, chiefly in bone marrow, to enhance endogenous circulating EPC levels[30]. While there is still much work to be done in validating these approaches, regenerative therapies hold great promise for vascular repair in diabetic retinopathy.

ELECTRONIC MEDICAL RECORDS, CLOUD COMPUTING AND BIG DATA

Widespread adoption of computerised medical records and the utilisation of cloud computing resources is the way of the future of healthcare. Digital records allow for standardised collection of key data, such as diabetic retinopathy screening outcomes, and for almost instantaneous sharing with members of the healthcare team. In an increasingly complex health environment, the centralisation of medical records is pivotal to co-ordinated and comprehensive care. The exponential growth in medical data, due to the increasing complexity of medical tests and the popularity of wearable fitness trackers and health recording technology, presents a tremendous opportunity for detailed environmental modelling and risk profiling. Analysis of the huge resultant datasets poses significant computing challenges. Artificial intelligence computing systems and image analytics platforms, such as IBM's Watson Health and Apple's Research Kit, are set to revolutionise health data analysis[98,99]. Accordingly, computer-assisted clinical decision-making will be inevitable if the clinician is to make sense of the vast array of biometric and health data that will soon be available. Such systems will facilitate the implementation of contemporary evidence-based medicine in an individualised manner for optimal health outcomes. Advances in medical diagnostic and imaging systems and more informed health consumers will mean that many consumers will play much more active roles in their own healthcare. The ubiquity of mobile computing technology and expanding wireless internet access will make the digital health community truly global. There is no doubt that security in the digital health age will be of great importance. Defining the limits of artificial intelligence will be an ongoing and significant societal challenge.

CONCLUSION

In the blur of technological advancement that is transforming the detection and management of diabetic retinopathy it is crucial for clinicians, and patients alike, not to lose sight of the fundamental importance of controlling the key systemic risk factors for diabetes complications: hyperglycaemia, hypertension, dyslipidaemia, physical inactivity and smoking. Controlling these factors remains the most effective means we currently have of preventing the development and progression of microvascular and macrovascular complications of diabetes. This is particularly true as our ability to effectively manage the ophthalmic complications of diabetes continue to improve; treating retinopathy is just one of many priorities in comprehensive diabetes care.

REFERENCE

Please visit www.wiley.com/go/scanlon/diabetic_retinopathy

18 Other retinal conditions in diabetes

Stephen J. Aldington & Peter H. Scanlon

[1]Gloucestershire Hospitals NHS Foundation Trust, UK; University of Warwick Medical School, UK
[2]Harris Manchester College, University of Oxford; Medical Ophthalmology, University of Gloucestershire, UK

HYPERTENSION

Systemic hypertension is all too frequently co-existent with diabetes mellitus, meaning that it is often difficult or impossible to clearly differentiate which is the cause of a particular retinal lesion. To further complicate the matter, many of the observable early retinal changes caused by systemic hypertension, such as arterial sclerosis and changes to arteriovenous crossing points, are very similar to those found in the common ageing processes. In younger patients it can usually be assumed that visible arteriolar narrowing and attenuation are likely to be hypertensive in origin, whereas in older patients this may not be so clear cut.

Hypertensive retinopathy shares several common lesions with diabetic retinopathy, principally retinal haemorrhage, cotton wool spots, hard exudates and apparent vascular occlusions. Microaneurysms, intraretinal microvascular abnormalities (IRMA) and venous beading are not, however, features commonly associated with hypertension. In the absence of widespread 'dot and blot' retinopathy, hypertensive retinopathy can usually be differentiated as nerve-fibre layer 'streak' or 'flame-shaped' haemorrhages frequently surrounding and pointing towards the optic disc and associated (nerve-fibre layer) cotton wool spots, also surrounding the optic disc. The presence of these features, when observed with co-existent widespread arteriolar constriction, is usually associated with prolonged chronic exposure to systemic hypertension.

In acute systemic hypertension however, while the major retinal arterioles are usually relatively unaffected, there is almost always a far more aggressive microvascular manifestation with severe flame- and even deep retinal haemorrhage, widespread peripapillary cotton wool spots and the presence of middle layer hard exudates. It is not uncommon to also observe quite marked swelling of the optic nerve head in these cases and, in its most severe manifestation, hard exudate development and coalescence in the form of a partial or full hypertensive macular exudate star.

Case History 18.1: Malignant hypertension

A 46-year-old man presented to eye clinic with blurring of vision in his right eye with visual acuities of right 3/60 (1.3 LogMAR), left 6/9 (0.1 LogMAR). He was incorrectly diagnosed but presented to eye clinic 3 days later with a drop in vision in his left eye and VAs of right 3/60 (1.3 LogMAR), left 3/60 (1.3 LogMAR). His retinal photographs appear slightly out of focus (Fig. 18.1a, b) due to the oedema in the disc and macular area with subretinal fluid on OCT in both macular areas (Fig. 18.1k, l). His blood pressure was 230/140 and this was gradually brought under control by the physicians and his retinal appearance improved. As the oedema cleared, exudates formed in both macular areas (Fig. 18.1c, d, m, n). It took approximately 6 weeks (Fig. 18.1e, f) for the subretinal fluid to clear, with only a very small amount remaining in the right eye at 6 weeks (Fig. 18.1o, p), although his visual acuity had improved to 6/9 (0.1 LogMAR) in each eye by 2 weeks. The exudate gradually cleared with a small amount remaining after 6 months (Fig. 18.1g, h) and 12 months (Fig. 18.1i, j).

A Practical Manual of Diabetic Retinopathy Management, Second Edition.
Edited by Peter Scanlon, Ahmed Sallam, and Peter van Wijngaarden.
© 2017 John Wiley & Sons Ltd. Published 2017 by John Wiley & Sons Ltd.
Companion Website: www.wiley.com/go/scanlon/diabetic_retinopathy

Other retinal conditions in diabetes 229

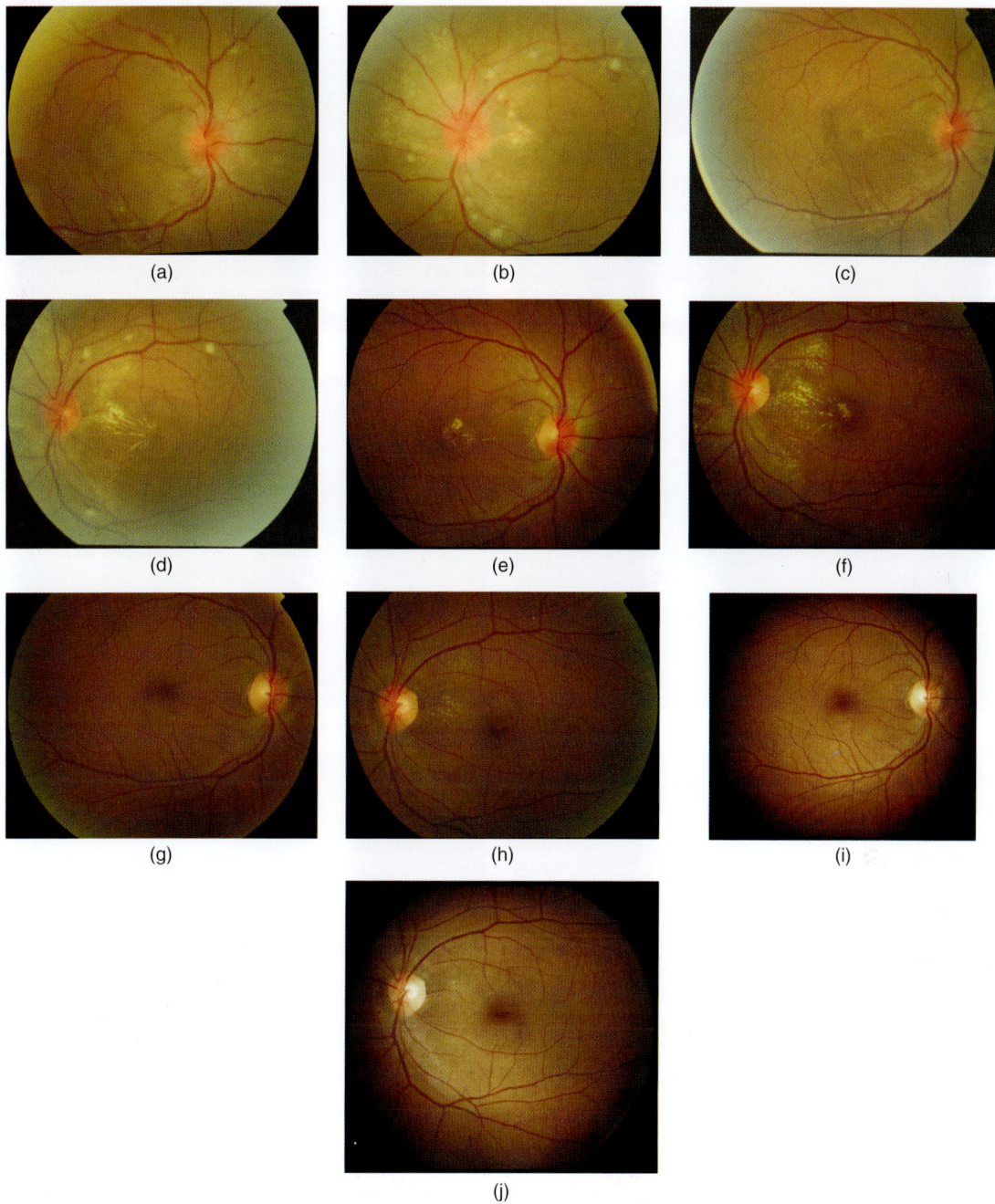

Fig. 18.1 Acute systemic hypertensive retinopathy: (a) right and (b) left eye day 1; (c) right and (d) left eye day 14; (e) right and (f) left eye 6 weeks; (g) right and (h) left eye 6 months; and (i) right and (j) left eye 12 months. OCT hypertensive retinopathy: (k) right and (l) left eye day 1; (m) right and (n) left eye day 14; (o) right and (p) left eye 6 weeks

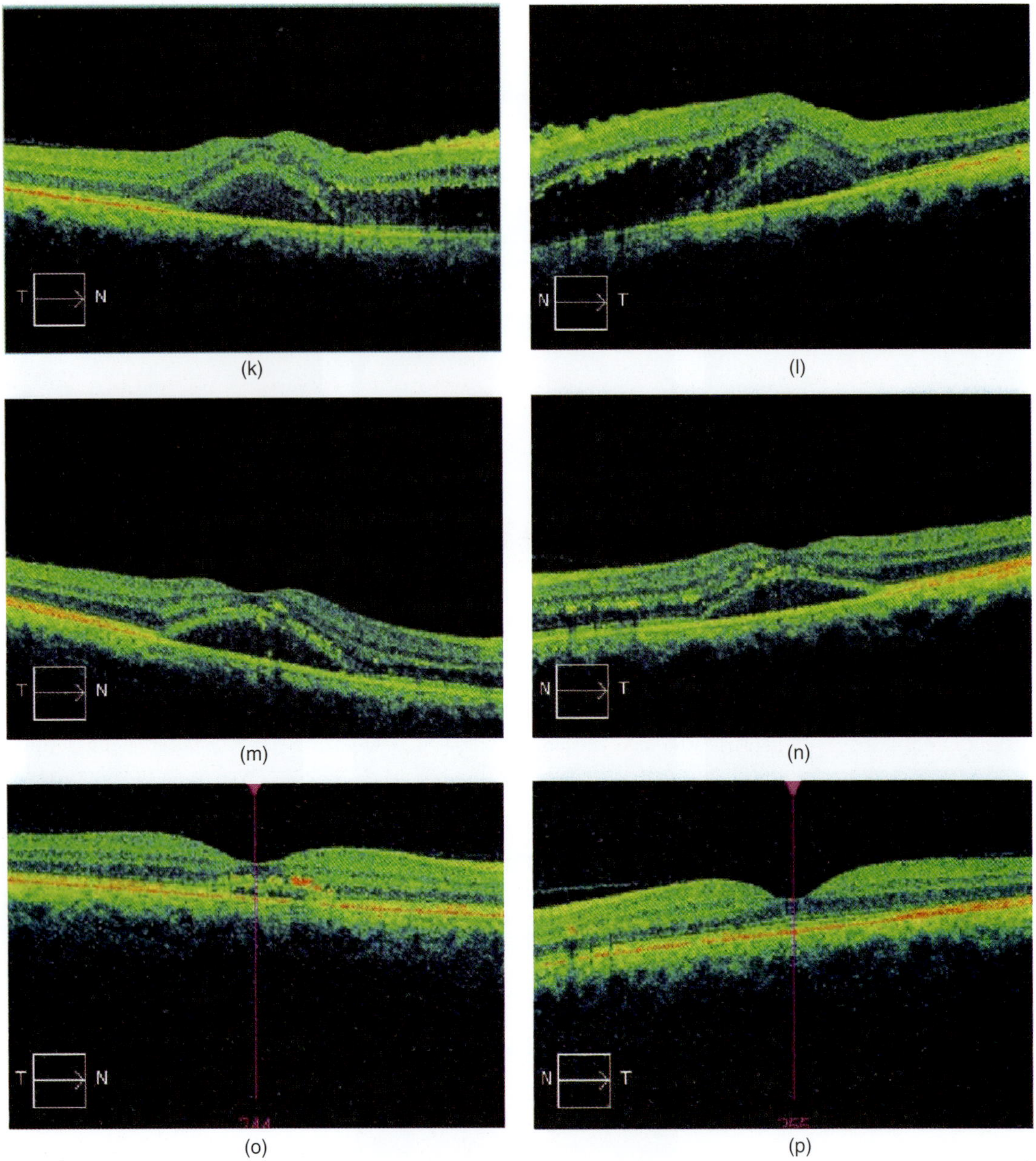

(k)

(l)

(m)

(n)

(o)

(p)

Fig. 18.1 (*Continued*)

RETINAL ARTERIAL OCCLUSIONS

The occlusion of a retinal artery can have acute, profound and long-lasting effects on visual function. When the occlusion is limited to a relatively small artery or arteriole, the damage and effect will be localised and indeed may not be sufficient to be symptomatic, at least not initially. Occlusion of larger arteries which deliver blood to quadrants or entire superior or inferior hemifields of the eye or, worse still, occlusion of the central retinal artery itself is always symptomatic and visual loss of some degree is usually inevitable.

Patients presenting with retinal arterial occlusions almost always do so complaining of just one affected eye (at that time). However, reoccurrence or subsequent occlusion of vessels in the fellow eye is common.

Clinical examination of the fundi and colour imaging are the common investigative techniques. Fluorescein angiography can be used although this is of little additional diagnostic value, particularly in cases of central retinal artery occlusion (CRAO). Fluorescein transit times would be significantly greater, if they can be assessed at all. Major arteries usually do become perfused to some degree eventually, although the majority of this is likely to come about through retrograde flow from the venous and capillary networks with little from residual direct arterial flow.

In all cases of vascular, particularly arterial, occlusion, a careful assessment of associated underlying systemic clinical conditions such as diabetes, temporal arteritis, hypertension or atherogenic diseases is necessary. Investigations such as full blood count, erythrocyte sedimentation rate, blood glucose and carotid ultrasonography are often indicated.

Case History 18.2: Arteriolar occlusion in diabetes associated with hypertension

This 65-year-old woman, with type 2 diabetes (diagnosed at age 59 years) controlled with tablets and a history of hypertension controlled with perindopril 8 mg o.d. and bendrofluazide 2.5 mg o.d., presented with a sudden onset of a blob in front of the central vision of her right eye and a visual acuity (VA) reduced to 6/24 (20/80 or logMAR 0.6). Figure 18.2a and b shows a colour photograph with a cotton wool spot on the superior aspect of the right macula and a fluorescein angiogram photograph taken at 57 s, showing some mild leakage of fluorescein from capillaries above the right fovea.

The cause of these changes is a small arteriolar occlusion leading to a small area of ischaemia, giving rise to the cotton wool spot demonstrated on the colour photograph. The cotton wool spot gradually cleared over the next 2 months, but unfortunately the vision remained at the reduced level of 6/24 (20/80 or logMAR 0.6).

Central retinal artery occlusion (CRAO)

Occlusion of the central retinal artery (CRAO) is most frequently caused by blockage of the artery by either local thrombosis or emboli originating from either the heart or carotid artery. Occlusion in younger adult patients, although less frequent, is more likely associated with cardiovascular instability while that occurring in the elderly population is more commonly associated with arteriosclerosis.

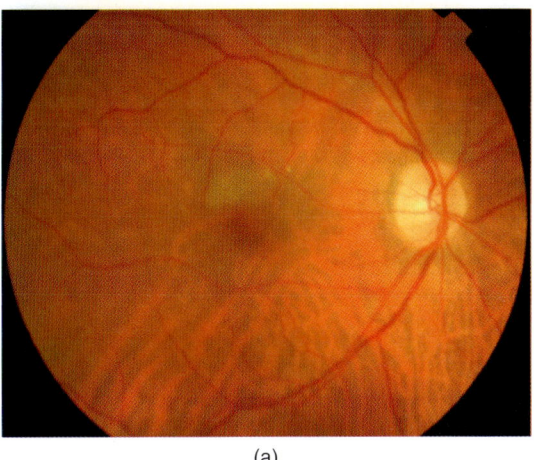
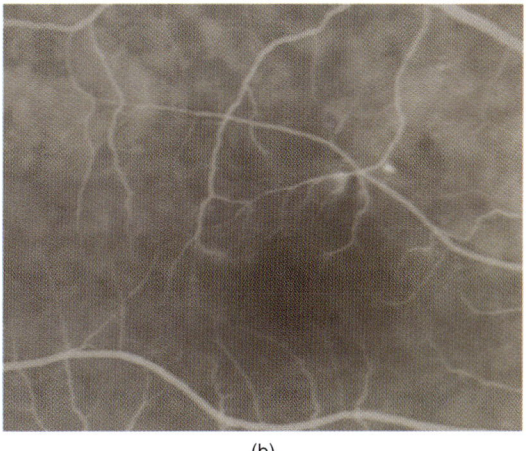

(a)   (b)

Fig. 18.2 (a) Colour photo right macular area showing CWS just above right central fovea due to small arteriolar occlusion. (b) Fluorescein right macular area 57 s after injection of dye.

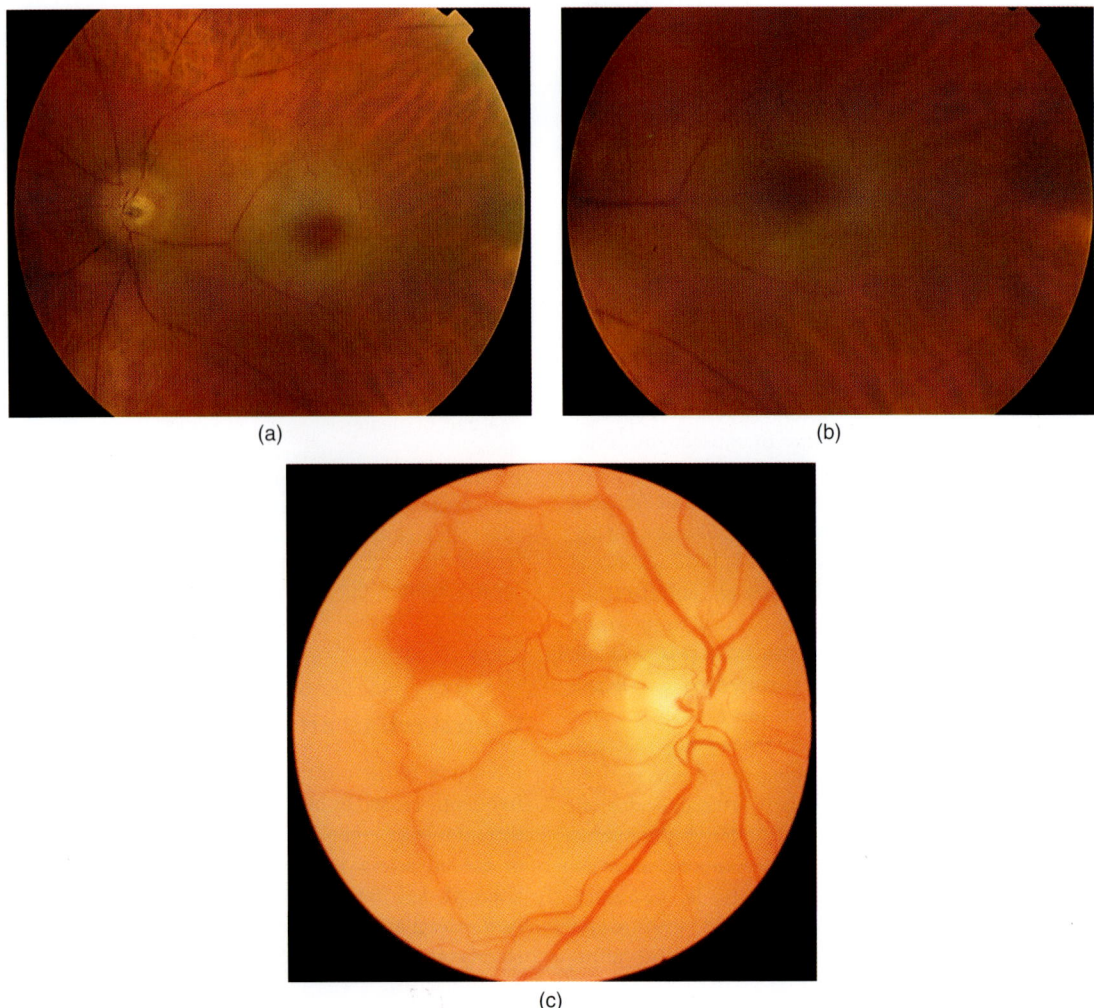

Fig. 18.3 (a) Central retinal artery occlusion. (b) Cherry red spot. (c) CRAO with a pre-existing cilioretinal artery supplying the macular region.

Occlusion of the central artery requires the blockage to have occurred in the retrobulbar region of the eye, before bifurcation of the central artery as it enters the visible globe. As such, the occlusion is in itself not visible to the examining observer. Much less frequently, CRAO is caused by vascular spasm of the artery itself, although this diagnosis is often controversial as rarely is a patient seen clinically while the spasm is occurring and indeed spontaneous return to normality is quite common. However relatively rare such cases of arterial spasms may be, recurrence is not uncommon and potential permanent occlusion is often the outcome, with resultant very severe visual loss in the affected eye.

Clinically, the appearance is one of a very pale yellowish retina, cloudy and with increased general opacity and gross swelling of and around the optic disc (Fig. 18.3a).

A classic characteristic of CRAO, however, is the often marked 'cherry-red spot', delineating the fovea. This is caused by the contrast between the redness of the still-patent choroidal capillary circulation serving the fovea against the whiteness of the totally occluded retinal arterial circulation in the surrounding region and the associated retinal oedema. Retinal arteries frequently appear thin and attenuated (Fig. 18.3b).

While total visual loss in an eye compromised by CRAO is not always inevitable the final outcome in that eye may, at best, be reduction of visual function to a level of simple perception of light. Indeed, such a reduction in visual function occurs very quickly, within minutes or certainly hours, of the actual arterial occlusion. Patients complain of visual loss in the affected eye which frequently takes the appearance of a total dimming and contraction of visual perception from the periphery towards the visual axis, usually over the course of just a few minutes. The longer a CRAO remains undiagnosed but potentially treatable, the greater the risk of permanent severe visual loss.

In some cases of CRAO, a significant amount of central vision may actually be retained due to the fortunate co-existence of one or more cilioretinal arteries. These are found in upwards of 15% or otherwise normal eyes. They are arterial vessels arising from the posterior ciliary circulation, that is, before the origination of the central retinal artery, and as such are independent of that retinal vascular supply route. If a pre-existing cilioretinal artery happens to supply the macular region, the patient may be fortunate enough to retain posterior pole blood supply and hence some macular function (Fig. 18.3c).

While acute CRAO can be diagnosed through sudden visual changes and by retinal examination of the affected eye, previously 'resolved' CRAO is often more difficult to diagnose on examination. Key visible features may include asymmetric vascular appearance between the affected and fellow eye, marked persistent attenuation of vessels in the affected eye and often a residual pale optic disc. Detection of lipid-like deposits along arterial walls is another not uncommon finding.

Branch retinal artery occlusion (BRAO)

As for the central retinal artery, there can be occlusion of a branch retinal artery (BRAO). As these occur in vessels within the visible retinal circulation, their point of actual occlusion can usually be determined and directly observed.

Small arteriolar branches, major branches, quadrants or indeed entire hemifields of the eye may be affected depending on the exact point of occlusion. In cases where the occlusion is caused by an embolus, the relative size of the embolus will usually determine how far along the retinal arteriolar circulation the blockage will occur. Local thrombosis or vessel wall-spasm-induced occlusions can however occur largely anywhere along the arterial tree.

On examination, the retinal appearance is dependent on the size of the arterial vessel compromised by the occlusion. Occlusions following the first or second bifurcations of the central retinal artery within the margins of the optic disc would affect an entire hemifield or one quadrant, respectively (Fig. 18.4a, b). More distal arterial occlusions would usually affect progressively smaller regions of the retinal circulation.

The classical appearance would be of marked whitening of the affected retinal region. Some smaller arterioles within affected areas may still appear to be patent, but this is due to retrograde filling of the end arterioles from the uncompromised venous circulation. The actual point of occlusion can often be clearly determined.

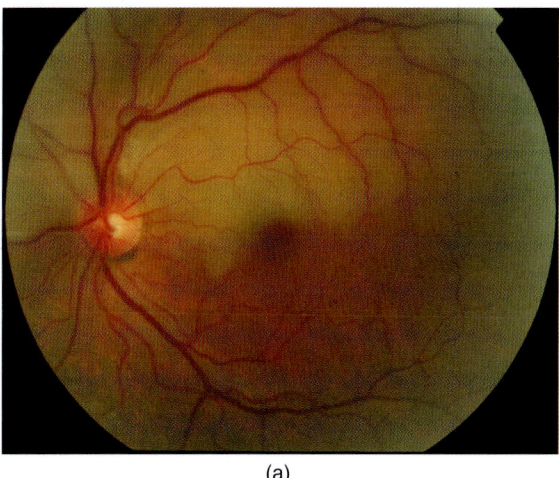
(a)

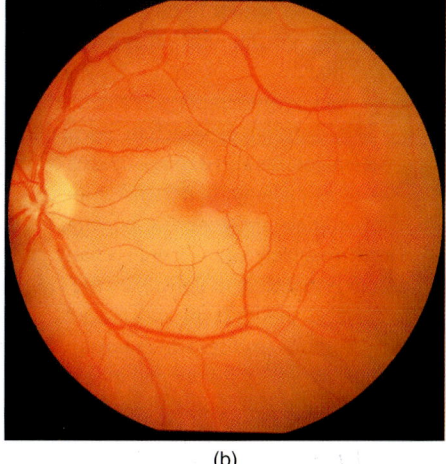
(b)

Fig. 18.4 (a) Left superior branch retinal artery occlusion. (b) Left infero-temporal branch retinal artery occlusion.

Arterial emboli

Circulating microemboli are relatively common. Should one of these find its way to the ocular circulation it will inevitably become trapped, frequently causing damage, and often it can be detected and imaged.

Emboli are formed from a variety of sources although cholesterol/fibrin or platelet emboli are by far the most common. Small emboli frequently travel considerable distances through the retinal arterial tree before lodging and causing a localised occlusion (Fig. 18.5a–f). Most emboli are asymptomatic and cause no noticeable visual defect, although transient uniocular or short-term visual loss is most likely to be embolitic in cause, even if the culprit is no longer detectable on examination.

Larger emboli can, and do of course, cause occlusion of major arterioles and arteries, with the effects on vision as noted in the preceding sections.

RETINAL VENOUS OCCLUSIONS

As diabetic retinopathy is classically associated with disease and early damage to the venous blood supply, incidence of retinal venous occlusions is higher in patients with diabetes than in age-matched non-diabetic persons. However, retinal vein occlusion, even in the non-diabetic population, is a common cause of retinal pathology and subsequent visual loss.

As for retinal arterial occlusions, the extent and severity of retinal damage in venous occlusions is largely dependent on the size of the vein occluded and whether partial or total occlusion has occurred. Retinal vein occlusions are most commonly seen affecting one or more quadrants of the eye and most commonly the superior or inferior temporal quadrant, but almost always affect only one eye at a single presentation.

The usual uniocular presentation of a patient with vein occlusion is a key criterion on which to base a differential diagnosis. Retinal lesions and damage caused by systemic conditions such as diabetes, hypertension or age-related macular degeneration are generally bilateral and affect both eyes with relatively equal vigour at any particular point in time. It is therefore not only the type and severity of lesions, but also the location and indeed absence of some abnormal retinal features which must be taken into account when arriving at a differential diagnosis.

In many cases of co-existent diabetic retinopathy and vein occlusion (particularly of a branch vein), it proves to be impossible to differentiate whether any particular retinal lesion or feature is likely to be caused by the effect of systemic diabetes or by localised venous occlusion. This is usually of little relevance in a clinical context, however.

It is important to note that venous occlusions are not caused by emboli; to do so, the embolus would have had to traverse the entire branching and reducing arterial system and cross through the capillary bed before affecting the venous side of the circulatory system.

Central retinal vein occlusion (CRVO)

Central retinal vein occlusion (CRVO) is a severe or total outflow obstruction to the main vein leaving the eye. This occurs out of sight of the observer and happens within the confines of the retrobulbar region of the optic disc. The acute and chronic damage done by a CRVO is, however, clearly visible.

In older patients, CRVO is commonly associated with diabetes, hypertension and arteriosclerosis. In some cases the entering central retinal artery, lying in close association to the leaving central retinal vein, can create sufficient pressure on the vein to cause a near- or total occlusion. In younger patients, occlusion is sometimes associated with systemic conditions such as sarcoidosis, Behçet's disease or a general phlebitis, causing an inflammatory response. In many case, particularly in the young, the exact cause remains unclear.

Severe or total occlusions affecting the central retinal vein have a marked appearance on clinical examination of the retina. Most common findings include large quantities of very dark red retinal haemorrhage surrounding the optic disc. These peripapillary haemorrhages are usually flame-shaped with their principal axis pointing to the centre of the optic disc as they are haemorrhages involving the superficial, nerve-fibre layer. Moving outwards towards the retinal periphery, the appearance is of large numbers and clusters of deep dark blot haemorrhages, indicating substantial damage also to the deeper retinal layers. Multiple retinal infarcts and ischaemic retina can usually also be seen and gross venous engorgement is commonplace. Should the macular region actually be visible (through retinal haemorrhaging), oedematous swelling is a common feature. The optic disc may well be swollen. Visual loss is common (Fig. 18.6a–d).

> **Case History 18.3: Central retinal vein occlusion in diabetes**
>
> This 58-year-old man with type 2 diabetes diagnosed 8 years previously was controlled on metformin 1000 mg

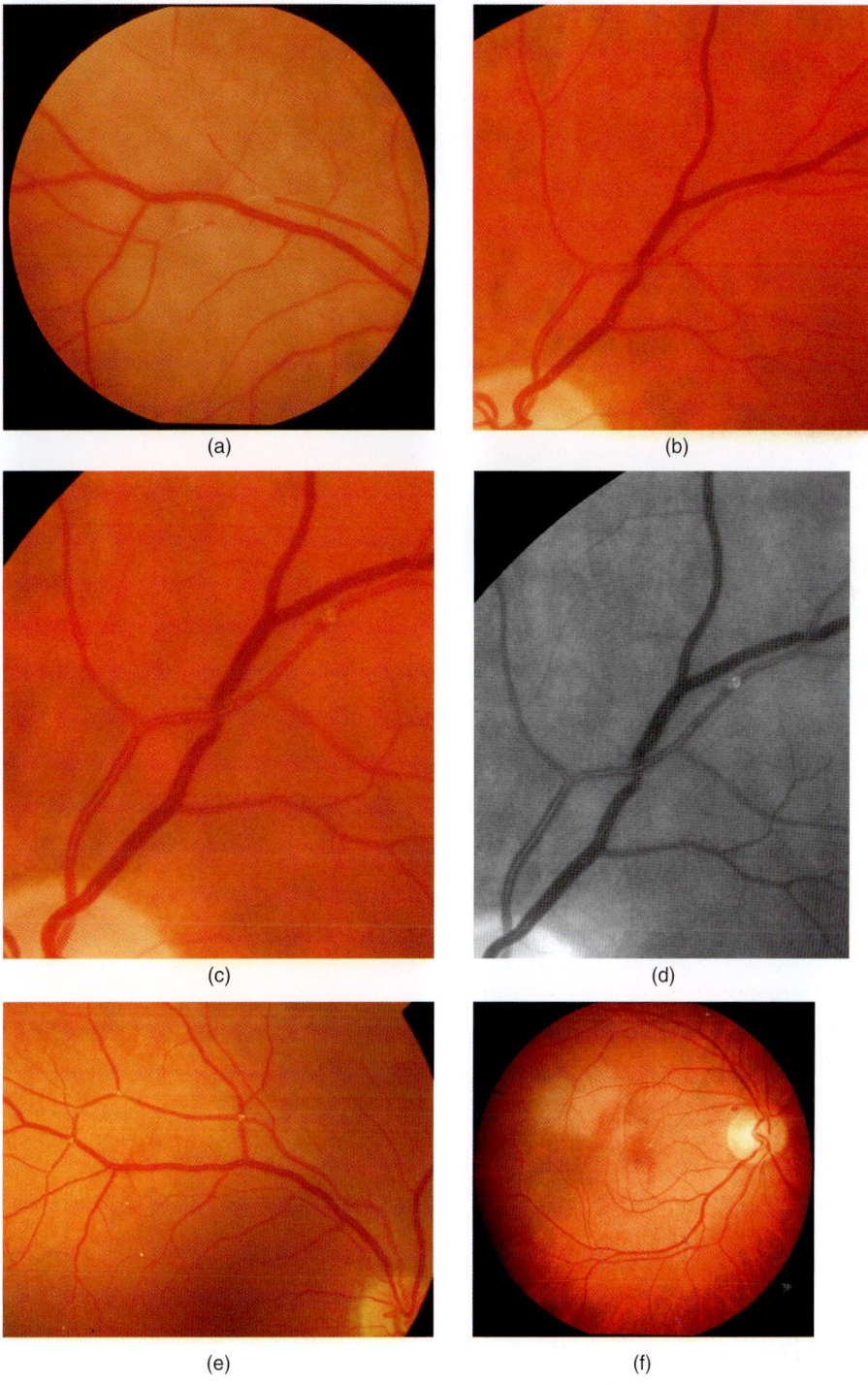

Fig. 18.5 (a) Fibrino-platelet arterial embolus. Left macular appearance (b) before and (c) after asymptomatic cholesterol emboli. (d) Red-free photograph of left macular appearance after asymptomatic cholesterol emboli. Multiple emboli (e) lodging at junctions in arterial tree and (f) causing pale areas of oedema in areas of retinal ischaemia.

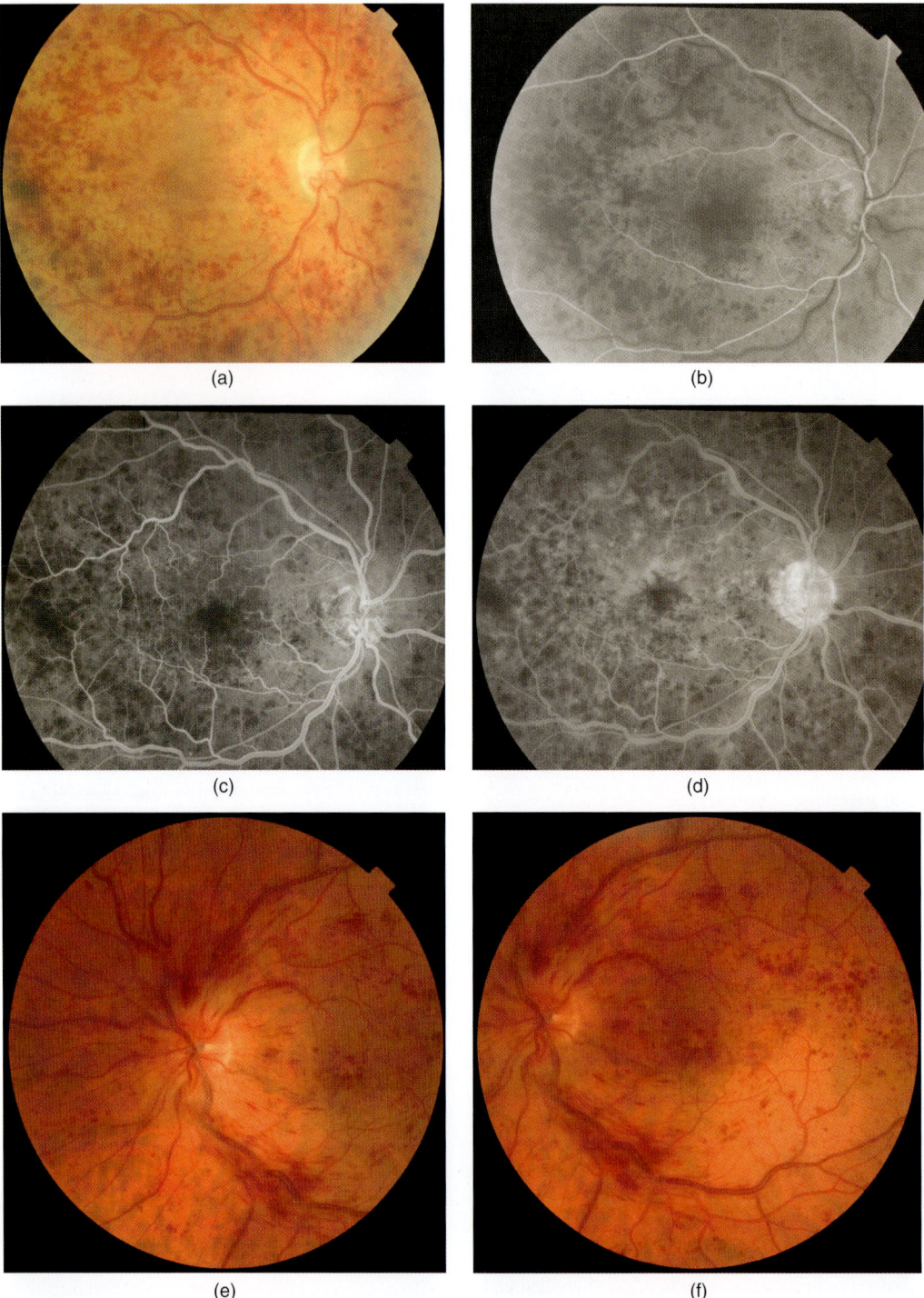

Fig. 18.6 Right CVRO: (a) colour photograph; fluorescein (b) 29 s; (c) 45 s; and (d) 4 min 5 s after injection. (e) Disc-centred view of multiple haemorrhages caused by a CRVO in a left eye and (f) macula-centred view of the same left eye showing multiple haemorrhages caused by a central retinal vein occlusion.

t.d.s. and gliclazide 40 mg b.d. added more recently. Over the previous 5 years his diabetes had been poorly controlled, with typical HbA1c values of 10.5–12% (91.3–107.7 mmol/mol) but the most recent value following the introduction of gliclazide had been 6.3% (45.4 mmol/mol).

He had a left phacoemulsification of cataract at the age of 57 years, and 1 week postoperatively his vision was good at 6/9 (20/30 or logMAR 0.2) unaided. However, 1 month postoperatively he developed a left central retinal vein occlusion with a reduced VA of 6/24 (20/80 or logMAR 0.6). The photographs show the signs of central retinal vein occlusion in his left eye (Fig. 18.6e and f). The timing of the central retinal vein occlusion 1 month after the cataract operation was felt to be coincidental.

In situations where the central retinal vein is not totally occluded, the retinal appearance is usually rather quieter. Some venous engorgement is still usually present, but fewer peripheral deep blot and considerably fewer nerve-fibre layer haemorrhages are visible. Infarcts as cotton wool spots are not particularly common and areas of apparent retinal ischaemia are fewer. In the early stages and in partial CRVO, noticeable visual loss may not have occurred.

In some cases, while the central retinal vein actually is mostly or totally occluded, some outflow from the affected eye is maintained through new collateral or existing cilioretinal vessels on the optic disc, linking the retinal circulation to that of the choroid and providing some outflow from the eye via the vortex veins. Development of true collateral vessels is usually a feature of long-standing vein occlusion however, and these tortuous remnants on the optic disc are often the sole remaining visible feature of a long-resolved CRVO (that and reduced visual acuity in the affected eye).

Visual loss from CRVO is generally caused either by extensive retinal capillary closure and ischaemia, with or without subsequent neovascularisation, or by subsequent macular oedema. Some improvement of visual function over time is common, particularly in cases of macular oedema, although the individual outcome varies considerably. What is however essential is continued monitoring of the patient and assessment of both the affected and fellow eye, both the posterior and crucially the anterior segments. Central retinal vein occlusion, through widespread retinal ischaemia, is frequently associated with subsequent development of iris neovascularisation and ultimately rubeotic glaucoma. With the common co-existing insult of diabetes-induced retinal ischaemia, such patients must receive long-term follow-up and monitoring.

Clinical examination and colour retinal imaging for recording purposes are always appropriate. Fluorescein angiography is an added advantage, although in profound cases little retinal detail may be visible due to overlying haemorrhage. In cases of suspected macular oedema, OCT investigations are particularly beneficial as they are not affected by other retinal lesions.

No direct or effective treatment is currently available for CRVO, although attention to any underlying systemic condition is essential. Anticoagulants such as heparin and aspirin have been tried but with little general effect. Treatment may however be required for complications that may develop, such as retinal or iris neovascularisation.

Branch retinal vein occlusion (BRVO)

Occlusion of a retinal branch vein (BRVO) is a relatively common finding, particularly in patients with diabetes, most frequently affecting the superior or inferior temporal arcades to create a quadrant occlusion. An occlusion involving the major vein immediately prior to the last bifurcation (actually re-joining) at the optic disc causes a defect which affects either the entire upper or lower hemifield of the eye. The unaffected portions of the eye are usually relatively, if not totally, normal.

Branch vein occlusions affecting a quadrant of the eye most commonly occur at an arteriovenous crossing point close to the optic disc. Arterial compression, with the artery usually crossing over the related vein, can cause relative or total venous occlusion. Occlusion of smaller retinal venules causes damage to a more restricted region with much more localised lesions.

Another cause of venous occlusion, particularly in the nasal retina, is when the vein becomes severely constricted due to it passing over the steep edge of the optic rim in cases of deeply cupped glaucomatous discs. Occlusion of smaller and more peripheral veins is thought to be linked to phlebitis or other inflammatory insults, although the susceptible arteriovenous crossing cannot be ruled out even in these cases.

Clinical examination of a branch vein occlusion in an otherwise normal eye (i.e. in absence of any other confounding features) reveals retinal lesions and features which are very localised and are restricted to the retinal area drained by the affected vein (Fig. 18.7a–g).

Laser treatment is indicated if neovascularisation develops in the distribution of an occluded vein. Focal

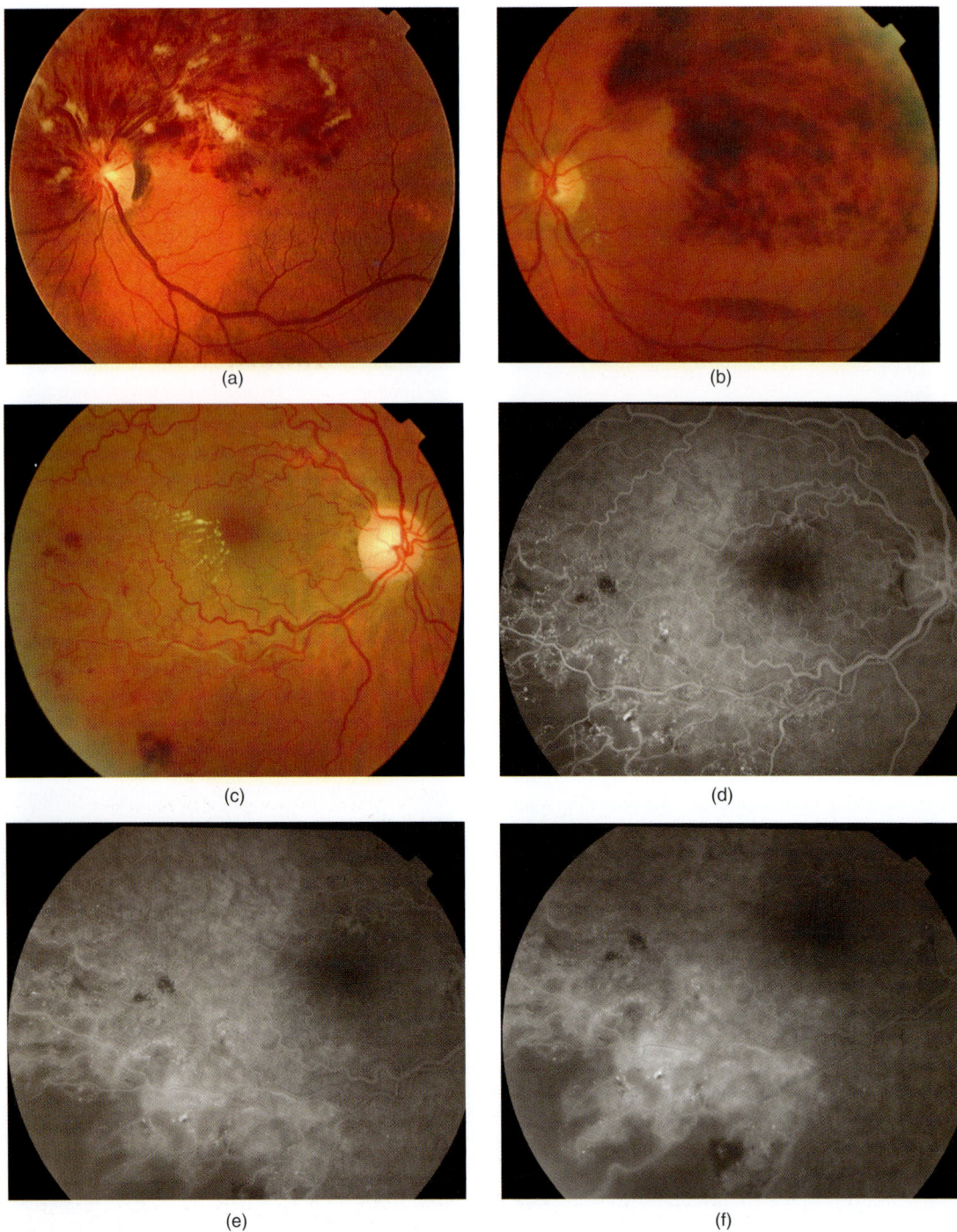

Fig. 18.7 (a) Recent left superior BRVO and (b) with haemorrhage in macular area. Older right infero-temporal BRVO: (c) with some collaterals; fluorescein angiogram (d) 37 s after injection, showing ischaemia in distribution of occluded vein; (e) 1 min 58 s after injection, showing ischaemia and leakage in the distribution of occluded vein; and (f) 3 min 31 s after injection, showing ischaemia and leakage in the distribution of occluded vein.

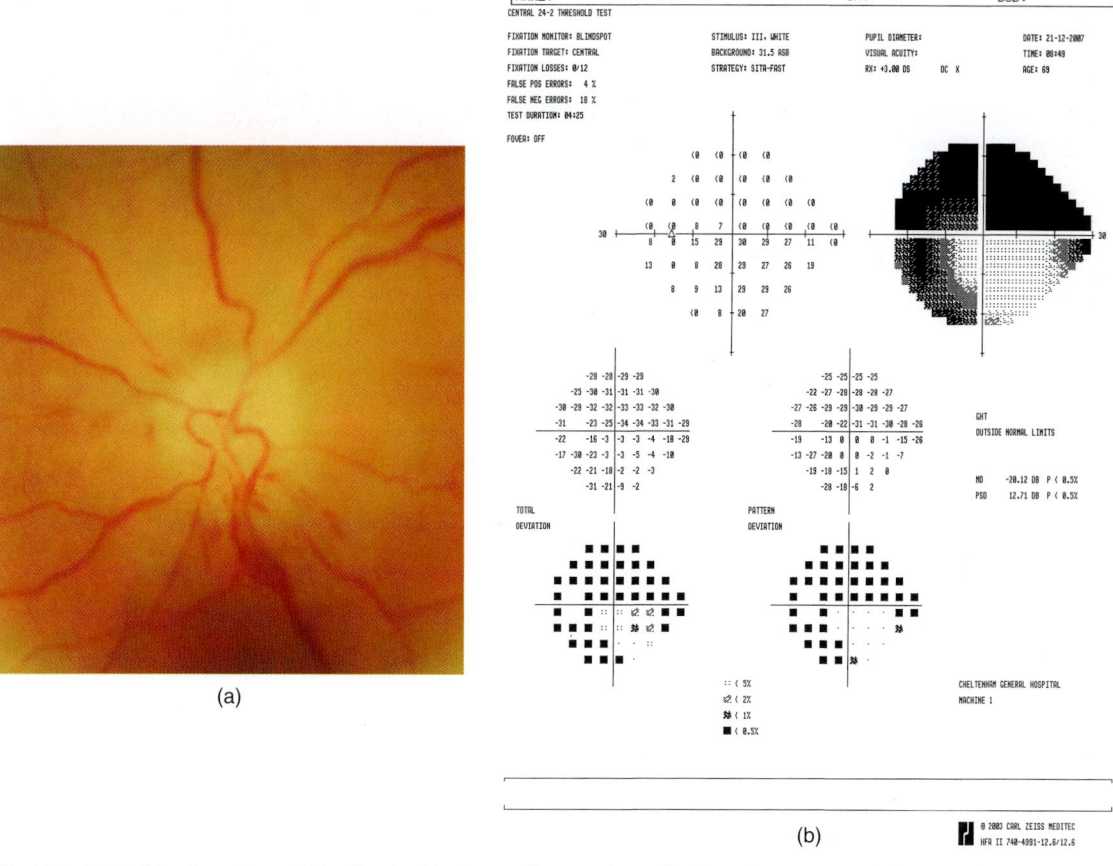

Fig. 18.8 AION: (a) colour photo of disc showing blurring and haemorrhage of inferior disc margin and (b) visual field demonstrating superior and inferonasal field loss.

laser treatment may be indicated for persistent macular oedema.

ANTERIOR ISCHAEMIC OPTIC NEUROPATHY

Anterior ischaemic optic neuropathy (AION) usually causes a sudden loss of vision because of ischaemia of the anterior part of the optic nerve. It is more common in people with diabetes and/or hypertension. It needs to be differentiated from temporal arteritis, which is an arteritic cause requiring urgent treatment to prevent involvement of the other eye.

Patients should be advised to pay careful attention to their blood pressure control and to avoid smoking.

> **Case History 18.4: Anterior ischaemic optic neuropathy in diabetes**
>
> A 64-year-old man with type 2 diabetes controlled with metformin 1000 mg b.d. and a history of hypertension controlled with atenolol 100 mg once daily noticed a sudden loss of vision in his left eye when he started to shave one morning. On examination his VA was found to be 6/12 (20/40 or logMAR 0.3) and the optic disc shows oedema, more marked inferiorly, with splinter haemorrhages at the disc margin (Fig. 18.8a).
>
> Within 2–3 months the optic disc swelling resolved spontaneously and the disc became pale. The left visual field shows loss of the superior field and some nasal loss inferiorly (Fig. 18.8b).

ASTEROID HYALOSIS

Asteroid hyalosis is a primarily unilateral disorder (bilateral in only 9%), occurring more frequently in men (almost twice the frequency) and in older patients. The condition is usually asymptomatic and only mildly affects visual acuity, even when it is difficult for the ophthalmologist to get a good view of the retina.

On examination, refractile yellow-white particles (asteroid bodies) are seen in the vitreous; they are composed of a mixture of calcium, phosphorus and oxygen showing a composition similar to those found for hydroxyapatite with the presence of chondroitin-6-sulphate at the periphery of asteroid bodies[1].

An association between asteroid hyalosis and diabetes mellitus was suggested by Cockburn[2] and, in a large study of 12,205 patients, Bergren et al.[3] found diabetes mellitus in 29 of the patients with asteroid hyalosis (29%), as compared to 10 of 101 (10%) control subjects ($p=0.0007$). However, this association has been disputed by Moss et al.[4] in the Beaver Dam Eye study, where they found an association with greater body mass ($p=0.02$) and higher alcohol consumption ($p=0.03$) but not with diabetes.

Asteroid hyalosis is a benign condition in itself and never leads to severe vision loss; the presence of asteroid hyalosis therefore usually only needs to be documented. Any significant visual loss in a person with asteroid hyalosis requires further investigation and treatment of any associated condition.

Interestingly, although the retinal view may be limited when using slit-lamp biomicroscopy or colour photography, one often finds a surprisingly good view is obtained on fluorescein angiography.

Case History 18.5: Macular oedema in a patient with asteroid hyalosis in diabetes

This 75-year-old man with type 2 diabetes for 11 years, controlled with insulin, noticed a gradual loss of vision in his right eye which was known to have asteroid hyalosis. On examination, the VA was reduced to 6/60 (20/200 or logMAR 1.0) and scattered haemorrhages and microaneurysms were noted in his right fundus, but the macular area was difficult to view adequately because of the asteroid hyalosis. His blood pressure was 181/64 and his HbA1c was 8.5% (69.4 mmol/mol).

Colour photographs (Fig. 18.9a and b) show the asteroid bodies on the anterior view and demonstrate the difficulty in obtaining a clear colour photograph of the macular area. A fluorescein angiogram demonstrates that good fluorescein pictures can often be obtained in patients with asteroid hyalosis and that, in this particular case, marked cystoid macular oedema was observed in the later stages of the angiogram (Fig. 18.9c and d).

MACROANEURYSM

Retinal macroaneurysms are dilatations of a retinal artery or an arteriole that is larger than the diameter of the vein as it crosses the optic disc margin. They are more common in diabetes, but because they are generally not regarded as microvascular pathology they do not come under a strict definition of diabetic retinopathy. They are often associated with systemic hypertension as well as diabetes. They are often asymptomatic but can be associated with leakage that threatens the macular area or bleeding producing intraretinal or vitreous haemorrhages. Four examples are given below of macroaneurysms that leaked and this leakage threatened the macular area and hence the central vision.

Case History 18.6: Macroaneurysm in type 1 diabetes

This 41-year-old man with type 1 diabetes since the age of 2 years presented at the age of 29 years with exudates threatening the left macular area due to leakage from a macroaneurysm. The VA was good at 6/6 (20/20 or logMAR 0.0). Figure 18.10a shows leakage from the macroaneurysm.

He was treated with 45 laser photocoagulation burns, 100 micron size, power 180–220 mW, 0.1 s, Area Centralis lens, with approximately 20 burns having been applied directly to the macroaneurysm and 25 burns to the surrounding thickened retina. The photographs taken within a few minutes of treatment show the pale laser burns on the macroaneurysm and some within the surrounding area of exudation (Fig. 18.10b and c).

Four months after treatment, there had been considerable clearing of the exudates and thrombosis of the macroaneurysm as shown in Figure 18.10d, and 14 years later this improvement had been maintained (Fig. 18.10e).

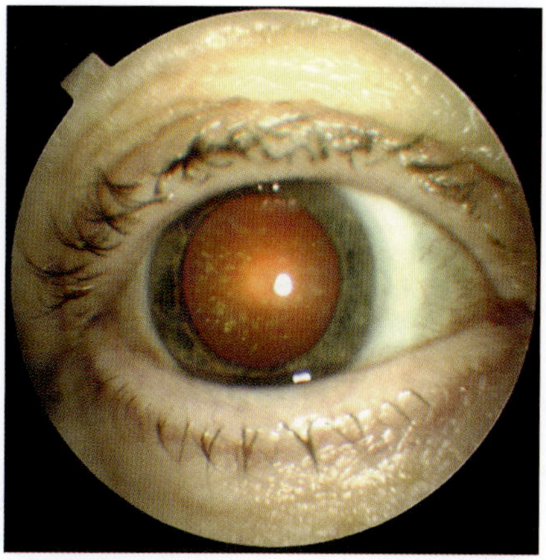

Other retinal conditions in diabetes 241

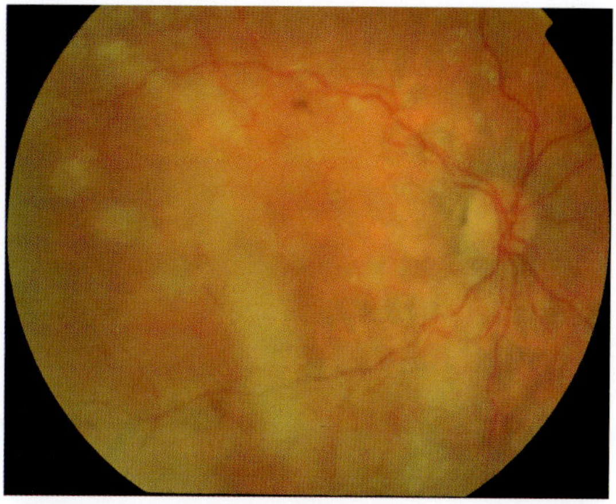

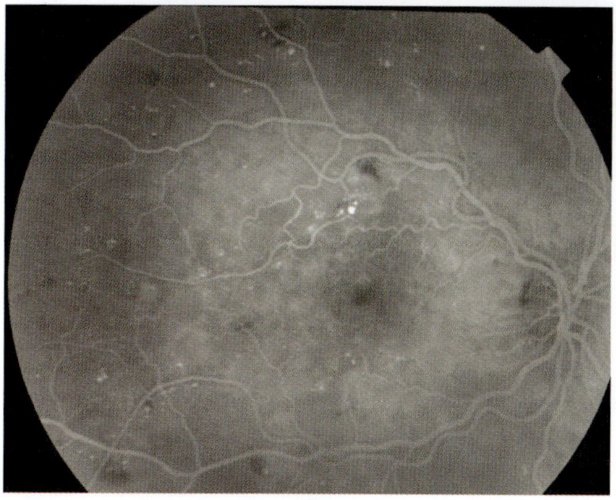

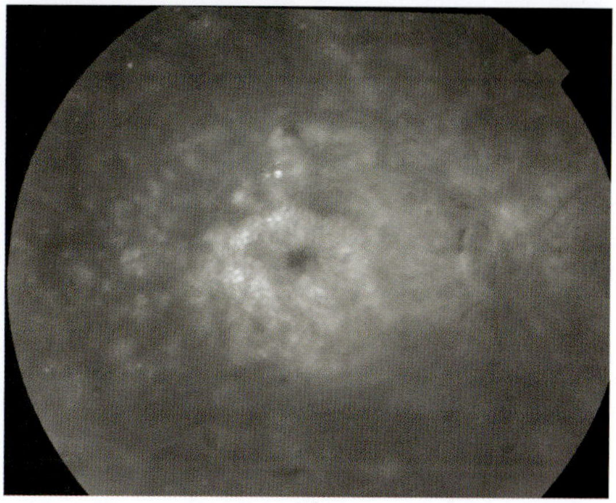

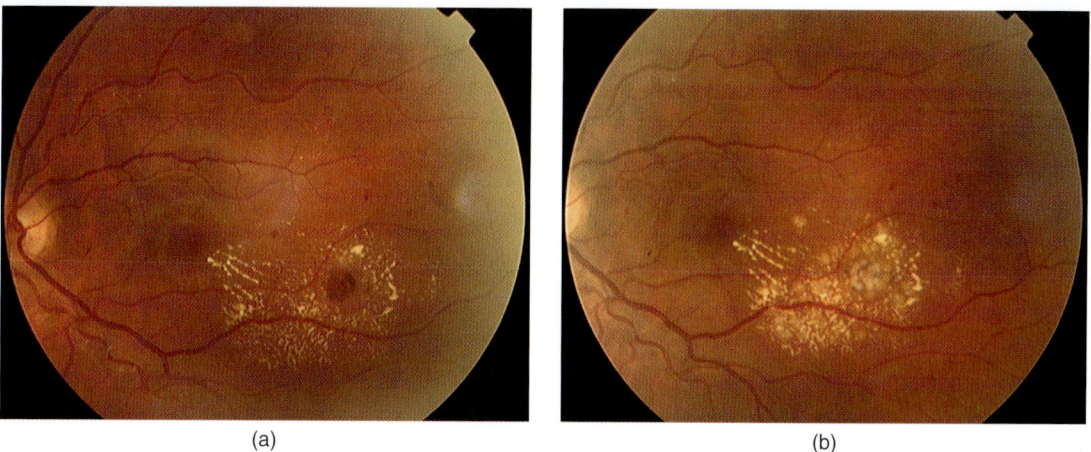

Fig. 18.9 Asteroid hyalosis: (a) right anterior and (b) macular colour; fluorescein angiogram (c) 47 s and (d) 3 min 30 s after injection of dye, showing cystoid macular oedema.

Fig. 18.10 Macroaneurysm (a) leaking, threatening left macular area; (b, c) immediately after treatment; (d) 4 months after treatment, showing clearing of most of the exudates; and (e) 14 years after treatment.

(c)

(d)

(e)

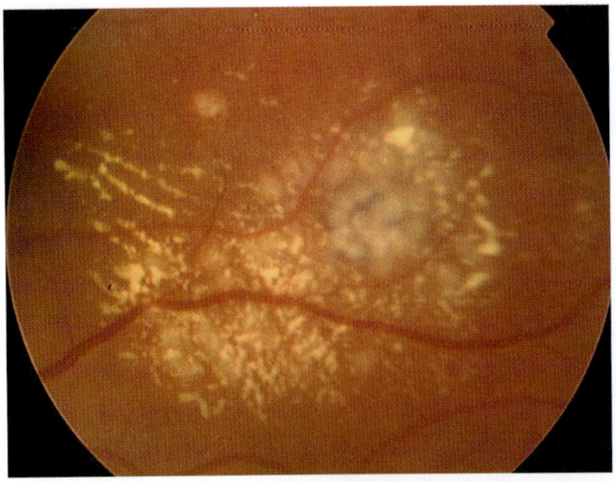

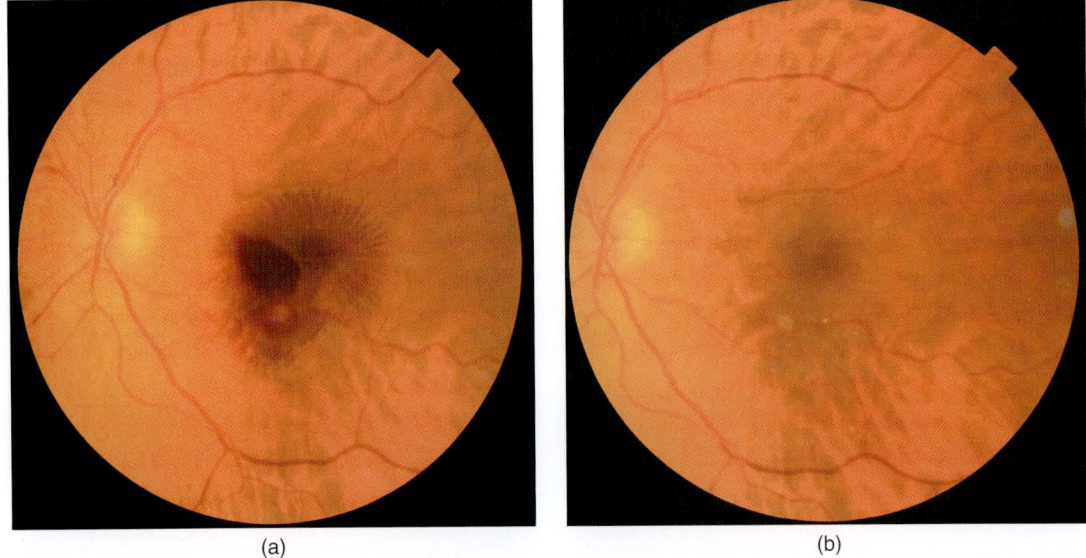

Fig. 18.10 (*Continued*)

(a)

(b)

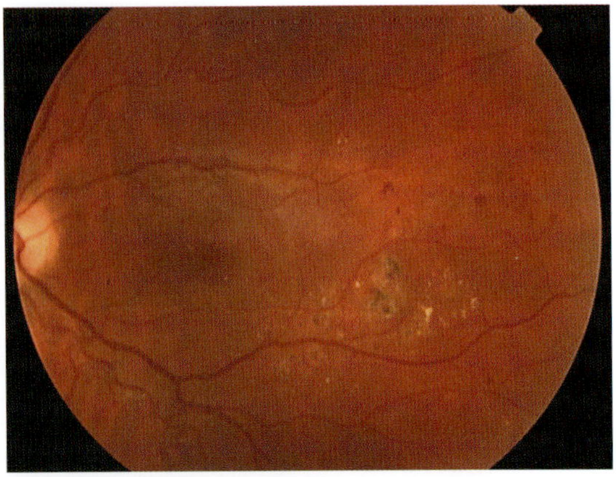

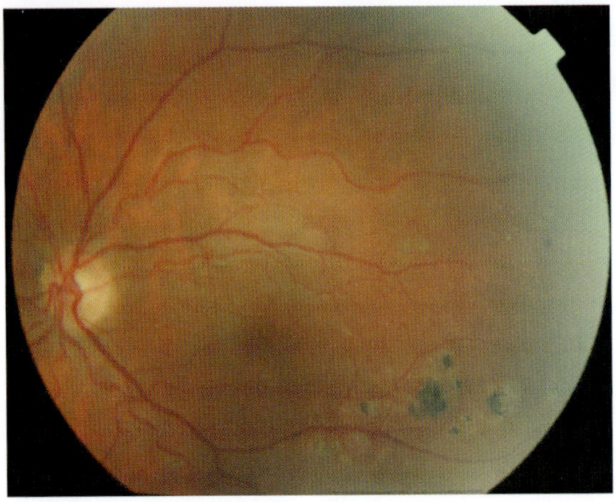

Fig. 18.11 (a) Macroaneurysm leaking blood in the left macular area. (b) Left macular colour photograph 7 months later.

Other retinal conditions in diabetes 243

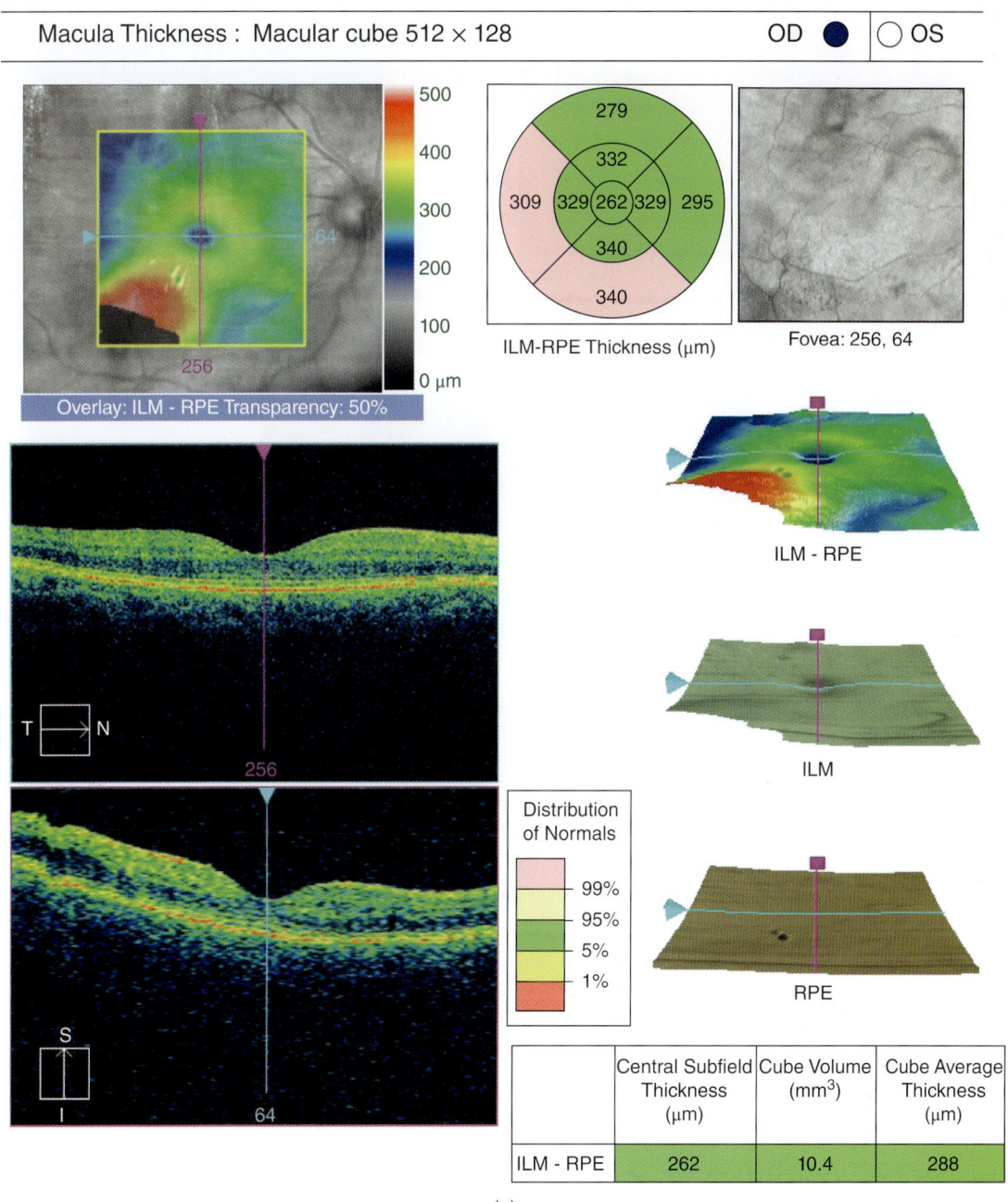

(a)

Fig. 18.12 (a) Colour photograph showing a macroaneurysm infero-temporal to the right central fovea. (b) OCT showing leakage from a macroaneurysm infero-temporal to the right central fovea. Fluorescein angiogram showing the macroaneurysm (c) 41 s and (d) 7 min 31 s after injection.

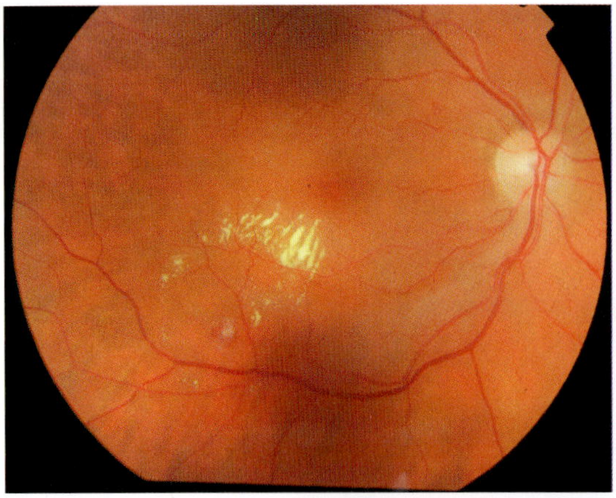

(b)

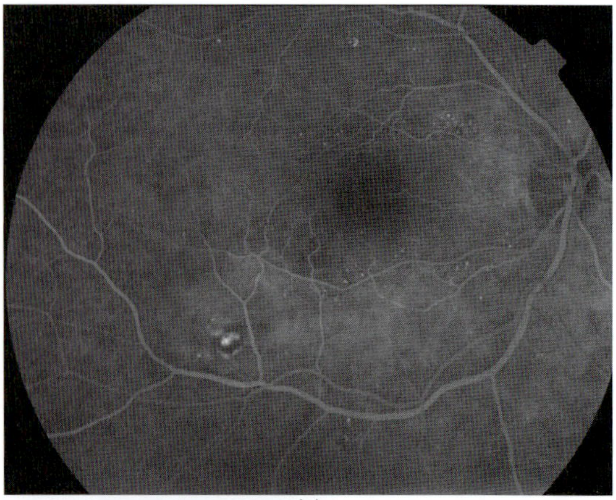

(c)

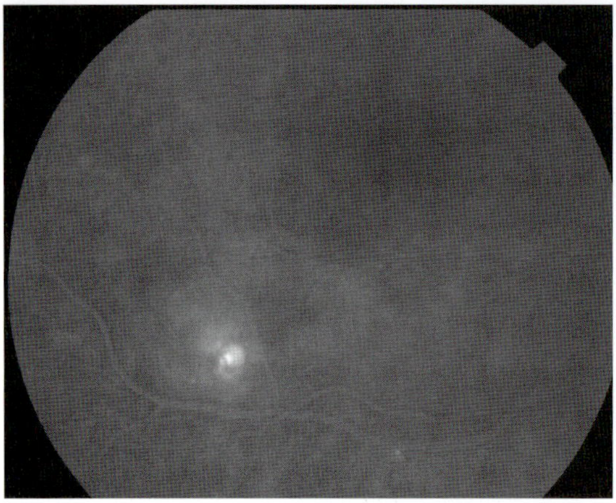

(d)

Fig. 18.12 (Continued)

Case History 18.7: Macroaneurysm in type 2 diabetes

This 84-year-old woman with type 2 diabetes diagnosed 15 years ago, controlled on tablets and with a history of hypertension treated with bendrofluazide 2.5 mg o.d., presented with sudden loss of vision in her left eye which was reduced to hand movements. Colour photographs demonstrate a haemorrhage from a macroaneurysm in her left macular area (Fig. 18.11a) which gradually cleared over the next 7 months (Fig. 18.11b), but unfortunately the final visual acuity only improved to a level of 6/36 (20/120 or logMAR 0.8) because of the damage to the cones in the left macular area caused by the blood in this area.

Imaging patients with macroaneurysms

In patients with macroaneurysms, OCT and fluorescein angiography are useful to demonstrate leakage that might threaten the central macula and consequently the vision. Two examples in patients with macroaneurysms are shown in Figure 18.12a–d. Figure 18.13a–d provides similar examples from another patient.

Other retinal conditions in diabetes 245

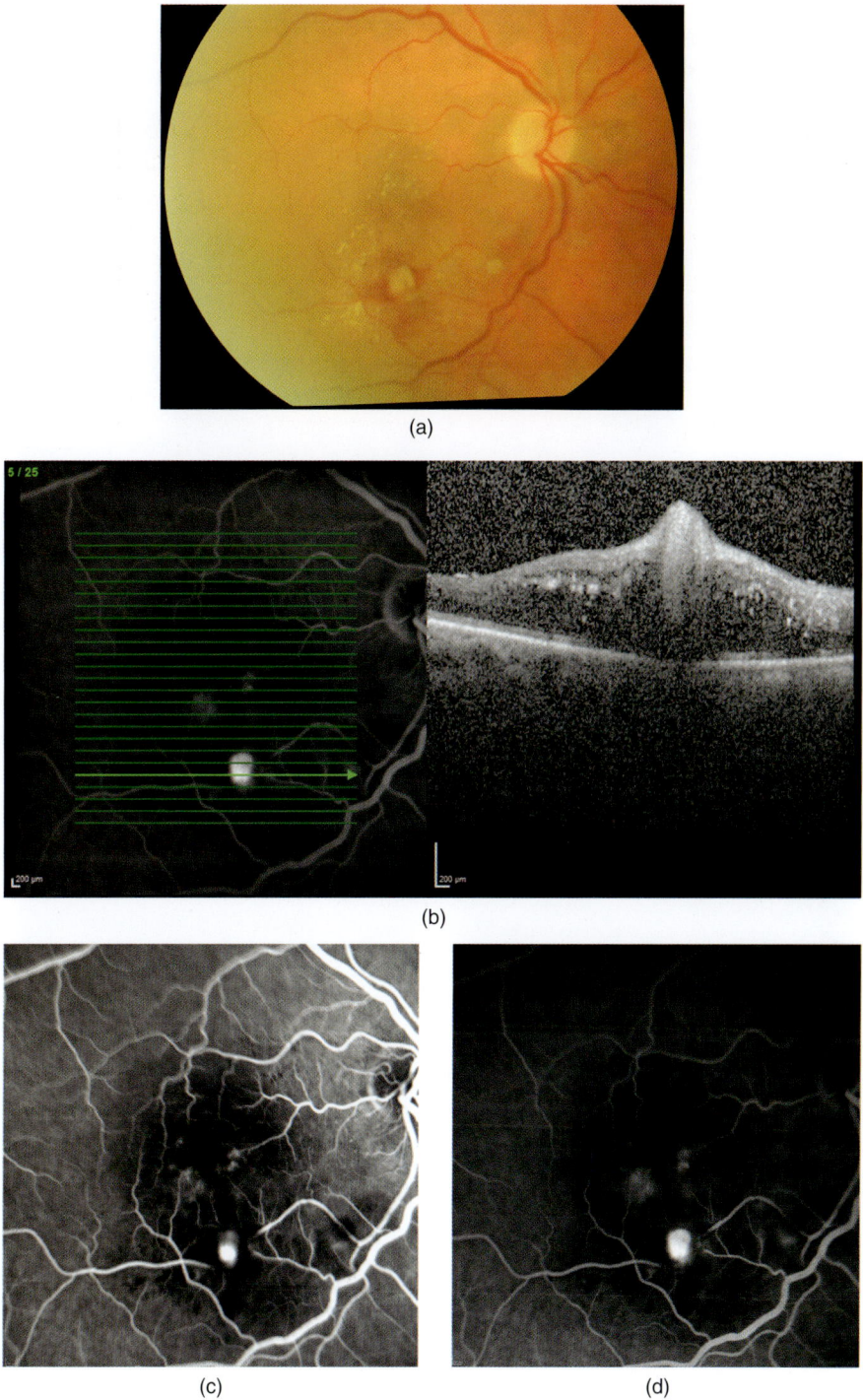

Fig. 18.13 (a) Colour photograph showing a macroaneurysm below the right central fovea. (b) OCT showing leakage from a macroaneurysm below the right central fovea. Fluorescein angiogram showing the macroaneurysm (c) 1 min 31 s and (d) 6 min 17 s after injection.

PRACTICE POINTS

Diabetic retinopathy is a microvascular disease. However, people with diabetes are also more liable to develop disease of the larger vessels (macrovascular disease) than a person without diabetes. Many of the conditions described in this chapter therefore also relate to diseases of the larger vessels.

REFERENCE

Please visit www.wiley.com/go/scanlon/diabetic_retinopathy

19 Conditions with appearances similar to diabetic retinopathy

Stephen J. Aldington[1] & Peter H. Scanlon[2]

[1] Gloucestershire Hospitals NHS Foundation Trust, UK; University of Warwick Medical School, UK
[2] Harris Manchester College, University of Oxford; Medical Ophthalmology, University of Gloucestershire, UK

DRUSEN AND AMD

One of the most frequently detected abnormal retinal features are drusen. Principally associated with general ageing, drusen are so common as to be present and detectable in most people over 50 years of age, particularly in the macular area. They are formed as deposits of lipofuscin, initially within the pigment epithelium and later as deposits between the basement membrane of the pigment epithelium and the inner layer of Bruch's membrane. On examination, they present as yellowish deposits varying in size and appearance from tiny, almost crystalline, individual hard 'druse' (a common American term for single drusen), to large, soft, less-defined yellowish-white drusen, each often more than twice the diameter of a major vein. Large soft drusen are frequently seen in near-confluent regions around the macula and in the posterior pole generally (Fig. 19.1).

It is important to make a differential diagnosis between drusen (particularly scattered hard drusen) and the presence of any retinal hard exudates which are diabetic in origin. While exudates are caused by leakage of lipid-rich plasma within the middle retinal layers, they are frequently associated with other (usually diabetic) retinal features such as microaneurysms; drusen are located much deeper in the eye, are usually less distinct and are unrelated to other (diabetic) retinal lesions. Drusen can of course be present in an eye also affected by intraretinal hard exudates.

While they are individually asymptomatic and not causative of visual loss, drusen directly affecting the macula are an early feature of age-related macular degeneration (AMD). A full explanation of the development, treatment and outcomes of AMD is beyond the scope of this book. Briefly, however, two main forms of AMD are identified: the 'dry' atrophic type where drusen ultimately cause pigment epithelium atrophy along with associated pigment clumping and possible RPE detachment; and the 'wet' type which leads to significant damage to Bruch's membrane and ultimately to subretinal neovascularisation.

AMD presence is most usually bilateral, although the pace of development may be very unequal in the two eyes. Visual loss in one eye has an approximate 12–15% chance of being followed by visual loss in the fellow eye within a year.

MYELINATED NERVE FIBRES

The normal adult human eye possesses usually unobservable superficial retinal nerve fibres, connecting the photoreceptors ultimately to the visual cortex. Retinal nerve fibres, unlike those within the optic nerve itself, are usually devoid of a myelin sheath. On occasions however, foetal and very early postnatal development causes the normal myelination to the optic nerve to extend forwards beyond its normal stopping point of the lamina cribrosa (situated within the optic disc), to involve some of the peripapillary retinal nerve fibres.

On examination, myelinated nerve fibres (MNFs) can be seen as highly reflective whitish-yellow opaque patches surrounding the optic disc with marked striations (caused by the fibres themselves) (Fig. 19.2). These patches are usually physically connected to the disc margin, although on occasion they can occur as an isolated island development some distance from the margin. It is quite common for the areas of MNF to effectively prevent or obscure an observer's view of retinal vessels in the affected area.

A Practical Manual of Diabetic Retinopathy Management, Second Edition.
Edited by Peter Scanlon, Ahmed Sallam, and Peter van Wijngaarden.
© 2017 John Wiley & Sons Ltd. Published 2017 by John Wiley & Sons Ltd.
Companion Website: www.wiley.com/go/scanlon/diabetic_retinopathy

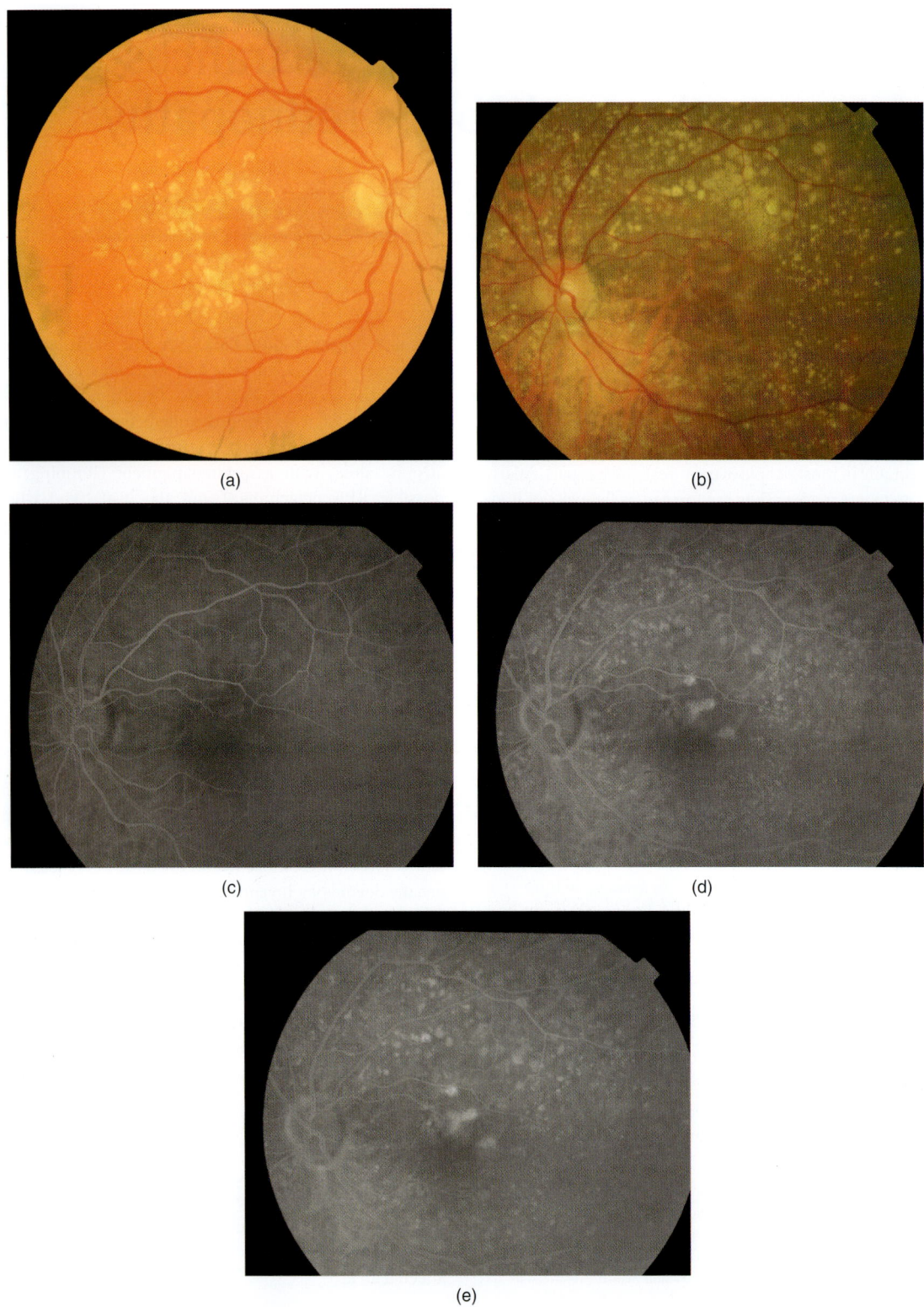

Fig. 19.1 Drusen: (a) surrounding the central foveal area; (b) scattered throughout the retina; Fluorescein from same patient showing minimal uptake of fluorescein by drusen at (c) 19 s; (d) 58 s and (e) 3 min 49 s.

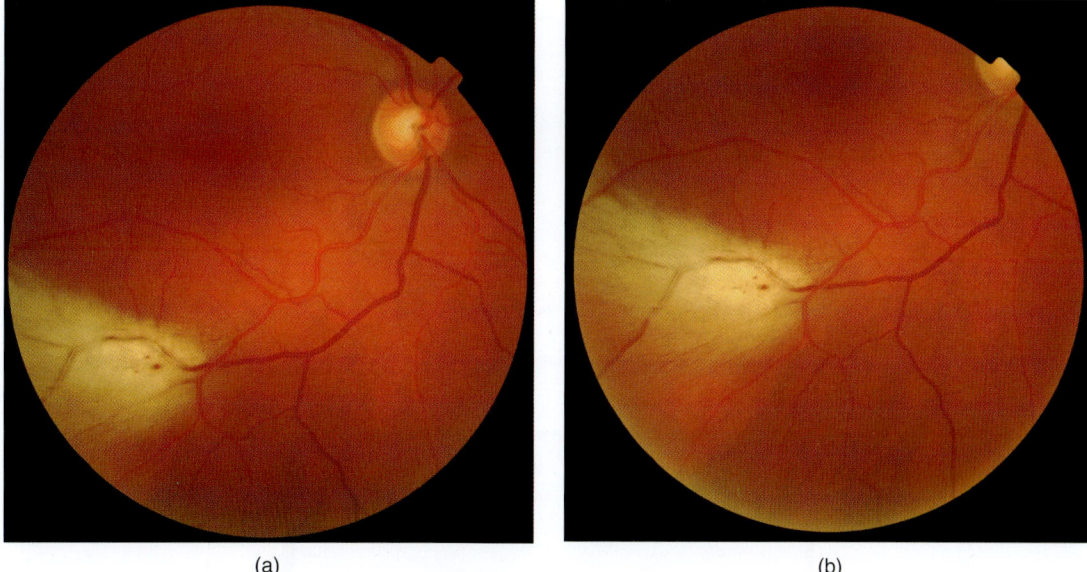

Fig. 19.2 (a, b) Myelinated nerve fibres: right infero-temporal colour.

Large areas of myelinated nerve fibres can cause field defects although, as these are congenital or at least immediate postnatal in terms of longevity, they are effectively asymptomatic and detailed field testing is required to detect their presence and influence.

The correct identification of patches of MNF is important in order to differentiate these from cotton wool spots, hard exudates and, in some cases, even retinal oedema.

SICKLE CELL RETINOPATHY

Sickle cell disease is an inherited blood disorder that affects red blood cells. People with sickle cell disease have red blood cells that contain mostly haemoglobin S, an abnormal type of haemoglobin. Sometimes these red blood cells become sickle-shaped (crescent-shaped) and have difficulty passing through small blood vessels.

The different kinds of sickle cell disease and the different traits are found mainly in people whose families come from Africa, the Caribbean, the Eastern Mediterranean, Middle East and Asia. A comparison between normal red blood cells and those that have become sickle-cell-shaped is shown in Figure 19.3a–c.

Ischaemia of the peripheral retina due to sickle cell retinopathy can result in neovascularisation and the primary aim of treatment is to prevent visual loss from the complications of the neovascularisation.

Although one might expect that peripheral vascular occlusion and ischaemia resulting in neovascularisation might be more common in homozygous sickle cell disease (SS genotype), it is in fact more common in adults with SC disease[1] (SC genotype). A number of classifications[2–4] have been developed to describe the progression of sickle cell retinopathy. In the publication by Sayag et al.[3], an extension of the original classification proposed by Goldberg[4] is described:

- Stage 1: peripheral arteriolar occlusion is present;
- Stage 2: peripheral arteriovenous anastamosis;
- Stage 3: neovascular and fibrous proliferations, subdivided by Sayag et al.[3] into 3A–E, depending on clinical and angiographic characteristics;
- Stage 4: intravitreal haemorrhage; and
- Stage 5: retinal detachment.

Laser treatment to ischaemic areas of peripheral retina may be required. A colour photograph of the left eye of a patient with sickle cell retinopathy, who presented with a vitreous haemorrhage requiring peripheral scatter laser treatment and who subsequently developed fibrotic bands in the peripheral retina, is shown in Figure 19.3d and e.

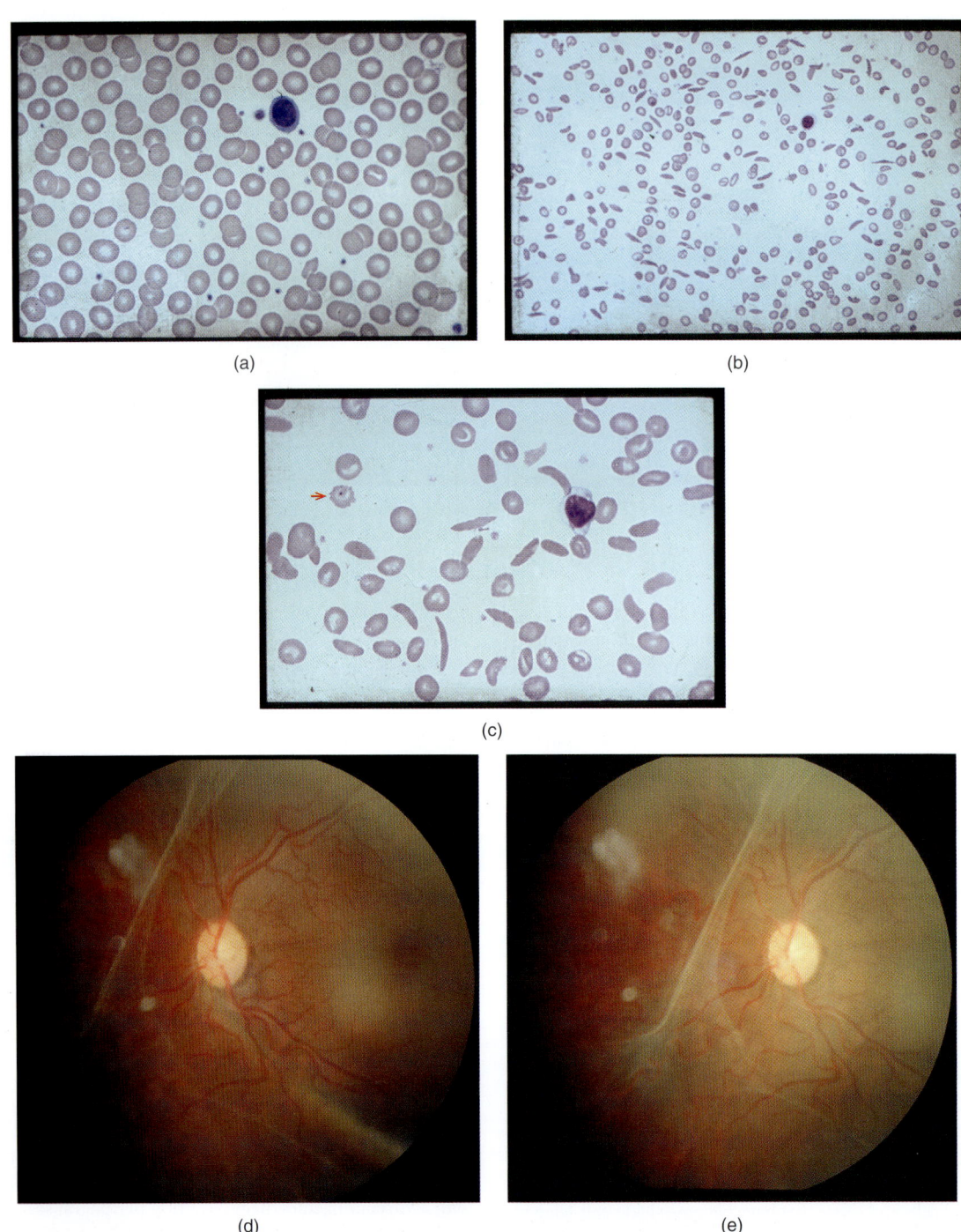

Fig. 19.3 (a) Normal red blood cells (high power): compare red blood cell size with that of lymphocyte. Sickle cell crisis: (b) low power, sickle cells and target cells and (c) high power, one red blood cell (arrowed) contains a Howell–Jolly body. (d, e) Fibrotic bands in the retinal periphery of a patient with sickle cell retinopathy.

COATS' DISEASE

Coats' disease is an idiopathic retinal telangiectasia first described by the Scottish ophthalmologist George Coats in 1908. It usually affects only one eye (unilateral) and occurs predominantly in young males, with the onset of symptoms generally appearing in the first decade of life.

A large series of 150 patients referred to the Wills Eye Hospital in Pennsylvania was described by Shields et al.[5] in 2001. In the 150 patients, Coats' disease was diagnosed at a median age of 5 years (range 1 month–63 years), occurred in 114 males (76%) and was unilateral in 142 patients (95%). The first symptom or sign was decreased visual acuity (VA) in 68 cases (34%), strabismus in 37 (23%), leukocoria in 31 (20%) and 13 patients (8%) were asymptomatic. VA at presentation was 20/200 to no light perception in 121 eyes (76%).

Shields et al.[6] later described the following stages:
- Stage 1: telangiectasia only;
- Stage 2: telangiectasia and exudates;
- Stage 3: subretinal or retinal detachment; and
- Stage 4: total retinal detachment and glaucoma.

Treatment for stages 1 and 2 is usually with laser therapy or cryotherapy. An example of a fluorescein angiogram of a patient who presented to the eye department at the age of 25 years with blurring of vision in his right eye is shown in Figure 19.4. This angiogram shows the retinal telangectasia and exudation in the peripheral retina and some central changes of cystoid macular oedema.

RADIATION RETINOPATHY

Radiation retinopathy is occasionally seen in the eye clinic. Amoaku and Archer[7] described the fluorescein angiographic features, natural course and treatment of radiation retinopathy in a publication in *Eye* in 1990. They described the following grades of severity.
- Grade 1: Small foci of dilated and irregular retinal capillaries with clusters of microaneurysms.
- Grade 2: Multiple foci plus capillary closure plus leakage of dye from defective capillaries.
- Grade 3: Widespread capillary dilatation, telangiectatic-like channels, microvascular incompetence and significant areas of capillary closure. IRMA at the borders of non-perfused areas. Significant macular oedema.
- Grade 4: Widespread disorganisation of the retinal microvasculature with extensive retinal ischaemia.

In a further publication Archer[8] suggested that the following doses and risk factors may give rise to radiation retinopathy.
- The minimum amount administered by teletherapy that will give rise to retinal vasculopathy is unknown; estimates vary from 1500 cGy to 6000 cGy.
- It is unusual for <2500 cGy to be given in fractions of less than 200 cGy.
- There is a higher risk with diabetes and concomitant chemotherapy.

Parsons et al.[9] studied the effect of the high dose radiotherapy on the normal eye in 157 patients followed for a minimum of 3 years treated for primary extracranial tumours.
- Radiation retinopathy developed in 27 eyes of 26 patients.
- The mean time of onset was 2.8 years.
- The risk increased steadily above 45 Gy, especially if fractions were greater than 1.9 Gy.
- There was an increased risk with diabetic and chemotherapy.

Takeda et al.[10] described late retinal complications in a retrospective study of 43 eyes of 25 patients treated with radiation therapy for nasal and paranasal malignancies.
- Radiation retinopathy developed in 7 eyes.
- The mean duration was 32 months (range 16–60 months).
- There were no retinal complications in patients receiving less than 50 Gy in fractions of 2 Gy.

Case History 19.1: Radiation retinopathy

A 45-year-old man had radiotherapy to his right temple for a recurrence of a basal cell carcinoma, and 9 months later presented with a blurring of vision in his right eye.

The colour photographs and fluorescein angiogram show the effect of radiation on the right retina and a normal left retina (Fig. 19.5). The right eye images show new vessels forming supero-temporally and infero-temporally, and areas of vascular occlusion and leakage. These changes are similar to those found in diabetic retinopathy and panretinal photocoagulation was required to treat the right eye.

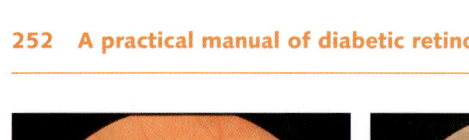

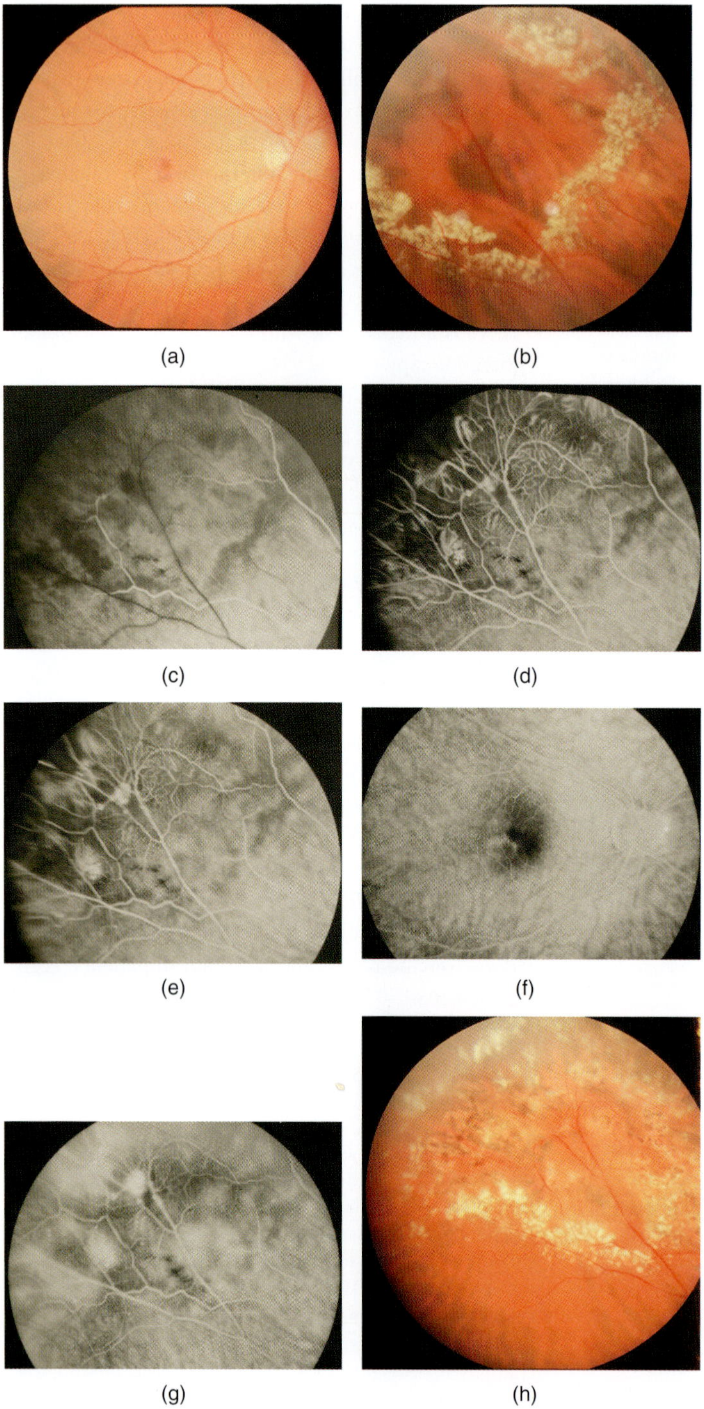

Fig. 19.4 Coats' disease: (a) right macula colour photo; (b) right peripheral retinal colour photo; fluorescein peripheral retina showing peripheral aneurysms and vascular patterns in (c) arterial phase and (d) arteriovenous phase. Fluorescein (e) peripheral retina showing leakage from peripheral aneurysms in early venous phase; (f) macular area showing some secondary oedema in the macular area and (g) peripheral retina showing leakage from peripheral aneurysms in late venous phase. (h) Right peripheral retinal colour photo showing some clearing of exudate 3 months after first laser treatment.

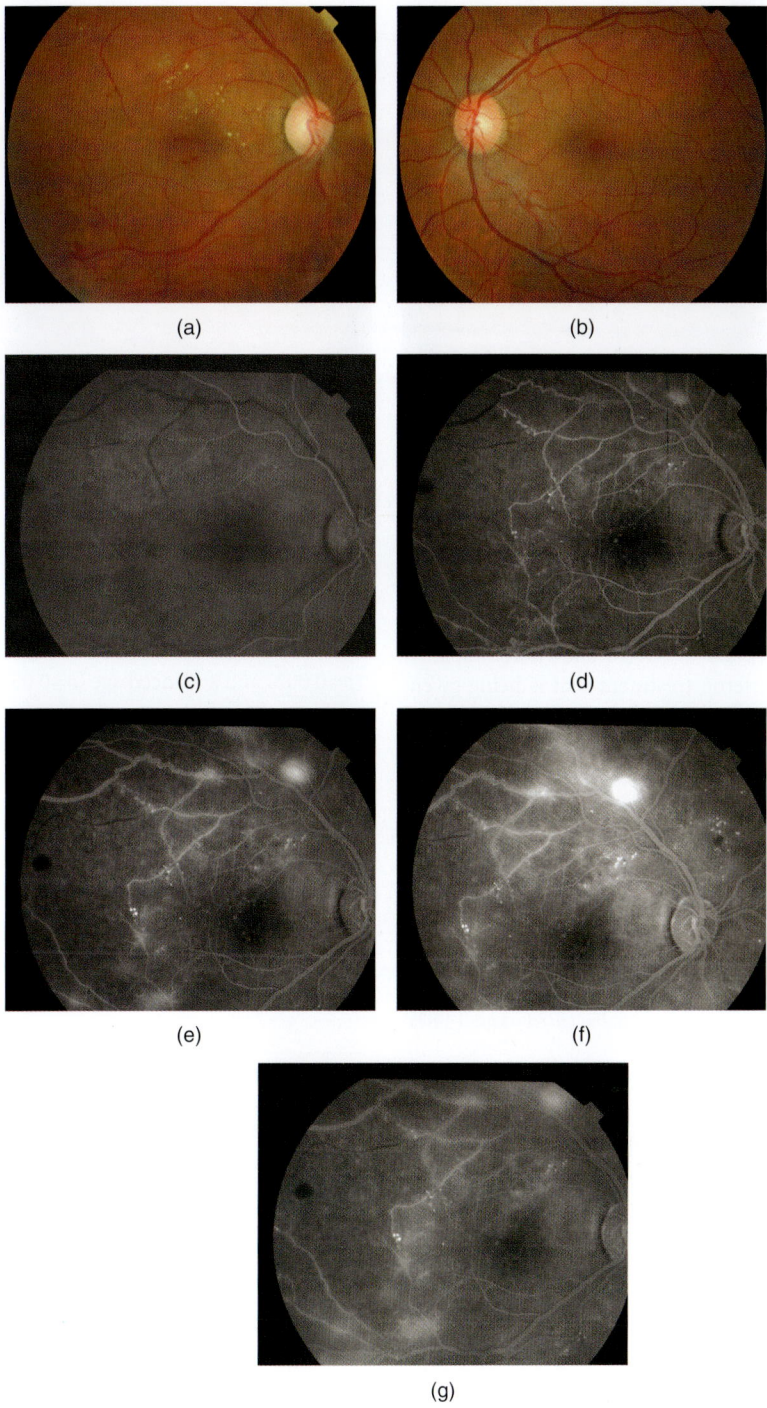

Fig. 19.5 Radiation retinopathy. (a) Right and (b) left macular colour photo. Fluorescein angiogram (c) 23 s; (d) 33 s; (e) 1 min; (f) 3 min 45 s; and (g) 4 min 11 s post injection.

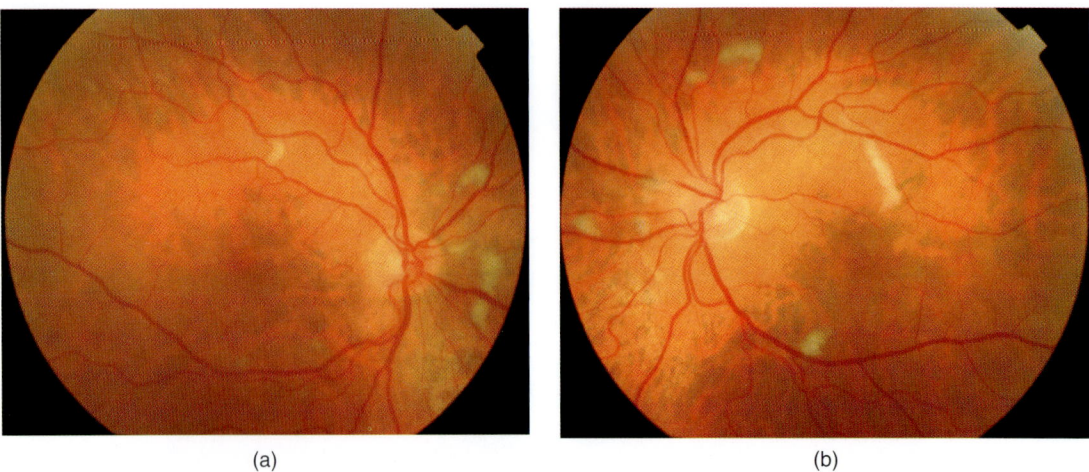

Fig. 19.6 (a) Right and (b) left macular view, showing cotton wool spots in both eyes in a person treated with interferon.

INTERFERON RETINOPATHY

Recent literature reports[11-13] have shown retinopathy associated with interferon treatment that is being given for conditions such as chronic hepatitis C, and these patients are beginning to appear in ophthalmology clinics in areas where interferon is being used.

In a prospective study of 81 patients, Saito et al.[12] found that 34.6% (28/81) of the patients treated with interferon-alpha therapy for chronic hepatitis C showed cotton wool spots, minor retinal haemorrhage or both lesions during therapy, but these lesions were reversed during or after interferon therapy. The occurrence rates of cotton wool spots alone, retinal haemorrhage alone and both lesions were 13.6% (11/81), 6.2% (5/81) and 14.8% (12/81), respectively.

In a prospective study of 107 chronic hepatitis C patients receiving systemic interferon treatment, Kawasaki[13] reported that retinopathy developed in 40 patients (37%) after an average of 77 days of treatment. The incidence of retinopathy was 28% in males and 51% in females, 75% in diabetics and 34% in non-diabetics, and 24% in persons below 55 years of age. They identified the following risk factors: females ($p=0.04$), diabetes ($p=0.002$) and advanced age ($p=0.05$).

Figure 19.6 shows an example of retinopathy developing in a patient being treated with interferon-alpha therapy for chronic hepatitis C who did not have diabetes. The patient developed multiple bilateral cotton wool spots that resolved during continuation of the interferon therapy.

PRACTICE POINTS

The conditions described in this chapter can produce lesions very similar to those described and found in diabetic retinopathy.

REFERENCE

Please visit www.wiley.com/go/scanlon/diabetic_retinopathy

Glossary

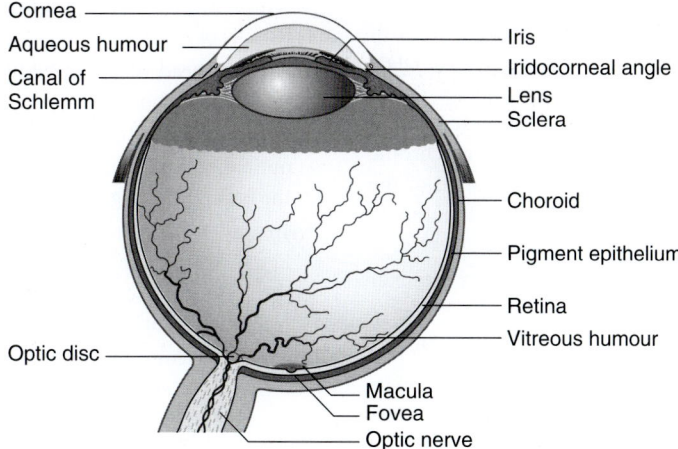

Anterior chamber: the space in the front portion of the eye between the cornea and the iris and lens, which is filled with aqueous humour.

Aqueous humour: the clear, watery fluid that fills the anterior chamber and the posterior chamber in the front part of the eye and provides nutrients to structures in the anterior chamber.

Arteriolar sheathing: opacification of the arteriolar wall.

Arterio-venous nipping: narrowing of the venous diameter where it is crossed by a branch artery. It is often a feature of hypertension.

Binocular indirect ophthalmoscopy: an examination technique of the retina involving a light source and viewing apparatus placed on the ophthalmologist's head and an indirect lens held between the light source and the eye, with the patient usually lying on a couch.

Blindness: WHO definition: visual acuity that does not exceed 20/200 in the better eye with correcting lens.

Choroid: the middle layer of the eye containing a large and highly vascular bed that provides nourishment to the other parts of the eye, especially the retina.

Ciliary body: a ring of tissue between the iris and the choroid consisting of muscles and blood vessels that changes the shape of the lens and produces the aqueous humour.

Conjunctiva: tissue that lines the inside of the eyelids and covers the front part of the eye except the cornea.

Contact lens biomicrosopy: examination technique using a slit-lamp biomicroscope to examine retinal detail through a diagnostic fundus contact lens applied to the cornea.

Cornea: the clear curved structure that comprises the front of the eye, a refractive surface through which light enters.

Cotton wool spots: fluffy white opaque areas caused by an accumulation of axoplasm in the nerve fibre layer of the retina.

A Practical Manual of Diabetic Retinopathy Management, Second Edition. Edited by Peter Scanlon, Ahmed Sallam, and Peter van Wijngaarden. © 2017 John Wiley & Sons Ltd. Published 2017 by John Wiley & Sons Ltd. Companion Website: www.wiley.com/go/scanlon/diabetic_retinopathy

Glossary

Diabetes mellitus: the chronic condition where there is an excess of glucose circulating in the bloodstream.

Diabetic retinopathy: the microvascular complication of diabetes affecting the eye.

Exudates (or hard exudates): small white or yellowish-white deposits with sharp margins, typically located in the outer layers of the retina but they may be more superficial, particularly when retinal oedema is present.

Fluorescein angiography: an examination technique involving the injection of fluorescein dye in the arm and taking a series of photographs over approximately the next 5 min using a blue light source entering the eye and a yellow filter allowing only fluorescent light to be captured leaving the eye on a monochrome sensor. This enables photographs to be taken of the passage of the fluorescein dye through the retinal vasculature.

FPD: fibrous proliferations on or within one disc diameter (1DD) of the disc margin.

FPE: fibrous proliferations 'elsewhere'.

Haemorrhage: a red spot which has irregular margins and/or uneven density, particularly when surrounding a smaller central lesion considered to be a microaneurysm. Flame haemorrhages are superficial haemorrhages just under the nerve fibre layer and blot haemorrhages are deeper haemorrhages.

HMa: a small haemorrhage or microaneurysm.

Iris: coloured circular membrane that is in front of the lens and controls the size of the opening at its centre (pupil), thereby regulating the amount of light entering the eye.

Intraretinal microvascular abnormality (IRMA): tortuous intraretinal vascular segments varying in calibre.

Laser: light amplification by simulated emission of radiation. Different types of laser are used in the diagnosis and treatment of many eye disorders.

LogMAR: logarithm of the minimum angle of resolution. This is a modern method used for measurement of visual acuity that has the same number of letters on each line.

Low-vision aids: optical devices that usually magnify the image to enable people with visual impairment to see print, objects or people at near or far that is not possible with the usual prescription lenses.

Macula: a rod-free area at the centre of the retina that surrounds the fovea and is responsible for best central vision.

Microaneurysm: as a red spot less than 125 microns (approximate width of vein at disc margin) and sharp margins.

MODY: maturity-onset diabetes of the young.

NVD: new vessels at the optic disc or within one disc diameter (1DD) of the optic disc margin.

NVE: new vessels > 1DD from the optic disc margin.

OCT: optical coherence tomography, an imaging technique that interprets the 'time of flight' and intensity of reflected optical waves via interferometry using wavelengths of 600–2000 nm.

Optic disc: head of the optic nerve where it meets the retinal nerve fibres.

Optic nerve: nerve of sight beginning in the retina at the optic disc, which carries messages from the retina to the brain, resulting in visual images.

Perimetry: is the systematic measurement of differential light sensitivity in the visual field by the detection of the presence of test targets on a defined background in order to map and quantify the visual field.

Posterior vitreous detachment (PVD): a common condition of the eye in which the vitreous humour separates from the retina.

Preretinal haemorrhage: boat-shaped haemorrhages and roughly round, confluent or linear patches of haemorrhage just anterior to the retina or under the internal limiting membrane.

PRP: panretinal photocoagulation is the type of scatter laser treatment that is given to patients with high-risk proliferative diabetic retinopathy and usually involves 1200–2000 burns of 500 micron spot size to an oval area of retina defined by a line passing two disc diameters above, temporal to and below the centre of the macula, and 500 microns from the nasal one-half of the disc margin.

Pupil: the opening in the centre of the iris that appears as a black dot and through which light enters the eye.

Retina: innermost layer of the eye containing photoreceptor cells and fibres connecting with the brain through the optic nerve, nourished by a network of blood vessels.

Sclera: the outermost layer of most of the eye, which is the tough protective 'white' of the eye.

Slit-lamp biomicroscopy: an examination technique using a slit-lamp biomicroscope to examine the anterior segment directly or retinal detail through an indirect lens held between the slit-lamp beam and the eye.

Type 1 diabetes: characterised by the absolute deficiency of insulin.

Type 2 diabetes: characterised by the relative deficiency of insulin associated with insulin 'resistance'.

Ultrasound B-scan examination: a means of visualising the eye and retro-bulbar region involving the placement of a high-frequency 10 MHz probe onto the eye or eyelid and taking a series of scan sections of the eye.

Venous loop: is an abrupt curving deviation of a vein from its normal path.

Venous reduplication: dilation of a pre-existing channel or proliferation of a new channel adjacent to and approximately the same calibre as the original vein.

Venous sheathing: opacification of the venous wall.

Visual acuity: measurement of the ability of the eye to perceive the shape of objects in the direct line of vision and to distinguish detail; generally determined by finding the smallest symbol on an eye chart that can be recognised at a given distance.

20/20 vision: the ability to correctly perceive an object or letter of a designated size from a distance of 20 feet; normal visual acuity.

6/6 vision: the ability to correctly perceive an object or letter of a designated size from a distance of 6 feet; normal visual acuity.

Vitreous body: transparent colourless mass of soft, gelatinous material filling the globe of the eye between the lens and the retina.

Vitreous haemorrhage: a haemorrhage that is in the vitreous gel, having penetrated through the internal limiting membrane.

Index

A
A-scan ultrasonography   60, 62, 63
ABCC8 (SUR1) gene mutations   20
abortive neovascular growths (ANO)   128
ACE inhibitors   100
acromegaly   21
aflibercept   107
age of diagnosis, risk factor for diabetic retinopathy   24–25
age-related macular degeneration (AMD)   89–90, 247
American Academy of Ophthalmology (AAO)   207
aminoguanidine   225
anaesthesia for retinal laser   143–144
angiopoietin-1 and -2   106
angiotensin I-converting enzyme gene   25
angiotensin receptor blockers   100
anterior ischaemic optic neuropathy (AION)   239
   case history   239
anterior segment neovascularisation   134
anti-angiogenic therapies, future developments   224–225
antioxidants   200
anti-VEGF (vascular endothelial growth factor) treatment   144, 146–147
   and laser treatment   151–159
   case histories   108–109, 110
   for DMO   106–111, 115
   future developments   224–225
   intravitreal   192–193
   predictors of visual outcome   109–111

aqueous humour   86, 87
argon blue-green laser   12, 13–14
argon ion laser   13
arterial emboli   234, 235
arteriolar abnormalities   33
arteriolar narrowing   33
arteriolar wall opacification (sheathing or 'white threads')   33
arterio-venous nipping   33
artificial intelligence   226
asteroid hyalosis   240, 241
   macular oedema in a patient with (case history)   240, 241
autoimmune aetiology of type 1 diabetes   17–18
automated static perimetry   7–8, 9–10
Avastin®   107

B
B-scan ultrasonography   60, 62, 64–66
background diabetic retinopathy, grading   116–119
Berlin Retinopathy Study   41
beta cell failure
   causes of   20–21
   in type 2 diabetes   19
bevacizumab   107, 192–193
Big Data   226
binocular indirect ophthalmoscopy (BIO)   5–6
biomarkers of retinopathy   221–223
blindness
   definition in the UK   207
   definition in the USA   207
   rates in the USA   207
blindness caused by diabetic retinopathy   207–218

advanced proliferative DR with left macular traction (case history)   213, 214–215
associated with macular ischaemia (case history)   213, 216
causes of loss of vision in diabetes and DR   213–218
chronic DMO prior to VEGF inhibitor treatments (case history)   213–214, 217
costs of   210–211
costs of treatment for DR   211
following cardiac arrest in a patient treated for PDR (case history)   216, 217–218
initiative to reduce   xiii–xiv
practice points   218
rates in Europe   210
rates in the USA   207–208
blood biomarkers of retinopathy   221–222
blood glucose control
   and improvement in retinopathy (case history)   22, 23
   and risk of diabetic retinopathy   21–22
   effects on retinopathy progression   xii
   evidence for benefit   42
blood pressure (BP)
   elevation risk factor for diabetic retinopathy   22, 23
   evidence for benefit of control   42
   influence on retinopathy progression   xii–xii
blood–retinal barrier   89
blot haemorrhages   26, 29

A Practical Manual of Diabetic Retinopathy Management, Second Edition.
Edited by Peter Scanlon, Ahmed Sallam, and Peter van Wijngaarden.
© 2017 John Wiley & Sons Ltd. Published 2017 by John Wiley & Sons Ltd.
Companion Website: www.wiley.com/go/scanlon/diabetic_retinopathy

BMI and risk of type 2 diabetes   19
branch retinal artery occlusion (BRAO)   233
branch retinal vein occlusion (BRVO)   237–239
brimonidine   225
bromofenac   192
Bruch's membrane   86, 89

C

candidate genes for diabetic retinopathy   25
cataract pathogenesis in diabetes   183–184
   osmotic stress pathway   183
   oxidative stress pathway   183–184
   types of cataract in patients with diabetes   183
cataract surgery in the diabetic eye   183–196
   adjunctive panretinal photocoagulation laser   194–195
   adjunctive pre- and intraoperative pharmacotherapy   191–194
   anaesthesia   185
   and vitrectomy   172
   anterior capsular contracture following (case history)   186
   anterior capsulorrhexis   186
   anterior segment evaluation   184
   anterior segment inflammation   188–189
   challenges of   183
   control of diabetes and associated systemic co-morbidities   184
   corneal epithelium and endothelium protection   185–186
   diabetic macular oedema (case history)   190–191
   endophthalmitis   191
   incidence of cataract in patients with diabetes   183
   indication for surgery   184
   iris neovascularisation   189
   macular oedema following cataract surgery   189–190
   operative considerations   185–188
   phacodynamics   186
   phacoemulsification technique   183
   posterior capsule rupture   186
   posterior segment evaluation   185
   postoperative considerations   188–191
   post-vitrectomy surgery cataract   188
   practice points   195–196
   preoperative considerations   184–185
   progression of diabetic retinopathy   189
   pseudophakic macular oedema (PMO)   189–190
   pseudophakic macular oedema (PMO) (case history)   191
   pupil management   186, 187
   risk of postoperative complications   183, 188
   silicone oil droplets on the back surface of silicone IOL (case history)   188
   subtle neovascularisation of the iris (case history)   185
   type of intraocular lens (IOL) implant   186–188
   visual outcome   195
central retinal artery occlusion (CRAO)   231–233
central retinal venous occlusion (CRVO)   234, 236–237
   case history   234, 236–237
China, incidence and prevalence of diabetes   ix
choroid   86, 87
choroidal circulation   90
ciliary body   86, 87
classification of diabetic retinopathy lesions   26–39
clinically significant diabetic macular oedema (CSMO)
   photocoagulation treatment   xiii
   incidence   xii
cloud computing   226
CO_2 laser   13
Coats' disease   251, 252
colour vision   89
   assessment   2
cone photoreceptors   89
confocal scanning laser ophthalmoscopy (cSLO)   55–56, 61, 62
confocal scanning laser ophthalmoscopy (cSLO) angiography   62–63
cornea   86, 87
corticosteroids, intravitreal treatments for DMO   111–114
costs of blindness caused by diabetic retinopathy   210–211
costs of treatment for diabetic retinopathy   211
cotton wool spots (soft exudates)   29–30, 116–118
Cushing's disease   21

D

dexamethasone intravitreal implant   111–112, 194
diabetes
   advances in management   xii–xiii
   aetiopathology   17–21
   classification   15
   complications of   1
   definition   15
   distinction between type 1 and type 2   15–17
   effects of hyperglycaemia   15
   epigenetic factors   220
   insulin resistance   15
   macrovascular complications   21
   maturity-onset diabetes of the young (MODY)   15, 19–20
   microvascular complications   21
   projected prevalence by 2035   ix, x
   rates of progression of diabetic retinopathy   xii
   retinopathy complication   21
   risk factors for type 2 diabetes   19
   scope of the worldwide epidemic   ix, x
   secondary diabetes   15, 20–21
   tissue complications   21
   type 1   15
      aetiopathology   17–18, 19
      with retinopathy (case history)   15–17
   type 2   15
      aetiopathology   18–19
      with neuropathy and retinopathy (case history)   17–18
   worldwide incidence and prevalence   ix, x
Diabetes Atlas   ix
Diabetes Control and Complications Trial (DCCT)   xii, 21, 22, 25, 42, 101, 130, 197, 220–221
diabetic ketoacidosis   15
diabetic macular oedema (DMO)
   anti-VEGF treatment   106–111, 115
   classification of diabetic maculopathy   93–97
   combination therapy   113, 115
   conventional laser treatment   103–104
   decision to use laser treatment   135–137

diffuse maculopathy 93, 95
diffuse maculopathy (case history) 102–103, 104
early worsening phenomenon (case history) 101–102
fluid accumulation patterns 93, 97–98
focal maculopathy 93, 94
focal maculopathy (case history) 102, 103
focal photocoagulation study 100–101
following cataract surgery 189–190
hypertension (case history) 98–100
incidence xii
intravitreal corticosteroids 111–114
ischaemic maculopathy 93, 96–97
laser treatment 100–106
limitations and adverse effects of conventional laser treatment 104
navigating laser treatment (Navilas) 105–106
optical coherence tomography (OCT) 93, 97–98
outcome of treatment 160–163
PASCAL (pattern scan argon laser) treatment 105
practice points 115
subthreshold micro-pulse laser (SMPL) photocoagulation 105
tomographic appearance (case history) 190–191
treatment of associated risk factors 98–100
treatment recommendations 115
vitrectomy 115, 177, 180
diabetic retinopathy (DR)
advances in management xiii–xiv
changes within the retinal capillary wall 26
definition 26
early detection initiatives xiii–xiv
English classification 37–39
ETDRS classification of progression 27
ETDRS classification of lesions 26–37
ETDRS maculopathy classification 27
International classification 37–39
lesion classification systems 26–39
rates of progression and regression xii
studies of incidence and prevalence ix–xii
systematic screening programmes xiii–xiv
worldwide incidence and prevalence ix–xii
Diabetic Retinopathy Study (DRS) xiii, 55, 130–132, 137
Diabetic Retinopathy Study Research Group 41
differential diagnosis for diabetic retinopathy 247–254
age-related macular degeneration (AMD) 247
Coats' disease 251, 252
drusen 247, 248
interferon retinopathy 254
myelinated nerve fibres 247, 249
practice points 254
radiation retinopathy 251, 253
sickle cell retinopathy 249–250
diffuse maculopathy 93, 95
case history 102–103, 104
digital retinal photography 54–59
diode laser 12, 13, 14
diplopia 3
direct ophthalmoscopy 4
as a screening test 42
Driver and Vehicle Licensing Agency (DVLA) visual field standard 8
driving, visual standards required for 8
driving field difficulties following treatment (case history) 134, 135–136
drusen 89, 247, 248
duration of diabetes, risk factor for diabetic retinopathy 24
dye laser 13

E
Early Treatment of Diabetic Retinopathy Study (ETDRS) xiii, 22, 24, 41, 55, 100–101, 132, 137
classification of lesions 26–37
grading of mild NPDR 116–119
maculopathy classification 27
early worsening phenomenon 101, 130
case history 101–102
electronic medical records 226
emmetropy (normal sight) 86
endophthalmitis 191
endothelial progenitor cells (EPCs) 226
English maculopathy classification 39
English retinopathy classification 37–39
Epidemiology of Diabetes Interventions and Complications (EDIC) study 22, 221
epigenetic factors in diabetic retinopathy 220–221
Esterman grid testing system 8, 12–13
ethnicity, risk factor for diabetic retinopathy 25
Europe
rates of blindness related to diabetes 210
rates of diabetes and diabetic retinopathy 208–210
excimer laser 13
Exeter standards 46
exudates (or hard exudates) 116, 118
eye, range of normal photographic appearances 90–92
eye anatomy 86–90
eye examination 2–6
assessment of colour vision 2
assessment of visual acuity 2
binocular indirect ophthalmoscopy (BIO) 5–6
direct ophthalmoscopy 4
inspection of external structures 2
intraocular pressure measurement 3
ocular movement 3
pupil dilation 4
pupillary reactions to light and accommodation 3
red reflex with an ophthalmoscope 3
routinely undertaken examinations 3
slit-lamp biomicroscopy of the eye 3
slit-lamp biomicroscopy of the retina 4–5
visual fields to confrontation 2–3
Eylea 107

F
Farnsworth-Munsell 100 hue discrimination test 2, 3
fenofibrate 22, 100
fibroblast growth factor-2 106
fibrous proliferations (FPD, FPE) 34
flame haemorrhages 26, 29
fluocinolone acetonide intravitreal inserts 112–113, 194
case history 113, 114
focal maculopathy 93, 94
case history 102, 103

fovea 88, 89
foveal avascular zone (FAZ) 93, 96
foveal hypoautofluorescence 59–60
foveola 89
fundus autofluorescence 59–60, 62, 63
fundus fluorescein angiography (FFA) 62–63, 66–71, 72, 73
  common causes of hypofluorescence and hyperfluorescence 66, 71, 72, 73
  sequence of events 66, 68–70
future advances in diabetic retinopathy management 219–227
  anti-angiogenic therapies 224–225
  Big Data 226
  biomarkers of retinopathy 221–223
  cloud computing 226
  electronic medical records 226
  genetic risk profiling and the role of epigenetics 220–221
  laser treatment 225–226
  potential of artificial intelligence 226
  predicting risk of DR and its progression 219–223
  regenerative therapies 226
  retinal neuroprotection 225
  role of endothelial progenitor cells (EPCs) 226
  targeting key pathogenic pathways 225
  timely detection of diabetic retinopathy 223–224
  treatment options 224–226

G

genetic factors in diabetes 18–20, 21
genetic predisposition for diabetic retinopathy 25
genetic risk profiling and the role of epigenetics 220–221
GKT137831 225
glaucoma 87, 128, 207
gliclazide 20
glucose homeostasis 15
glutamic acid decarboxylase antibodies (GADA) 17
Goldmann kinetic perimetry 7, 8, 9
Goldmann tonometer 3
Greenland effect 56
growth factors, overexpression in hyperglycaemia 106

H

haemochromatosis 21
haemorrhages, classification 26, 28, 29
hard exudates 26, 29
Heidelberg Spectralis system 59
Heidelberg UWF imaging system 56, 59
hemianopia 207
HMa (small haemorrhage or microaneurysm) 26, 28
HNF-1α abnormalities 19, 20, 21
HNF-1α MODY diabetes (case history) 20, 21
HNF-1β abnormalities 20
HNF-4α abnormalities 20
human lymphocytic antigens (HLA) 25
Humphrey visual field analyser 7–8, 9–11
hyperglycaemia
  and retinopathy xii
  effects in the eyes 106
  effects of 15
  epigenetic modifications induced by 220
  influence on retinopathy progression xii
hyperinsulinemia 15
hypermetropy (long-sightedness) 86
hypertension in diabetes xii–xiii, 228–230
  arteriolar occlusion in diabetes associated with (case history) 231
  arterio-venous nipping 33
  diabetic maculopathy risk factor 98–100
  malignant hypertension (case history) 228–230
  risk factor for diabetic retinopathy 22, 23
hypertensive retinopathy 228–230

I

Iluvien 112, 113
imaging, range of normal photographic appearances of the eye 90–92
imaging of DMO, optical coherence tomography (OCT) 93, 97–98
imaging techniques in diabetic retinopathy 54–85
  delivery of laser therapy 54
  digital retinal photography 54–59
  fundus autofluorescence 59–60, 62, 63
  fundus fluorescein angiography (FFA) 62–63, 66–71, 72, 73
  image registration technology 54
  indocyanine green (ICG) angiography 70, 71
  optical coherence tomography (OCT) 59, 73–83
  optical coherence tomography (OCT) angiography 83–85
  range of techniques 54
  retinal autofluorescence 59–60, 62, 63
  retinal photography 54–59
  stereoscopic photography 54–55, 56
  ultrasonography 60, 62, 63, 64–66
  ultra-wide-field angiography 71–73, 74, 75
  ultra-wide-field imaging 55–59, 60, 61, 62
indocyanine green (ICG) angiography 70, 71
infliximab 225
INS (insulin) gene mutations 20
insulin-dependent diabetes mellitus (IDDM) see diabetes, type 1
insulin-like growth factor-1 106
insulin resistance 15, 19
  causes of 20–21
interferon retinopathy 254
International classification
  grading of mild NPDR 116–119
  grading of moderate and severe NPDR 120–127
  maculopathy classification 39
  retinopathy classification 37–39
International Diabetes Foundation (IDF) ix, x
intraocular pressure 87
  measurement 3
intraretinal microvascular abnormalities (IRMAs) 30, 31, 32, 120, 122
intravitreal corticosteroids, for DMO 111–114
investigative techniques to assess diabetic retinopathy 7–8
IPF-1 abnormalities 20
iris 86–87, 88
iris hooks 186, 187
iris neovascularisation (case history) 134, 137
iris rubeosis 186
ischaemia, signs of 135, 137
ischaemic maculopathy 93, 96–97
Ishihara test 2
islet cell antibodies (ICA) 17

J

juvenile-onset diabetes *see* diabetes, type 1

K

krypton laser   12

L

laser iridotomy   12
laser subepithelial keratectomy (LASEK)   13
laser treatment
   anaesthesia for retinal laser   143–144
   and intravitreal anti-VEGF therapy   151–159
   evidence for effectiveness   41–42
   follow-up after panretinal photocoagulation   137
   for diabetic macular oedema   100–106
   for diabetic retinopathy   xiii–xiv
   for proliferative DR   129, 130–144
   future developments   225–226
   navigating laser treatment (Navilas)   140–141
   patient experiences of   143–144
   pattern argon laser   139–140
   proliferative diabetic retinopathy with maculopathy   150
   quantification of retinal ablation   137–138
   recommended settings for non-pattern argon laser   138–139
   targeted PRP laser   140
laser treatment scars   36–37
lasers
   active laser media   13
   application in diabetic retinopathy   8, 12, 13–14
   coherence of laser light   8
   gain medium   13
   light wavelengths produced by different lasers   13–14
   photoablation (photochemical effect)   13
   photocoagulation (photothermal effect)   12
   photodisruption (photoionising effect)   12
   types of laser–tissue interactions   12, 13
   types of lasers used   13–14
lens   86–88

lesion classification systems   26–39
lipid level
   evidence for benefit of control   42
   risk factor for diabetic retinopathy   22, 24
lipofuscin   59
Liverpool Diabetic Eye Study   46
LogMar visual acuity chart   2, 3
low-vision aids   212–213
low-vision assessments   212
low vision caused by diabetic retinopthy   207–218
   practice points   218
   quality of life effects   211–212
low-vision rehabilitation   212–213
Lucentis™   106
lutein   59, 89

M

macroaneurysm   240, 241–245
   imaging   243–245
   in type 1 diabetes (case history)   240, 241–242
   in type 2 diabetes (case history)   242, 244
macrovascular complications of diabetes   21
Macugen®   106
macula   89
macular oedema *see* diabetic macular oedema (DMO)
maculopathy
   ETDRS maculopathy classification   27
   English classification   39
   International classification   39
   types of diabetic maculopathy   93–97
   see also diabetic macular oedema (DMO); proliferative diabetic retinopathy with maculopathy
Malyugin ring   186, 187
maturity-onset diabetes *see* diabetes, type 2
maturity-onset diabetes of the young (MODY)   15, 19–20
metabolic memory   220–221
metformin   225
microaneurysms   26, 28, 116, 117
microRNAs (miRNAs)   220
microvascular complications of diabetes   21
mild non-proliferative diabetic retinopathy (NPDR) grading   116–119

minocycline   220
moderate non-proliferative diabetic retinopathy (NPDR)
   case history   123, 124
   grading   120–127
   practice points   127
multidisciplinary management of diabetic retinopathy   7
mydriasis   56
mydriatic digital photography, as a screening test   43–45
mydriatic imaging   56
mydriatic photography (35mm or polaroid), as a screening test   43
myelinated nerve fibres   247, 249
myopia (short-sightedness)   86

N

NADPH oxidase   225
National Diabetic Retinopathy Laser Treatment Audit   137–138
National Institute for Health and Care Excellence (NICE) UK   106
navigating laser treatment (Navilas)   105–106, 140–141
Nd:YAG lasers   12, 13
neovascular glaucoma   128
neovascularisation of the anterior segment   128
nepafenac   192
nephropathy complication of diabetes   21
neuropathy complication of diabetes   21
new vessels elsewhere (NVE)   34, 35, 36, 37, 128, 129, 130, 132
   and NVD with maculopathy (case histories)   150–152
   in superotemporal retina with some macular ischaemia (case history)   141, 143
   treated NVE proliferative DR (case history)   167–168
   treatment outcome   163, 167–170
   views on treatment of NVE that have not haemorrhaged   148–149
   with vitreous haemorrhage (case history)   147–148
new vessels on the disc (NVD)   34, 35, 36, 37, 128, 129, 130, 131, 132
   and NVE with maculopathy (case histories)   150–152
   severe NVD in both eyes (case history)   141, 142

new vessels on the disc (NVD) (continued)
  treated NVD proliferative DR (case histories)   167, 169–170
  treated with panretinal photocoagulation (case history)   141, 144
  treatment outcome   163, 167–170
  views on treatment of NVD less than one-quarter disc area   148
nitric oxide synthase (NOS2A and NOS3) genes   25
non-insulin dependent diabetes mellitus (NIDDM) see diabetes, type 2
non-mydriatic imaging   56
non-mydriatic photography, as a screening test   43
non-proliferative diabetic retinopathy (NPDR) grading
  mild   116–119
  moderate and severe   120–127

O

ocular fluid biomarkers of retinopathy   221–222
optic disc   88–89
optic disc neovascularisation treated with PRP laser and intravitreal anti-VEGF (case history)   147
optic nerve   87, 88–89
optical coherence tomography (OCT)   59, 73–83
  for DMO   93, 97–98
optical coherence tomography (OCT) angiography   83–85
optical coherence tomography (OCT)/photographic clinics   48–49
optometrist's slit-lamp biomicroscopy, as a screening test   42–43
Optos UWF imaging system   55–56, 60
osmotic stress pathway, cataract development   183
other retinal conditions in diabetes   228–246
  anterior ischaemic optic neuropathy (AION)   239
  asteroid hyalosis   240, 241
  hypertensive retinopathy   228–230
  macroaneurysm   240, 241–245
  practice points   246
  retinal arterial occlusions   231–234, 235
  retinal venous occlusions   234–239

outcomes see stable treated eye
oxidative stress pathway, cataract development   183–184
Ozurdex   111

P

Pacific Islands countries, rates of diabetes   ix
PAN-90806   225
pars plana vitrectomy   xiii
partial sight, definition   207
PASCAL (pattern scan argon laser)   14
  evidence behind its recommendation   139–140
  for macular oedema   105
pathogenesis of diabetic retinopathy, targeting key pathogenic pathways   225
patient experiences of laser treatment   143–144
patient history
  complications of diabetes   1
  diabetic history   1
  drug history   1
  family history   1
  past medical history   1
  past ocular history   1
  presenting complaint   1
  psychosocial history   1
pegaptanib sodium   106
perimetry   7–8, 9–13
perivenous exudates   32–33
phacoemulsification technique   183
phaeochromocytoma   21
photoablation (photochemical effect)   13
photocoagulation (photothermal effect)   12
  circinate maculopathy in diabetic retinopathy   xiii
  clinically significant diabetic macular oedema (CSMO)   xiii
photodisruption (photoionising effect)   12
photographic appearance of the eye, range of normal appearances   90–92
photopigments   59
photoreceptor cells   86, 87, 88, 89
photorefractive keratectomy (PRK)   13
pigment epithelium   86
pigmented epithelium-derived factor (PEDF) gene   25
PKC inhibitors   100

posterior vitreous detachment (PVD)   37
  with horseshoe-shaped tear (case history)   143, 146
post-maculopathy laser treatment, laser scars   36
post-scatter laser treatment for PDR, laser scars   36–37
practical assessment   1–6
  eye examination   2–6
  history of the patient   1
predicting risk of DR and its progression   219–223
pregnancy and the diabetic eye   197–206
  diabetic retinopathy in pregnancy (case history)   201, 203–205
  effects on retinopathy   21
  independent association with DR progression   197
  laser treatment   199
  postpartum regression of DR   201, 206
  practice points   206
  proliferative DR in pregnancy (case histories)   199–202
  recommendations for retinal assessment   199
  risk factors for DR progression   197–199
  treatment before and during pregnancy   199–205
pre-proliferative diabetic retinopathy, grading   120–127
preretinal haemorrhage (PRH)   34, 35, 130–131
presenting complaint   1
proliferative and advanced diabetic retinopathy   128–149
  abortive neovascular growths (ANO)   128
  adverse effects of laser treatment   132–134
  anaesthesia for retinal laser   143–144
  anti-VEGF treatments   144, 146–147
  development of new vessels   128, 129
  driving field difficulties following treatment (case history)   134, 135–136
  early worsening phenomenon   130
  factors other than high-risk characteristics influencing the decision to laser   134–137

fluorescein angiographic appearance of new vessels   128, 129
follow-up after panretinal photocoagulation   137
iris neovascularisation (case history)   134, 137
laser treatment for proliferative DR   129, 130–144
  multidisciplinary approach   130
  navigating laser treatment (Navilas)   140–141
neovascular glaucoma   128
neovascularisation of the anterior segment   128
new vessels elsewhere (NVE)   128, 129
  superotemporal retina with some macular ischaemia (case history)   141, 143
  with vitreous haemorrhage (case history)   147–148
  views on treatment of NVE that have not haemorrhaged   148–149
new vessels on the disc (NVD)   128, 129
  severe NVD in both eyes (case history)   141, 142
  treated with panretinal photocoagulation (case history)   141, 144
  views on treatment of NVD less than one-quarter disc area   148
optic disc neovascularisation treated with PRP laser and intravitreal anti-VEGF (case history)   147
patient experiences of laser treatment   143–144
pattern argon laser treatment   139–140
photographic appearance of new vessels   128
posterior vitreous detachment with horseshoe-shaped tear (case history)   143, 146
practice points   149
presentation   128
quantification of retinal ablation   137–138
recommended setting for non-pattern argon laser   138–139
relevant anatomy   128
risks for patients without high-risk characteristics   131–132
targeted PRP laser   140

treatment of associated risk factors   130
undertreated proliferative retinopathy (case history)   141, 145
views on treatment of NVD less than one-quarter disc area   148
views on treatment of NVE that have not haemorrhaged   148–149
vitrectomy surgery   147–149
vitreous haemorrhage   128
vitreous haemorrhage obscuring the retinal view   147–149
proliferative diabetic retinopathy (PDR)
  rates of progression to   xii
  worldwide incidence and prevalence   xi
proliferative diabetic retinopathy with maculopathy   150–159
  case histories   152–159
  laser treatment   150
  laser treatment and intravitreal anti-VEGF therapy   151–159
  NVD and NVE with maculopathy (case histories)   150–152
  practice points   159
protein kinase C-beta (PKC-beta) gene   25
pseudophakic macular oedema (PMO)   189–190
  tomographic appearance (case history)   191
pupil dilation for eye examination   4
pupillary reactions to light and accommodation   3

Q
quality of life effects of reduced vision   211–212

R
radiation retinopathy   251, 253
  case history   251, 253
ranibizumab   106–107, 193
reactive oxygen species   220
receptor for advanced glycation end products (RAGE) gene   25
red reflex with an ophthalmoscope   3
regenerative therapies   226
regorafenib   225
renal failure   137
retina, anatomy   86–89
retinal arterial occlusions   231–234, 235
retinal autofluorescence   59–60, 62, 63

retinal biomarkers for risk of retinopathy progression   222–223
retinal haemorrhages   116, 117, 120, 121
  classification   26, 28, 29
retinal neuroprotection   225
retinal photography   54–59
retinal pigment epithelium   59, 89–90
retinal venous occlusions   234–239
retinitis pigmentosa   207
retinopathy complication of diabetes   21 see also diabetic retinopathy
RetinoStat   224
risk factors for diabetic retinopathy   21–25
  age of diagnosis   24–25
  duration of diabetes   24
  elevated blood pressure   22, 23
  ethnicity   25
  genetic predisposition   25
  hypertension   22, 23
  lipid levels   22, 24
  modifiable risk factors   21–24
  non-modifiable risk factors   24–25
  poor blood glucose control   21–22
  practice points   25
  smoking   22
risk factors for type 2 diabetes   19
rod photoreceptors   89
Rubin laser   13
ruboxistaurin   225

S
Schlemm's canal   87
sclera   86, 87
screening for diabetic retinopathy   40–53
  advances in screening   46, 48–49
  automated analysis   48
  availability of a suitable screening test   42–45
  costs of screening and effective treatment   45–46
  definition of screening   40
  evidence for effective treatment   41–42
  extent of the public health problem   40–41
  grading of mild NPDR   116–119
  grading of moderate and severe NPDR   120–127
  optical coherence tomography (OCT)/photographic clinics   48–49
  practice points   49

screening for diabetic retinopathy (continued)
   principles of screening   40–46
   purpose of screening   40
   recognisable latent or early symptomatic stage   41
   risk-based screening intervals   46, 48
   sight-threatening diabetic retinopathy (case histories)   46, 47–48, 49–53
secondary diabetes   20–21
severe non-proliferative diabetic retinopathy (NPDR)
   case history   123, 125–127
   grading   120–127
   practice points   127
severely sight impaired, definition   207
sickle cell retinopathy   249–250
sight impaired, definition   207
sight-threatening diabetic retinopathy (STDR), incidence and prevalence   ix–xii
single venous loop   118
slit-lamp biomicroscopy
   of the eye   3
   of the retina   4–5
small haemorrhage or microaneurysm (HMa)   26, 28
smoking, risk factor for diabetic retinopathy   22
Snellen visual acuity chart   2
somatostatin   225
squalamine lactate   225
St Vincent Declaration on diabetes care and research   xiii–xiv, 208–210
stable treated eye   160–170
   following maculopathy treatment   160–163
   following NVD or NVE treatment   163, 167–170
   ischaemic maculopathy   163
   practice points   170
   treated centre-involving DMO with VEGF inhibitors (case history)   160–163
   treated centre-involving or diffuse DMO   160
   treated focal exudative or focal/multifocal oedema   160
   treated non-centre-involving DMO with focal laser (case history)   160, 164–166
   treated NVD proliferative DR (case histories)   167, 169–170
   treated NVE proliferative DR (case history)   167–168
stereoscopic photography   54–55, 56
stromal-derived factor-1   106
subthreshold micro-pulse laser (SMPL) photocoagulation, for DMO   105
sulphonylureas   19, 20

T
targeted PRP laser   140
tight junctions between retinal blood vessel cells   89
timely detection of diabetic retinopathy   223–224
tissue complications of diabetes   21
topical non-steroidal anti-inflammatory drugs (NSAIDs)   192
trabecular meshwork   87
treatment options, future advances   224–226
triamcinolone acetonide   192, 193
   intravitreal injection of   193–194
   intravitreal treatment for DMO   111
   posterior sub-Tenon injection   192
tropical calcific disease   21
tumor necrosis factor   106

U
ultrasonography   60, 62, 63, 64–66
ultra-wide-field angiography   71–73, 74, 75
ultra-wide-field imaging   55–59, 60, 61, 62
undertreated proliferative retinopathy (case history)   141, 145
United Kingdom Prospective Diabetes Study (UKPDS)   xii–xiii, 15, 22, 24, 25, 40, 41, 42, 220
United States
   definition of legal blindness   207
   rates of blindness and visual impairment   207–208
uveal layer   86

V
vascular circulation of the retina   89
vascular endothelial growth factor (VEGF)
   gene   25
   inhibitors   xiii
   overexpression in hyperglycaemia   106
   see also anti-VEGF
venous abnormalities   30–33
venous beading   32, 120–123
   sign of ischaemia   135, 137
venous dilation   32–33
venous loops and/or reduplication   30–32
venous narrowing   32–33
venous sheathing or 'white threads'   32–33
venous wall opacification   32–33
vision impairment, definition   207
vision-related quality of life   211–212
vision-threatening diabetic retinopathy (VTDR), incidence and prevalence   ix–xii
visual acuity assessment   2
vitrectomy (vitreous surgery)   xiii, 37, 147–149, 171–182
   for diabetic macular oedema   115
   for epiretinal membrane formation with macular traction   180, 182
   for macular off-tractional detachment (case history)   180, 181
   for severe vitreous haemorrhage and NVD (case history)   176–177
   for tractional retinal detachment and vitreous haemorrhage due to PDR (case history)   177–178
   goals of vitreous surgery   173
   indications in diabetic retinopathy   171–172
   intraocular tamponade   176
   post-operative complications   176
   post-vitrectomy surgery cataract   188
   practice points   180, 182
   preoperative use of intravitreal anti-VEGF treatment   172
   removal of fibrovascular tissue   174–175
   removal of vitreous haemorrhage and vitreous gel   173–174
   role of the posterior cortical surface (PCS) of the vitreous gel   171
   treating retinal breaks and detachments   175–176

treatment techniques for DMO   177, 180
treatment techniques for PDR   172–176
vitreous haemorrhage   34, 36, 128, 130, 131
  obscuring the retinal view   147–149
vitreous humour   86, 87
vitreous surgery *see* vitrectomy

W
Western Pacific, rates of diabetes   ix, x
wide-field scanning laser ophthalmoscopy, as a screening test   43
Wisconsin Epidemiological Study of Diabetic Retinopathy (WESDR)   xii, 24, 41, 116

World Health Organisation (WHO)   xiii, 40
  definition of legal blindness   207

Z
zeaxanthin   59, 89